RADIOLOGY FOR THE MRCP

RADIOLOGY FOR THE MRCP

John Curtis MB ChB MRCP FRCR DMRD

*Consultant Radiologist,
University Hospital Aintree, Liverpool, UK*

Graham Whitehouse MBBS FRCP FRCR DMRD AKC

*Professor of Diagnostic Radiology,
University of Liverpool, Liverpool, UK*

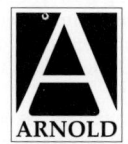

A member of the Hodder Headline Group
LONDON • SYDNEY • AUCKLAND
Co-published in the United States of America by
Oxford University Press Inc., New York

First published in Great Britain in 1998 by
Arnold, a member of the Hodder Headline Group,
338 Euston Road, London NW1 3BH

http://www.arnoldpublishers.com

Co-published in the United States of America by
Oxford University Press Inc.,
198 Madison Avenue, New York, NY10016
Oxford is a registered trademark of Oxford University Press

© 1998 John Curtis and Graham Whitehouse

All rights reserved. No part of this publication may be reproduced or transmitted in any form or by any means, electronically or mechanically, including photocopying, recording or any information storage or retrieval system, without either prior permission in writing from the publisher or a licence permitting restricted copying. In the United Kingdom such licences are issued by the Copyright Licensing Agency: 90 Tottenham Court Road, London W1P 9HE.

Whilst the advice and information in this book is believed to be true and accurate at the date of going to press, neither the author[s] nor the publisher can accept any legal responsibility or liability for any errors or omissions that may be made. In particular (but without limiting the generality of the preceding disclaimer) every effort has been made to check drug dosages; however, it is still possible that errors have been missed. Furthermore, dosage schedules are constantly being revised and new side-effects recognized. For these reasons the reader is strongly urged to consult the drug companies' printed instructions before administering any of the drugs recommended in this book.

British Library Cataloguing in Publication Data
A catalogue record for this book is available from the British Library

Library of Congress Cataloging-in-Publication Data
A catalog record for this book is available from the Library of Congress

ISBN 0340 71886 2

1 2 3 4 5 6 7 8 9 10

Commissioning Editor: Fiona Goodgame
Production Editor: Wendy Rooke
Production Controller: Sarah Kett
Cover Design: Terry Griffiths

Typeset in 9/12pt Helvetica by Saxon Graphics Ltd, Derby
Printed and bound in Great Britain by St Edmundsbury Press, Bury St Edmunds, Suffolk and J W Arrowsmith Ltd, Bristol

---

What do you think about this book? Or any other Arnold title?
Please send your comments to feedback.arnold@hodder.co.uk

To Juliet and Matthew (JC)

To Jacqueline, Richard and Victoria (GW)

Contents

Preface ix

Acknowledgements x

Questions and Answers 1–180 1–363

Appendix 364–373

Index 375

Preface

The supervision and interpretation of complex diagnostic imaging procedures are firmly in the ambit of the specialist radiologist. However, such is the accuracy and clarity of modern imaging modalities that they serve as an important means of teaching clinical and pathological manifestations of disease.

Diagnostic imaging is a well-established element of the MRCP examination. We attempt in this book to demonstrate radiological findings in a wide range of diseases, followed by a commentary on the important features of these conditions. The intent is that readers test their diagnostic acumen on the images and then use the text in the answer sections as a revision aid on the topic. As well as MRCP candidates, radiologists preparing for the Final FRCR examination should find this book useful.

In order to assist in image interpretation, we have included an Appendix showing differences between basic magnetic resonance imaging sequences and computed tomography. Also in the Appendix are most of the important M-mode echocardiograms likely to be encountered in the examination.

We are indebted to Mrs Joan Scott for all her hard work and patience in preparing the manuscript.

John Curtis and Graham Whitehouse
1998

ACKNOWLEDGEMENTS

We wish to thank our colleagues who provided material for this book:

Dr I. Brett, Dr M. Critchley, Dr R. Edwards, Dr H. Fewins, Dr R. Hammond, Dr M. Hughes, Dr S. King, Dr J. Ko, Dr G. Lamb, Dr M. Lombard, Dr K. Meakin, Dr H. Lewis-Jones, Dr G. Murphy, Dr T. Nixon, Dr V. Pellegrini, Dr D. Ritchie, Dr P. Rowlands, Dr S. Saltissi, Dr A. Smethurst, Dr D. White, Dr J. Wide, Mr S. Ellenbogen and Mr A. Wu.

We are grateful to the radiographic staff at The Royal Liverpool University Hospital, University Hospital Aintree and The Magnetic Resonance and Image Analysis Research Centre, University of Liverpool for their help in producing the images used in this book. We would also like to thank the Departments of Medical Illustration at The Royal Liverpool University Hospital and University Hospital Aintree for the preparation of the illustrations.

QUESTION 1

Sudden onset of chest pain, breathlessness and circulatory collapse in a 60-year-old woman. Three weeks later, a contrast-enhanced CT of the thorax (Figs 1.1a and 1.1b) was performed because of persisting abnormalities on her chest radiograph.

a What are the abnormalities on CT?
b What is the diagnosis?

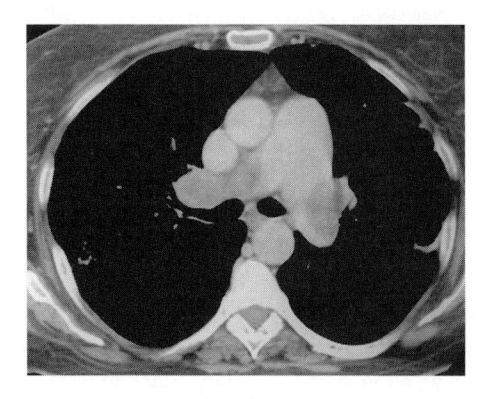

Fig. 1.1a
CT thorax on soft tissue settings.

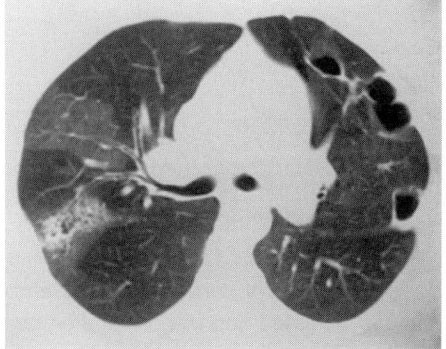

Fig. 1.1b
CT thorax on lung settings.

ANSWER 1

a i Filling defects in right and left pulmonary arteries (Fig. 1.1a).
   ii Most of both lungs are underperfused and appear hyperlucent (dark) on Fig. 1.1b. There are only two parts which appear well perfused, situated at the periphery of the right lung. This pattern is termed mosaic oligaemia.
   iii There are four peripheral lung cavities in the left lung (Fig. 1.1b).
b Bilateral pulmonary thromboembolic disease.

Discussion

Pulmonary thromboembolism (PE) is an important diagnosis to establish. On its own the chest radiograph is both insensitive and non-specific. Isotope lung scanning in conjunction with a chest radiograph provides the most commonly used investigation in the first instance for suspected PE. In difficult cases pulmonary angiography is performed, and occasionally contrast-enhanced CT for central emboli.

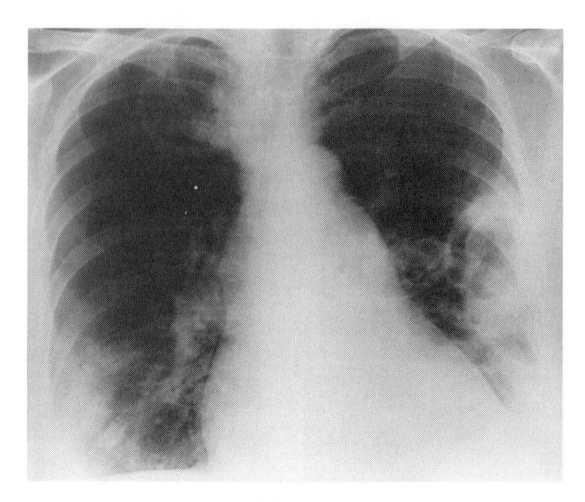

Fig. 1.2
Chest radiograph showing enlarged pulmonary artery with distal oligaemia. Note peripheral cavitary consolidation.

Approximately 15% of pulmonary emboli cause infarction. This is more likely when there is left-sided heart failure or if emboli lodge in the lung periphery. Cavitation within an area of infarction is rare, but usually occurs as a result of secondary infection or septic emboli. Aseptic cavitation can also occur and is more likely to do so when the infarct exceeds 4 cm in diameter.

The radiological features can be summarized as follows:

Chest radiography

PE without infarction: normal; oligaemia of the lung fields distal to the occluded vessel (Fig. 1.2); enlargement of the main pulmonary artery and/or the right and left pulmonary arteries; linear collapse and elevated hemidiaphragm.

PE with infarction: pleural-based rounded consolidation, called Hampton's hump when it occupies the costophrenic angle; pleural effusion and cavitating infarction (rare).

Isotope lung scanning

Perfusion defects *not* matched by ventilatory defects (Fig. 1.3).

Pulmonary angiography

This is the most accurate but most invasive imaging method.

CT

Large thrombi can be seen in the major pulmonary arteries during contrast-enhanced CT. Under-perfusion of the lung distal to the embolus gives rise to so-called mosaic oligaemia (Fig. 1.1b).

(a)

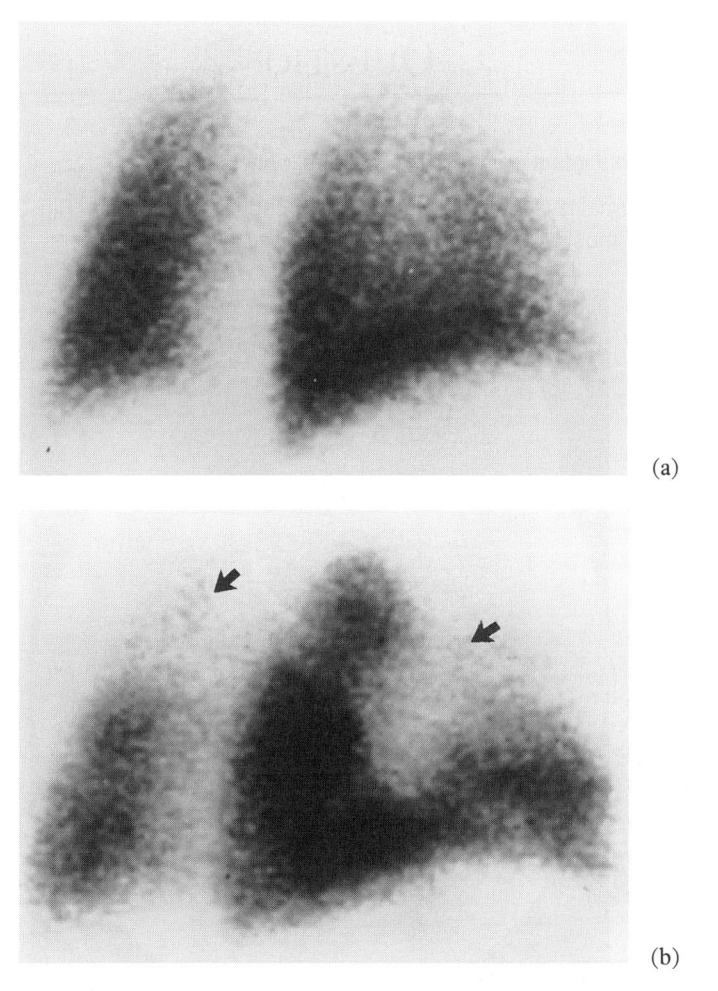

(b)

Fig. 1.3 a and b
Isotope (a) ventilation and (b) perfusion lung scan in another patient showing a mismatched perfusion defect (arrows).

QUESTION 2

This 6-month old infant presents with bilateral optic atrophy.

a What abnormality is visible on this unenhanced CT of the brain (Fig. 2.1)?
b What is the most likely diagnosis?

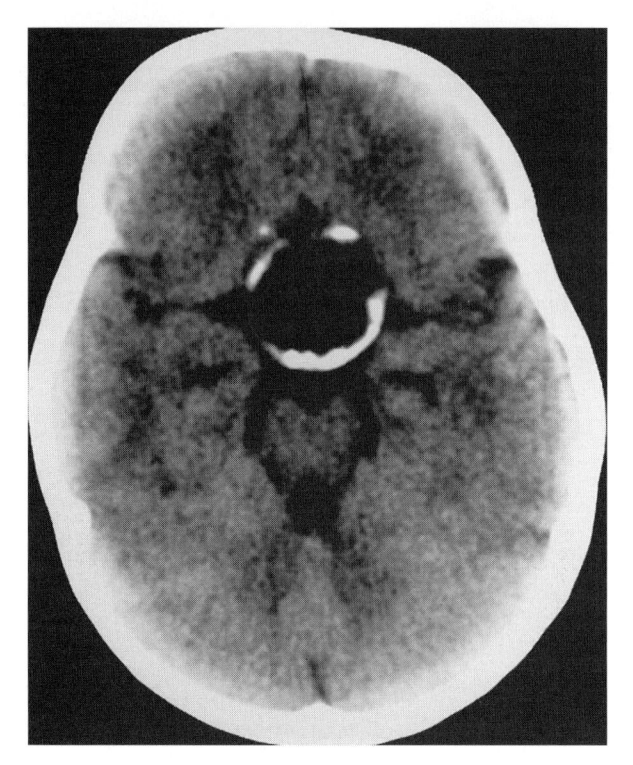

Fig. 2.1

ANSWER 2

a Low-attenuation spherical mass in the suprasellar region with peripheral curvilinear calcification.
b Craniopharyngioma (cystic variety).

Discussion

Craniopharyngiomas arise from Rathke's pouch or midline epithelial cysts in the suprasellar region, and mostly present in childhood. Calcification occurs in over 80% of cases, although this is less common in adults. The cysts contain cholesterol, lowering their attenuation value and making them appear dark. Approximately 15% of tumours extend into the pituitary fossa, causing enlargement of the sella (Fig. 2.2). In adults the differential diagnosis includes teratomas, partially thrombosed aneurysms, hypothalamic gliomas and cystic meningiomas.

In this patient the expansile craniopharyngioma had compressed the optic chiasm and caused bilateral optic atrophy. Other clinical presentations include bitemporal hemianopia, headache due to obstructive hydrocephalus at the level of the third ventricle and diabetes insipidus.

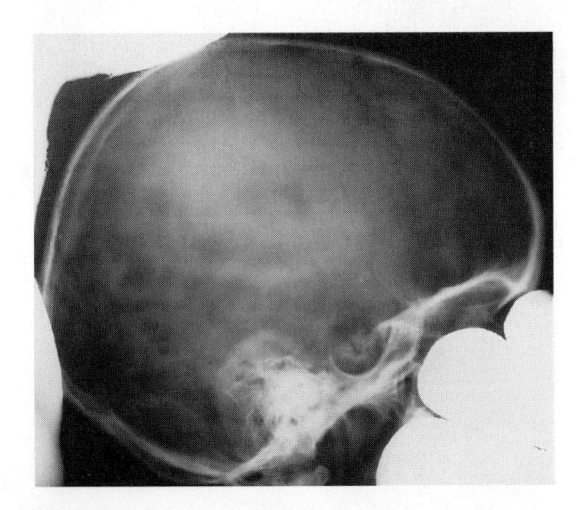

Fig. 2.2
Craniopharyngioma. Lateral skull radiograph in another patient showing enlargement of the pituitary fossa with erosion of the dorsum sellae and suprasellar calcification.

QUESTION 3

There is a 3-month interval between these two chest films (Figs 3.1a and 3.1b).
a What is the most likely diagnosis?
b List the possible causes.
c What investigation would confirm the diagnosis?

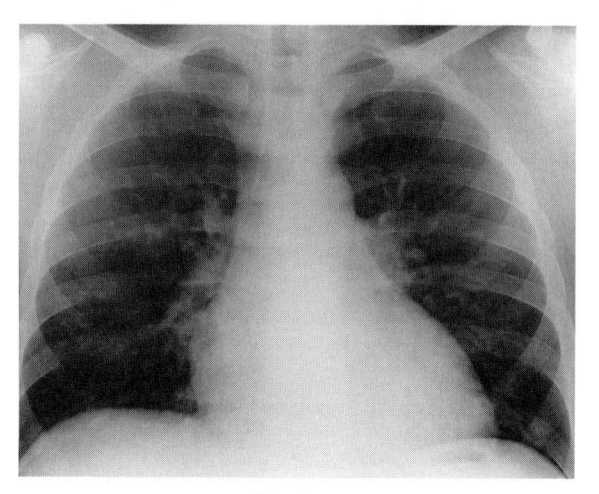

Fig. 3.1a
Baseline chest radiograph.

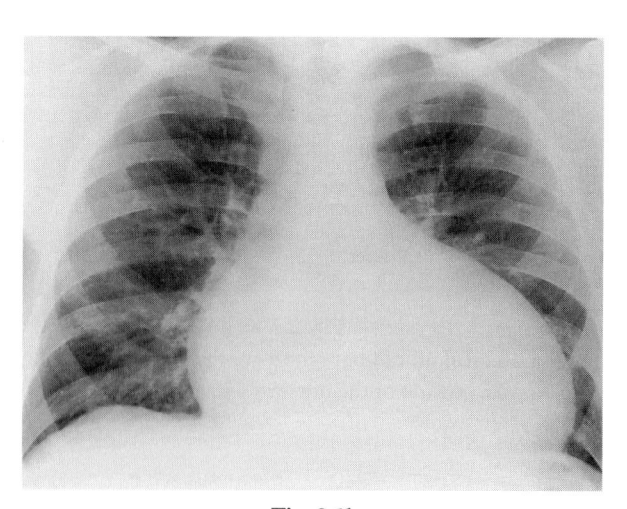

Fig. 3.1b
Chest radiograph 3 months later.

ANSWER 3

a Pericardial effusion.
b Viral pericarditis.
   TB pericarditis (often rapid in onset).
   Malignancy, especially bronchial carcinoma.
   Uraemia.
   Myocardial infarction, Dressler's syndrome.
   Trauma.
   Radiotherapy.
   Connective tissue disorders.
   Hypothyroidism.
c Cardiac ultrasound or echocardiography.

Discussion

The heart has a globular shape on the PA chest radiograph (Fig. 3.1b). The heart borders have a more distinct outline because the pericardial fluid 'cushions' movement from the cardiac pulsations. Despite the degree of cardiac enlargement, there is a normal pulmonary vasculature and no evidence of heart failure. There are numerous causes of pericardial effusions, so always review the chest radiograph for a possible aetiology. For example, erosions in the outer ends of the clavicles and shoulders would suggest rheumatoid arthritis, and a mastectomy or pulmonary mass lesion would suggest malignancy as the underlying cause. The cause in this man was uraemia secondary to chronic renal failure, although there were no secondary features on the chest radiograph to support this.

QUESTION 4

This is an unenhanced CT brain scan of a 73-year-old woman (Fig. 4.1).

a What is the diagnosis?

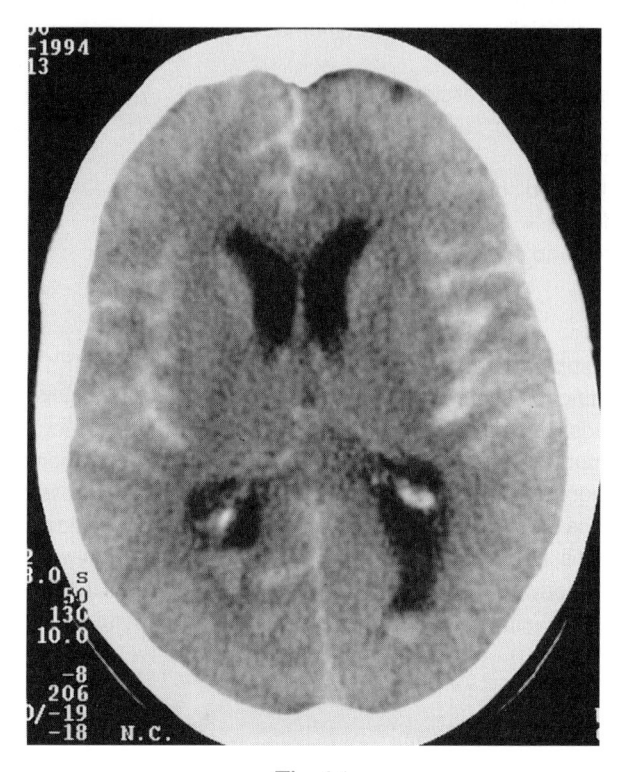

Fig. 4.1

ANSWER 4

a Subarachnoid haemorrhage with intraventricular extension.

Discussion

Subarachnoid haemorrhage is spontaneous or traumatic in origin. Spontaneous bleeding is caused by rupture of a berry aneurysm in 75% of patients, and arises from an arteriovenous malformation in 10%. The remainder have no known cause but probably arise from small berry aneurysms. The patients in this last group have a better prognosis. Berry aneurysms develop in medium-sized arteries at bifurcations. The common sites are at the anterior communicating artery (40%), internal carotid/posterior communicating artery (30%) and at the bifurcation of the middle cerebral artery (25%). Between 15 and 25% of berry aneurysms are multiple. Berry aneurysms are associated with polycystic kidneys, coarctation, Marfan's syndrome, Ehlers–Danlos syndrome, pseudoxanthoma elasticum and Osler–Rendu–Weber syndrome.

In this patient, high-attenuation areas are present in the Sylvian fissures. There is high-attenuating fluid, appearing white, in the dependent parts of the occipital horns of both lateral ventricles (Fig. 4.1). This is due to fresh blood in the subarachnoid space extending into the ventricles. A late complication is obstructive hydrocephalus occurring due to adhesions in the region of the aqueduct of Sylvius or third ventricle.

There is a high risk of rebleeding in the first week, and surgical intervention should be undertaken as soon as possible after the bleed. In unconscious patients and in those with a severe neurological deficit, clipping aneurysms is a potentially hazardous procedure. As carotid and vertebral arteriography should only be carried out when surgery is being contemplated, these investigations should only be applied to those patients who are conscious and have only minor neurological deficit (Fig. 4.2).

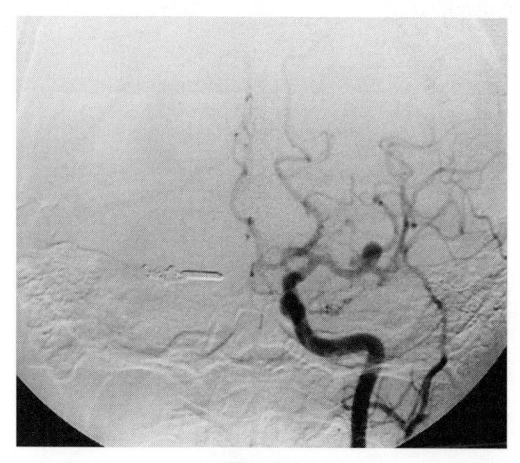

Fig. 4.2
Carotid arteriogram in another patient showing an aneurysm in the middle cerebral artery. Note the clip at the site of an aneurysm on the opposite side.

QUESTION 5

This 40-year-old man presented with diarrhoea, weight loss and backache (Fig. 5.1).

a List the radiological abnormalities.
b What is the most likely diagnosis?

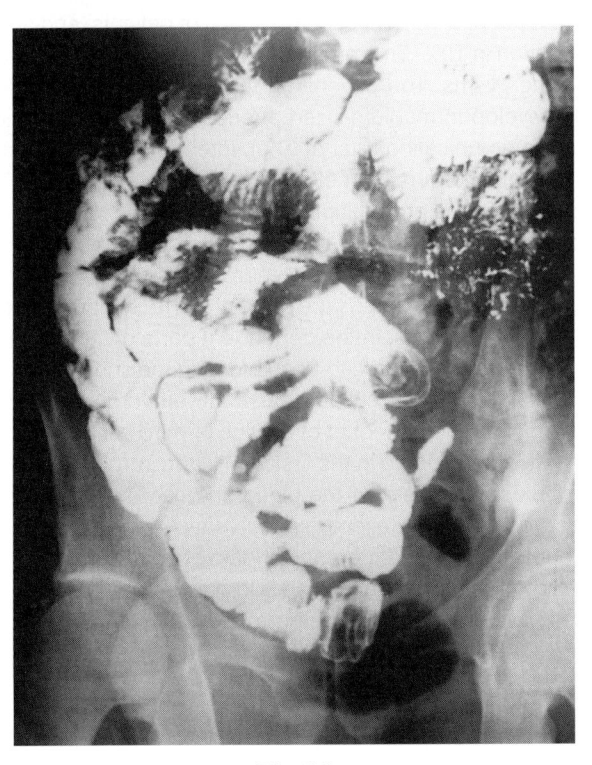

Fig. 5.1

ANSWER 5

a **i** Small bowel strictures separated by segments of normal bowel (skip lesions).
  ii Broad-based, pointed, penetrating ('rose-thorn') ulcers.
  iii Narrowing and erosion of the visible left sacroiliac joint with underlying sclerosis.
b Crohn's disease.

Discussion

Crohn's disease usually presents in young adults. The most common site of involvement is the terminal ileum. The small bowel is involved in 80% of cases, but any part of the alimentary tract, from mouth to anus, can be involved. Fifty per cent of patients have colonic involvement.

Crohn's disease is a transmural process. The earliest manifestation is the small aphthous ulcer, followed by deeper 'rose-thorn' ulcers. These intersect between oedematous islands of residual mucosa, giving a cobblestone pattern. Inflammatory thickening of the bowel wall causes stricture formation and bowel loop separation. Complications include fistulae, abscesses and, in individuals who are HLA-B27-positive, the development of ankylosing spondylitis. There is a higher incidence of sacroiliitis, although this is not related to HLA-B27 status. Crohn's disease is also associated with gallstones (due to malabsorption of bile salts from the terminal ileum), sclerosing cholangitis and oxalate urinary tract calculi.

When examining a radiograph from a small bowel series, always actively look for evidence of gallbladder disease (radiopaque stones or surgical clips in the right upper quadrant), sacroiliitis and ankylosing spondylitis.

QUESTION 6

This was an incidental finding in a 9-year-old girl.

a What abnormality is shown on the chest radiograph (Fig. 6.1)?
b What is the differential diagnosis?

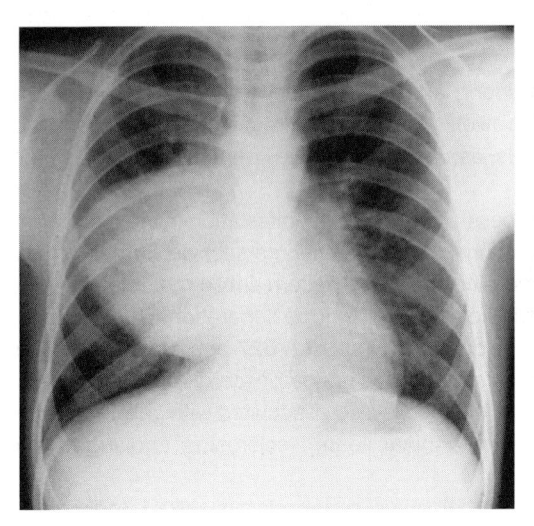

Fig. 6.1a
PA chest radiograph.

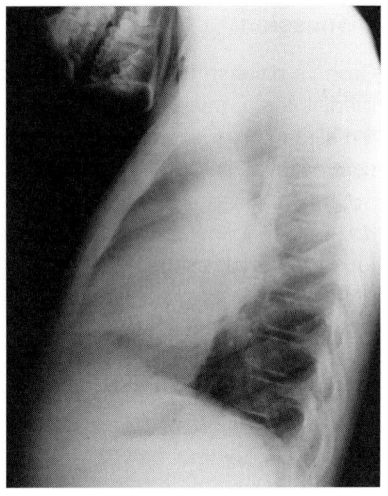

Fig. 6.1b
Lateral chest radiograph.

Answer 6

a The PA chest radiograph shows a large mass arising from the mediastinum. The right heart border is obscured, indicating that the mass lies anteriorly. This is confirmed on the lateral projection. The mediastinal mass has a lobulated margin and is of soft tissue density.

b The differential diagnoses for a mass in this position include teratoma, thymoma, lymphoma and also a pericardial or 'springwater' cyst.

Discussion

In this patient the diagnosis was a teratoma (benign cystic dermoid) confirmed on a CT examination of the thorax (Fig. 6.2). The mass abuts the right heart border, accounting for the loss of this silhouette on the PA chest radiograph.

Anterior mediastinal masses also include those situated at the cardiophrenic angle, such as pericardiac fat pads seen in the obese, diaphragmatic humps and Morgagni herniae.

Thymic tumours may also occur in the superior mediastinum. This causes obliteration of the retrosternal air space on a lateral chest radiograph. Other causes of superior mediastinal masses include thyroid masses and lymph node masses. In elderly subjects one should also consider tortuous great vessels and aneurysms of the ascending aorta as possible causes.

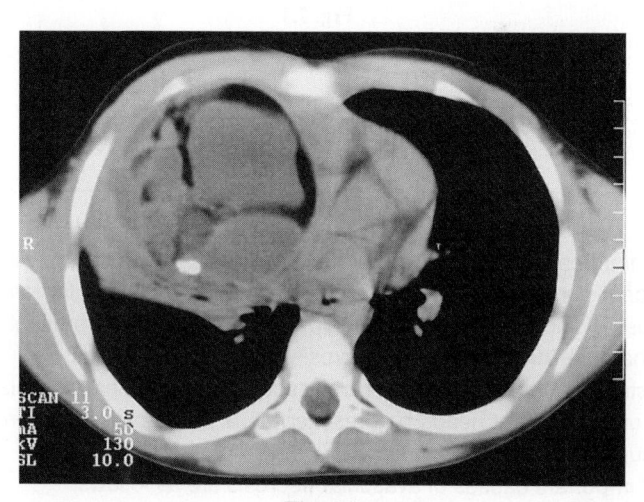

Fig. 6.2
CT of the thorax demonstrating a smooth, well-defined mass with elements of calcification (white), soft tissue (grey) and fat (black) densities. The appearances are those of a mediastinal teratoma (benign cystic dermoid).

QUESTION 7

a What are the radiological abnormalities in these hips (Fig. 7.1)? What is the underlying pathological process?
b Is there a clue as to the possible cause?
c What are the other causes of this condition?

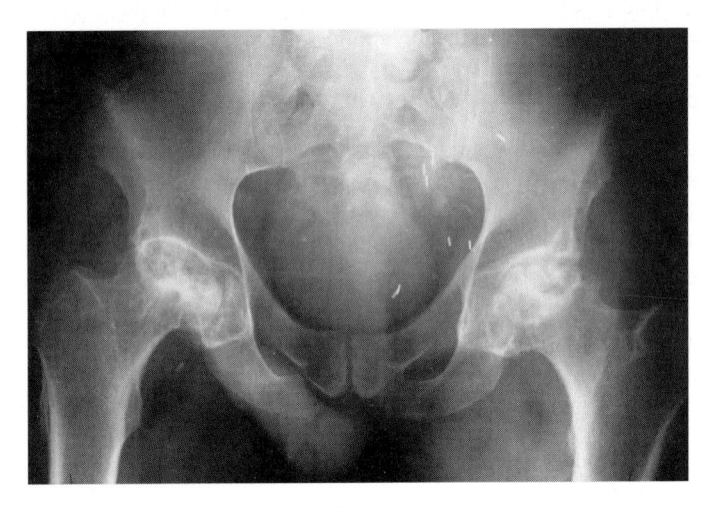

Fig. 7.1

ANSWER 7

a Both femoral heads show a mixture of sclerosis and radiolucency, with flattening of their superior surfaces. There is some fragmentation of the left femoral head. While there is loss of joint space in the right hip, no osteophytes are present. This appearance is characteristic of avascular necrosis of the femoral heads.
b Surgical staples in the left iliac fossa are associated with a renal transplant. Avascular necrosis of the femoral heads has resulted as a complication of steroid and other immunosuppressives.
c The most important causes of avascular necrosis are as follows:

Femoral neck and scaphoid fractures; Perthe's disease; chronic use of non-steroidal anti-inflammatory drugs; alcohol; radiotherapy; vasculitis associated with rheumatoid arthritis and systemic lupus erythematosus; diabetes mellitus; pregnancy; fat emboli following trauma, pancreatitis and hyperlipidaemia; sickle cell disease; polycythaemia rubra vera; Gaucher's disease; haemophilia; caisson disease seen in deep sea divers.

Discussion

Avascular necrosis is an important radiological finding and is a manifestation of a number of diseases. The clues to the underlying aetiology can be gained from careful examination of the film. For example, the association of avascular necrosis with an enlarged spleen would raise the possibility of portal hypertension secondary to alcohol excess, polycythaemia rubra vera or Gaucher's disease. In established sickle cell anaemia the spleen tends to be small due to infarction, but early disease may cause bony changes with mild splenomegaly. It is essential to look carefully at the film for evidence of the use of steroid or other immunosuppressive therapy. For instance, an ileostomy in the right iliac fossa for ulcerative colitis may indicate the prior use of steroids and/or other immunosuppressives. Calcification of the pancreas may suggest that the patient has chronic pancreatitis and/or diabetes, either of which could be implicated in the development of avascular necrosis.

When changes are seen on plain radiographs the ischaemic process is well established. The sclerosis is caused by reparative bone in response to the ischaemic process. Magnetic resonance imaging (MRI) is the most sensitive method for detecting early change, and will pick up changes earlier than either isotope scanning or CT. Figure 7.2 shows the typical MRI changes of avascular necrosis of both hips in the same patient as depicted in Fig. 7.1.

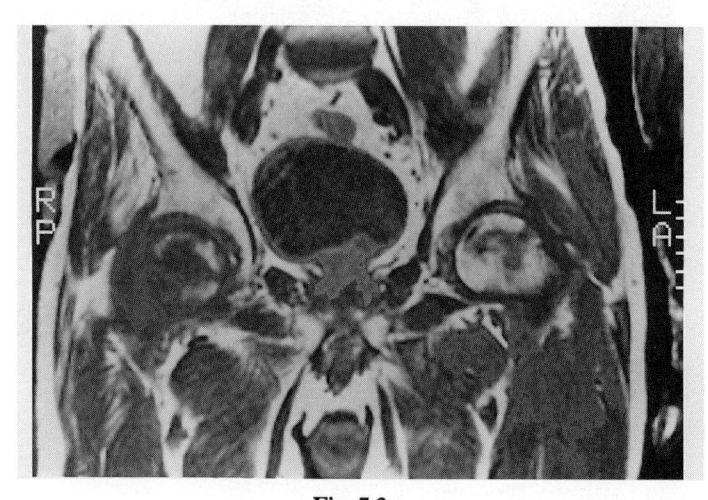

Fig. 7.2
Coronal T1-weighted MRI showing patchy low-signal change and fragmentation in both femoral heads.

QUESTION 8

A 60-year-old lady presented with diarrhoea, weight loss and a macrocytic anaemia.

a What is the investigation?
b What is the diagnosis?
c How do you explain the anaemia?

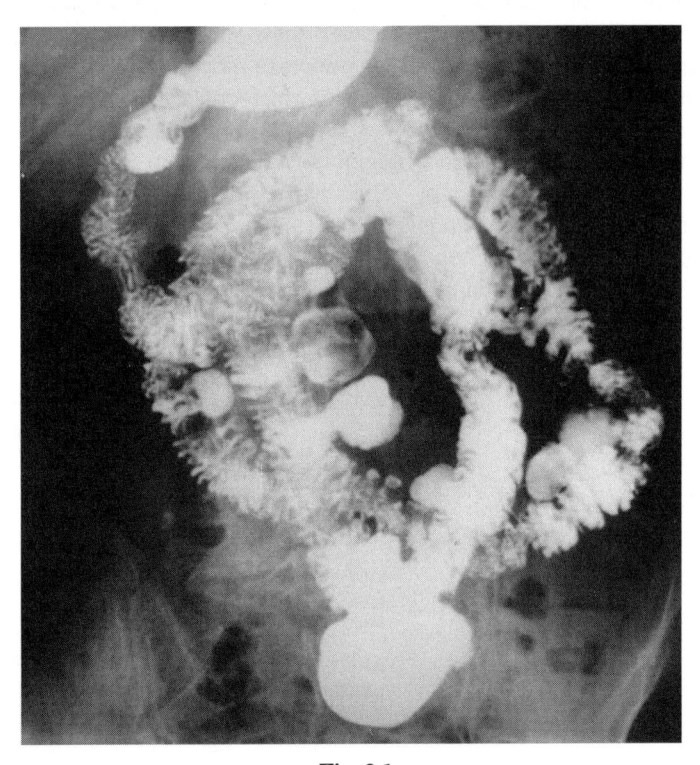

Fig. 8.1

Answer 8

a Small bowel meal.
b Jejunal diverticulosis.
c Vitamin B_{12} deficiency due to bacterial overgrowth.

(Multiple jejunal diverticula are outpouchings of bowel containing stagnant intestinal fluid. This results in bacterial overgrowth within the diverticula themselves. Anaerobic bacteria bind the cobalamin-intrinsic factor complex, making it unavailable for production of vitamin B_{12}. The resulting B_{12} deficiency is responsible for the development of megaloblastic anaemia in which the red cells are macrocytic.)

Discussion

Causes of small bowel bacterial overgrowth are structural or functional. Structural causes include the following: jejunal and duodenal diverticulosis; entero-enteric fistulae; small bowel strictures; afferent loop following partial gastrectomy and end-to-side anastomoses (blind loop). Functional causes include reduced intestinal motility leading to stagnation of intestinal contents, e.g. systemic sclerosis, diabetic autonomic neuropathy, intestinal pseudo-obstruction and amyloidosis. Another functional cause is gastric hypochlorhydria occurring after vagotomy or gastric resection, use of proton pump inhibitors and chronic atrophic gastritis.

Bacterial overgrowth will cause malabsorption not only of vitamins but also of fats, carbohydrates, proteins, bile salts and minerals. It is thought that this occurs in two ways. First, intraluminal metabolism is altered by the abundant abnormal bacteria and secondly, enterocytes lining the intestinal mucosa become damaged, leading to a loss of viable absorptive surface area.

QUESTION 9

This is an unenhanced axial CT scan through the orbits in a 72-year-old man.

a   What is the diagnosis?

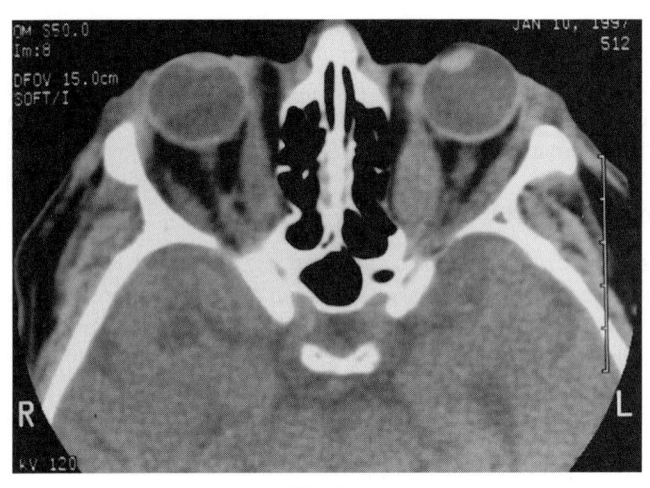

Fig. 9.1

ANSWER 9

a Graves' ophthalmopathy.

Discussion

The exact mechanism underlying the association of ophthalmopathy with Graves' disease is unknown. There is increasing evidence for a role of immunological cross-reactivity against thyroid and orbital tissue shared antigens. Patients are usually hyperthyroid, but eye involvement can be seen in both hypothyroid and euthyroid states.

Extra-ocular muscles are infiltrated by T-lymphocytes which stimulate fibroblasts and glycosaminoglycan production. These contribute to swelling of the muscle bellies due to water-binding. Eventually muscle fibrosis may result. The tendinous portions of the extra-ocular muscles are almost never involved. All extra-ocular muscles can be involved, but the inferior and medial recti are the most frequently affected. Diplopia tends to be worse when looking up, because of the swelling and restriction of the inferior rectus muscle.

There is oedema of the eyelids, which is typically worse on waking. On testing vertical eye movements, both lid retraction and lag are seen. Exophthalmos can be detected clinically by the absence of eyelid cover to that portion of sclera below the lower corneal margin. The exophthalmos is caused by hypertrophy of retrobulbar fat. The cornea may not be completely covered on blinking if protrusion is severe, causing abrasions and ulceration. The optic nerve can be compressed by swollen extra-ocular muscles at the orbital apex, leading to reduced visual acuity and even blindness. This complication is particularly well seen on MRI.

Question 10

a What is the diagnosis?

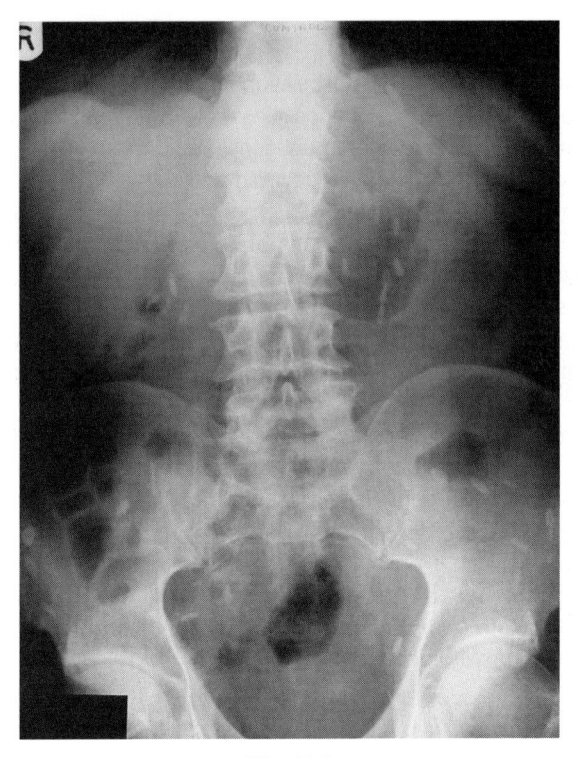

Fig. 10.1

Answer 10

a Cysticercosis.

Discussion

Cysticercosis is caused by the larval form of the pork tapeworm. *Taenia solium* in its adult form lives in the human small bowel. Ova are transferred to pigs feeding on contaminated human waste, who then become the intermediate host. Larvae penetrate the pig intestines and develop into cysts (cysticerci) in the brain and muscles of the animal. The cycle is completed when poorly cooked pork is eaten by the human host.

Cysticercosis occurs mainly in areas of poor hygiene, such as Central and South America, Africa, India and South East Asia.

Symptoms of cysticercosis may include epilepsy when there is brain involvement, visual disturbance with eye involvement and muscular discomfort when the cysticerci are situated in muscle. Inactive cysts calcify, giving characteristic radiological appearances in muscle – the cysts become compressed from side to side when they lie within muscle, such that their long axes align themselves parallel to the direction of the muscle fibres. Calcified cysts involving the brain (Fig. 10.2a and b) may be difficult to distinguish from tuberculomata or toxoplasmosis, and when uncalcified (active) they may be clinically and radiologically indistinguishable from small abscesses, metastases, toxoplasmosis or hydatid disease.

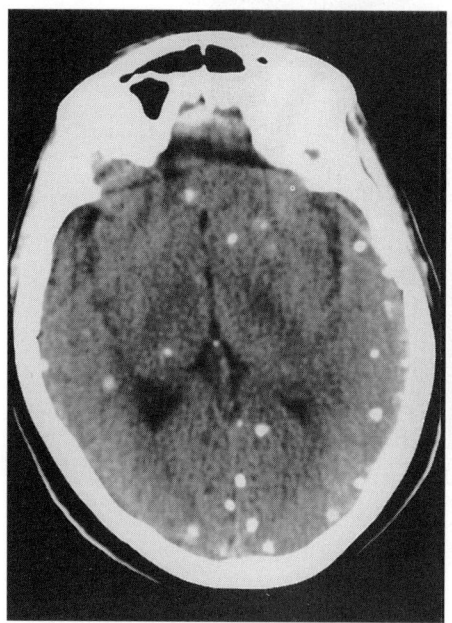

Fig. 10.2a
CT brain. Cysticercosis. Note the calcified spherical cysticerci throughout the brain.

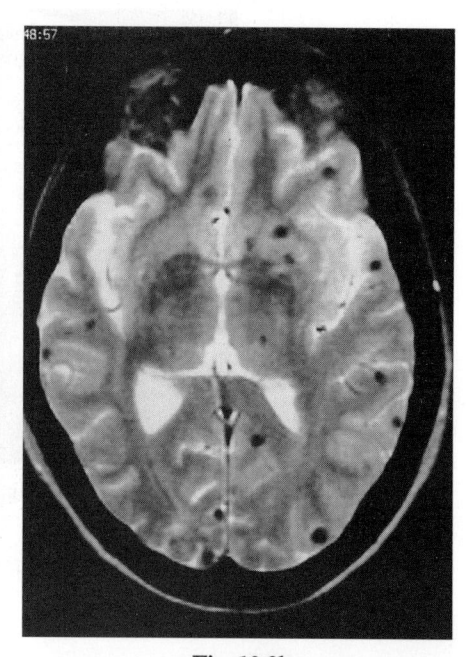

Fig. 10.2b
T2-weighted MRI brain. Cysticercosis. The calcified cysticerci are of uniformly low signal on all sequences.

QUESTION 11

A 30-year-old woman has a 7-day history of headache with sudden onset. Figure 11.1 shows a sagittal T1-weighted image from an MRI scan of her brain. No contrast medium has been given.

a What is the cause of her headache?
b Suggest a precipitating factor in **i** adults
 ii children.

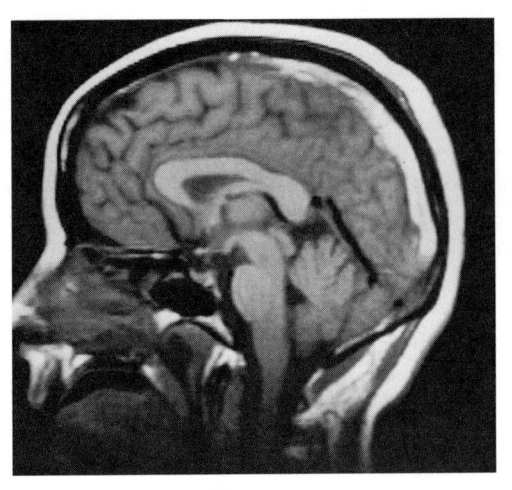

Fig. 11.1

ANSWER 11

a Superior sagittal sinus thrombosis.
b i Pregnancy.
   Use of oral contraceptives.
   Hypercoagulable states.
   Impaired venous return from the head and neck due to superior vena caval obstruction.
   ii Dehydration.
   Middle ear infection.

Discussion

The diagnosis can be simply made by obtaining a sagittal image of the brain on a T1-weighted sequence. The thrombosed dural sinus loses its 'flow void' and appears of high signal (white) instead of its normal low signal (black). Arteries and veins with flowing blood exhibit the so-called 'flow void' which appears black on a T1-weighted sequence.

If MRI is not available, the diagnosis of superior sagittal sinus thrombosis may be made on enhanced axial CT of the brain. This gives the so-called 'delta' sign of contrast-enhanced venous blood flowing at the periphery of the thrombosed and centrally unenhanced sinus. Thrombosis of the venous sinuses predisposes to haemorrhagic infarction of the brain substance, best imaged by CT.

Question 12

This young male has acute chest pain.

a What is this radiological feature called?
b List two possible causes for the appearance shown in Fig. 12.1.
c Give two possible causes of his chest pain.

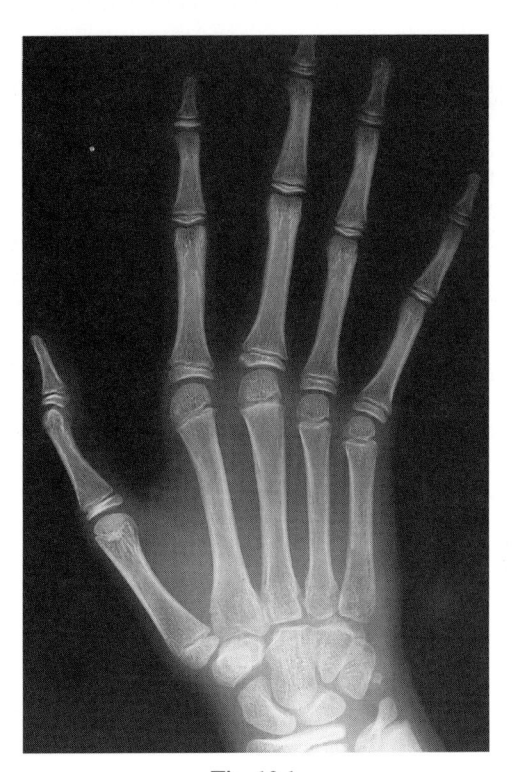

Fig. 12.1

ANSWER 12

a Arachnodactyly.
b Marfan's syndrome, homocystinuria.
c The chest pain is due to either pneumothorax or thoracic aortic dissection associated with Marfan's syndrome.

Discussion

In Fig. 12.1 the metacarpals and phalanges are gracile, demonstrating a high metacarpal index (ratio of length to width of the second to fifth digits is normally between 5.4 and 8). However, the metacarpal index is now thought to be unreliable for diagnosing Marfan's syndrome.

Marfan's syndrome is a multisystem connective tissue disorder with an autosomal dominant mode of inheritance of variable expression and high penetrance. Affected individuals are tall and slender. Their hands are spider-like in appearance (arachnodactyly). Joints are hypermobile due to ligamentous laxity. Marfan's syndrome is associated with dislocation of the lens of the eye and cataract formation. There is a high incidence of mitral and aortic regurgitation, mitral prolapse and aortic dissection due to cystic medial necrosis. Spontaneous pneumothorax is a recognized complication. Examination of the mouth may reveal a high arched palate, with dental crowding.

Homocystinuria is an autosomal recessive condition due to deficiency of cystathionine beta-synthetase. Marfanoid features are present in a third of cases. The key to the diagnosis is the presence of high plasma levels of homocystine and methionine and persistent urinary excretion of homocystine. Pectus excavatum and carinatum may occur in both Marfan's syndrome and homocystinuria. The latter predisposes to thromboembolic disease.

QUESTION 13

This 60-year-old lady has a cough.

a List two radiological abnormalities.
b What is the most likely diagnosis?
c What is the single most important further investigation?

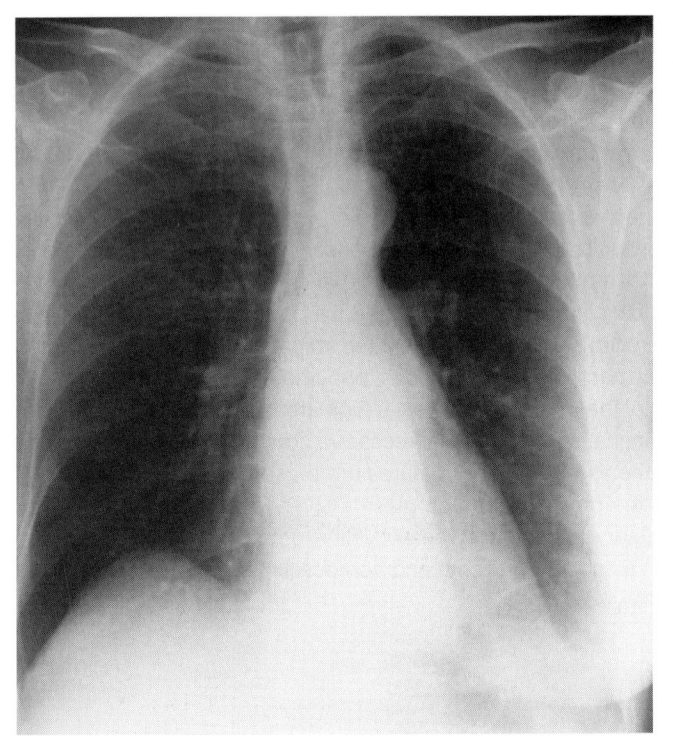

Fig. 13.1

ANSWER 13

a Right mastectomy.
   Triangular (sail-shaped) opacity projected through the heart shadow with loss of definition of the left hemidiaphragm.
b Left lower lobe collapse secondary to enlarged metastatic mediastinal lymph nodes from breast carcinoma.
c CT of the thorax.

The collapse could also be due to an endobronchial lesion rather than extrinsic compression. In these circumstances a primary bronchial neoplasm or an endobronchial metastatic deposit should be considered and bronchoscopy and/or biopsy performed.

Discussion

When the left lower lobe collapses it pulls the greater (or oblique) fissure backwards to the midline. This results in a triangular opacity behind the heart and downward displacement of the left hilum. The left upper lobe expands to occupy the space vacated by the collapsing lower lobe. The left hemithorax reduces its overall volume, but this may be a very subtle radiological sign. The left hemidiaphragm becomes less distinct since the left lower lobe abuts the diaphragm. Metastases to the walls of bronchi are unusual, occurring in only 2% of cases of death from solid tumours. Always check the bones for evidence of metastatic spread.

Always check the symmetry and presence of the breast shadows on chest radiographs in both sexes. Gynaecomastia in men is a useful radiological sign when associated with other signs. For instance, if there was an enlarged heart, think about digoxin treatment. Similarly, if the bones are sclerotic, think about metastatic prostatic carcinoma treated with stilboestrol. Gynaecomastia may be a physical sign in large cell cancers of the lung because of increased gonadotrophin production and in cirrhosis because of sex hormone imbalance with or without spironolactone therapy.

Do not be caught out in any examination by the presence of prosthetic breast implants. They have a characteristic radiographic appearance (Fig. 13.2).

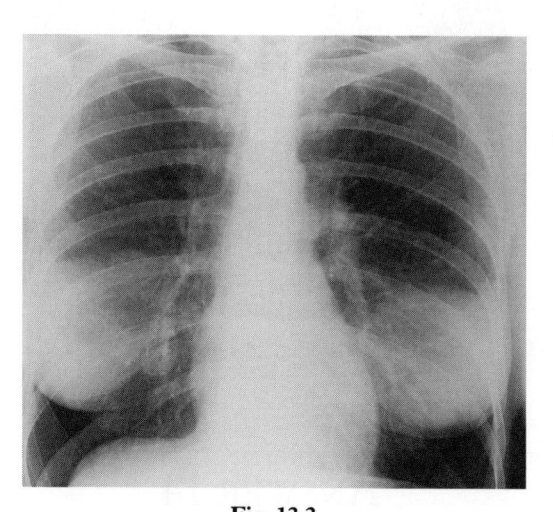

Fig. 13.2
Bilateral breast prostheses.

QUESTION 14

a What investigation has been performed?
b What is the radiological diagnosis, and with which underlying disease is this finding most likely to be associated?
c Which alternative imaging methods can be used to establish the cause of the symptoms in these patients?

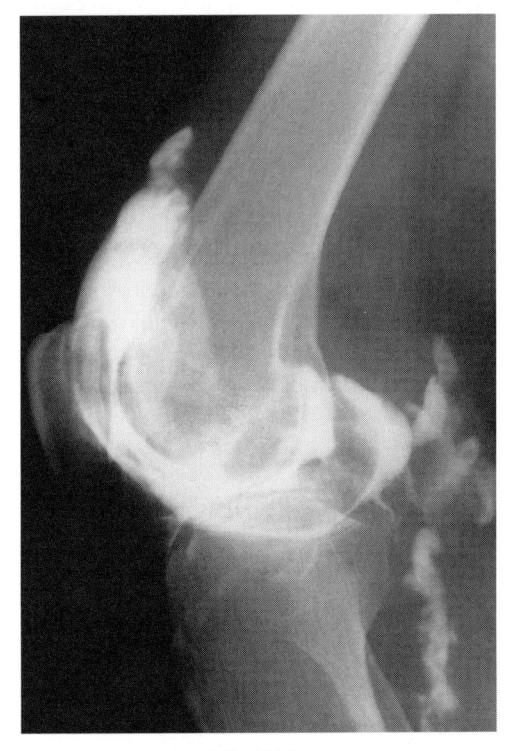

Fig. 14.1

ANSWER 14

a Knee arthrogram.
b Ruptured popliteal (Baker's) cyst associated with rheumatoid arthritis.
c Ultrasound for Baker's cyst. Venogram for deep vein thrombosis.

Discussion

In rheumatoid arthritis, the presence of an effusion in the knee causes stretching of the posterior portion of the joint capsule and increased intra-articular pressure. Eventually a sac is formed by extrusion of synovium through the least supported part of the capsule. Fluid enters this synovial sac but cannot return into the joint because of a valve mechanism, as the neck of the cyst is compressed between the gastrocnemius and semimembranosus muscles. If the cyst ruptures, synovial fluid dissects down through the calf muscles, causing sudden intense swelling, irritation and pain.

The presence of a popliteal cyst with or without this complication can be shown on arthrography or ultrasound. During arthrography, contrast medium enters the joint and communicates with the cyst. If a rupture is present, contrast medium will dissect through the calf muscles as shown in Fig. 14.1. Popliteal cysts are also associated with pigmented villonodular synovitis.

The signs and symptoms of a ruptured popliteal cyst can exactly mimic deep venous thrombosis; even a positive Homan's sign may be present. However, unlike a ruptured popliteal cyst, the onset of pain with calf thrombosis is often insidious. A venogram is diagnostic. Figure 14.2 shows fresh thrombus in the deep veins of the calf.

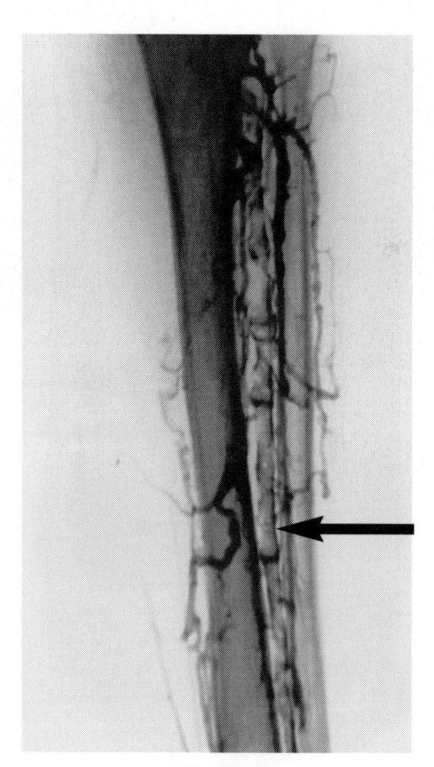

Fig. 14.2
Venogram showing fresh thrombus (arrow) in the deep veins of the calf.

QUESTION 15

This 60-year-old-man complains of severe upper thoracic pain.
a What is the diagnosis?
b What two investigations would you consider in order to influence the patient's management?

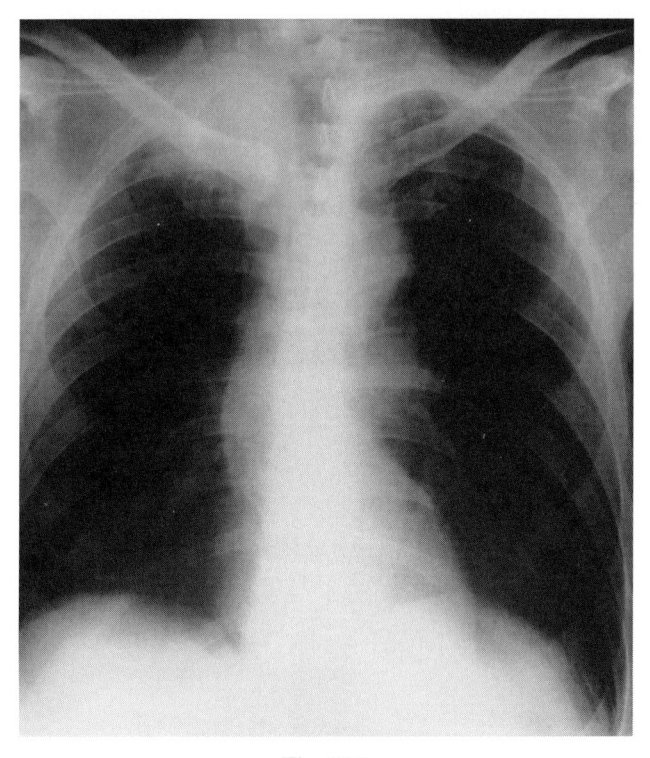

Fig. 15.1

Answer 15

a Right-sided Pancoast (or superior sulcus) tumour with destruction of the posterior second and third ribs and the first and second thoracic vertebrae.
b Sputum cytology. Fine-needle aspiration biopsy.

Discussion

Pancoast tumour occurs in 3% of bronchial carcinomas and involves the superior sulcus. Although the cell type of the tumour is usually squamous, any cell type may give rise to a Pancoast tumour. It is often appropriate to determine the cell type, especially if the tumour is inoperable, as in this case. The simplest and safest method is to obtain sputum cytology. If this is negative, a percutaneous fine-needle aspiration biopsy should be considered. A small-cell carcinoma is the only cell type which is likely to respond favourably to chemotherapy, although only palliation is possible.

If there is no evidence of bony destruction on plain radiography, and the patient has no pain, the next most useful investigation would be an MRI scan. MRI gives excellent soft tissue delineation. Invasion of the brachial plexus and adjacent structures by tumour can be well shown. However, pain arising from the chest wall or brachial plexus is a more sensitive marker of local invasion than MRI.

Pancoast syndrome is due to invasion of the brachial plexus and sympathetic stellate ganglion, and consists of ipsilateral arm pain, muscle wasting of the hand and Horner's syndrome.

Question 16

This 60-year-old woman has a low-grade fever, proximal muscle weakness and a purplish rash.

a What is the diagnosis?
b Name three non-skeletal complications of this disorder.

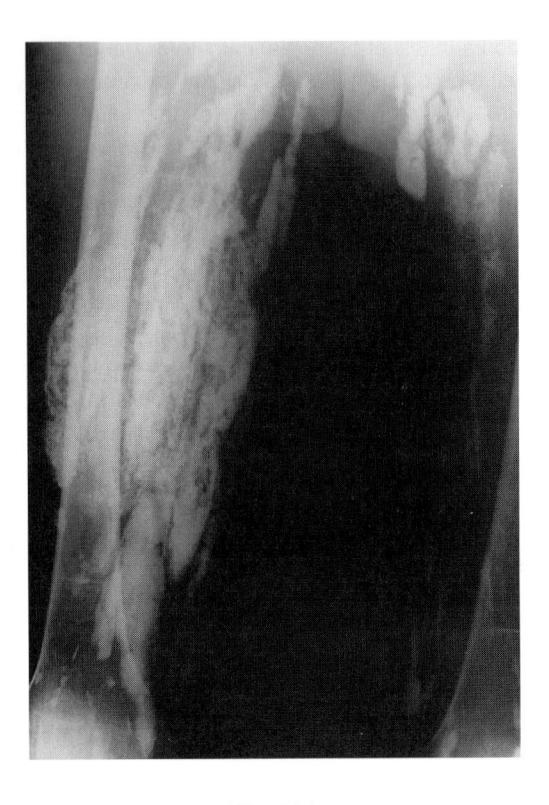

Fig. 16.1

ANSWER 16

a Dermatomyositis.
b i Disseminated pulmonary infiltrates and fibrosis.
  ii Atonic bowel leading to bacterial overgrowth, as in scleroderma.
  iii Association with malignancy (GI tract, ovary, lung, kidney and breast).

Discussion

Dermatomyositis is a humoral-mediated autoimmune syndrome caused by degeneration and inflammation of muscles in association with skin and mucous membrane involvement. Polymyositis, a lymphocyte-mediated process, is the term used when there is only muscle involvement.

Dermatomyositis may occur at any age, with a peak in middle age. In this age group there is a high incidence of malignant neoplasms in the lung and gastrointestinal tract. This association is much weaker in polymyositis patients. Clinically, acute inflammation of muscle causes proximal muscular pain and weakness with a rash on the limbs and trunk. Classically, a purplish rash may be found around the eyelids.

Radiologically, dermatomyositis causes linear confluent calcification in the soft tissues and muscles. This is more common in childhood disease. Rarely, patients may get a rheumatoid-like arthritis, pointing of the terminal phalangeal tufts and a myocarditis.

Pulmonary complications may occur in dermatomyositis. Weakness of the pharyngeal muscles leads to aspiration pneumonitis, and weakness of the diaphragm and intercostal muscles results in hypoventilation. Fibrosing alveolitis and fibrosis are rare complications. Bronchial carcinoma occurs with a higher incidence than in the general population.

Question 17

A 70-year-old woman developed suprapubic pain and fever.

a What are the two radiological abnormalities?
b What is the diagnosis?
c What underlying condition must be excluded?

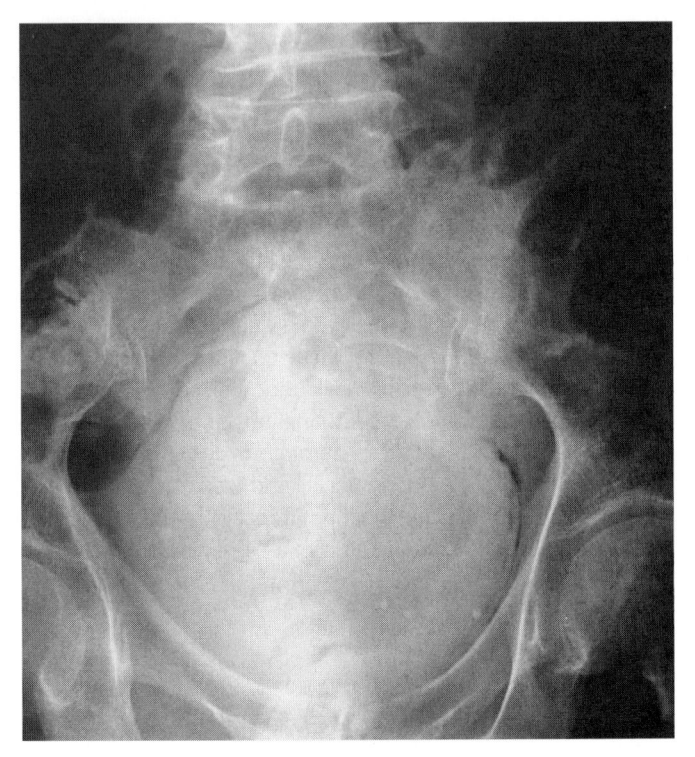

Fig. 17.1

Answer 17

a Gas in the bladder lumen and wall.
b The appearances are those of emphysematous cystitis.
c Diabetes mellitus.

Discussion

Infectious cystitis due to *Candida albicans* and *E. coli* can give rise to gas in the bladder lumen or wall. Patients are usually diabetic. A CT scan of the same patient is shown (Fig. 17.2). Emphysematous cystitis may be associated with bladder outflow obstruction, e.g. neuropathic bladder or prostatic enlargement.

Rarely, emphysematous pyelonephritis also occurs in diabetics and is often fatal.

Other causes of gas in the bladder include recent catheterization or instrumentation (commonest) and a vesico-enteric fistula. The latter is usually seen in diverticulitis, but may occur in other inflammatory conditions and in carcinoma of the bowel or bladder.

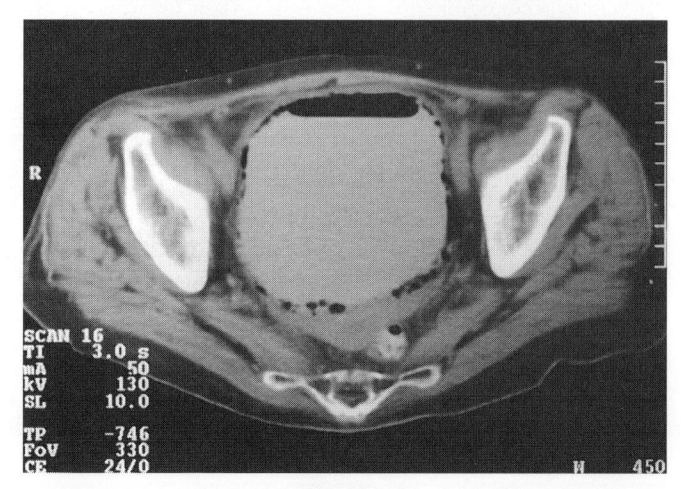

Fig. 17.2
CT scan of the bladder in the same patient, showing an air-fluid level in the bladder and gas in its wall.

QUESTION 18

This patient underwent a thoracic operation 30 years ago.

a What three radiological features are shown?
b What is the diagnosis?

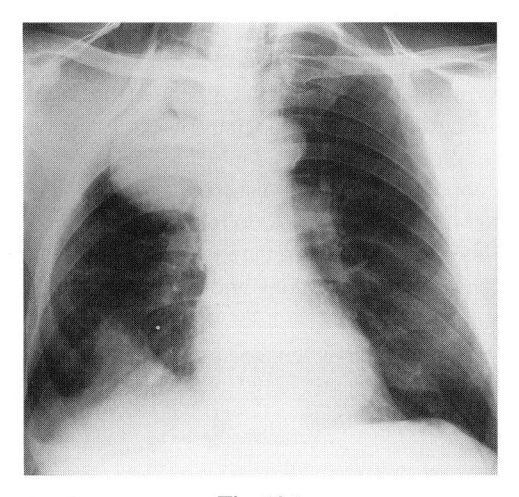

Fig. 18.1

Answer 18

a **i** Deformity of the upper right thoracic cage (thoracoplasty);
 ii Mass lesion with surrounding rim of lucency in the right upper lobe;
 iii Pleural thickening and 'tenting' of the right hemidiaphragm.
b The appearances are those of an aspergilloma (mycetoma) in an old tuberculous cavity in the right upper lobe.

Discussion

Aspergilloma is a term used when the fungus *Aspergillus fumigatus* colonizes a pre-existing pulmonary cavity. Other fungi may cause similar appearances but are much less common. The cavity is usually post-tuberculous, but may occur in other conditions causing cavitation or fibrosis with emphysema such as sarcoidosis, bullous lung disease, ankylosing spondylitis, chronic extrinsic allergic alveolitis or even carcinoma.

The patient is frequently asymptomatic but, when symptoms occur, may complain of cough with or without haemoptysis. Patients occasionally present with massive haemoptysis which requires surgery or bronchial artery embolization. Aspergillomata can be treated with systemic and topical antifungal therapy (i.e. by percutaneous cavity puncture). It may sometimes be difficult to distinguish an aspergilloma from a carcinoma. Characteristically an aspergilloma has a rim of air around it which moves on repositioning the patient. An aspergilloma has a characteristic appearance on CT (Fig. 18.2; see also Fig. 58.1).

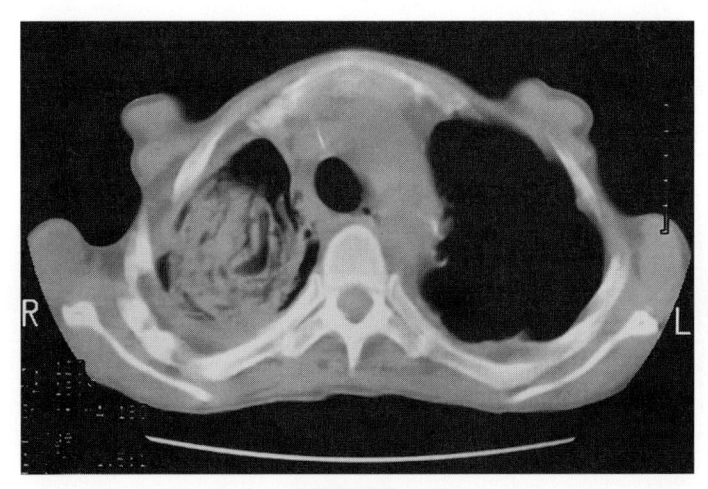

Fig. 18.2
CT thorax. Early stages of an aspergilloma right upper lobe. The mass of fungal hyphae has a 'whorled' appearance. Eventually the fungal mass condenses, producing the typical fungal ball within a cavity.

QUESTION 19

This 70-year-old former boilermaker has right-sided chest pain and weight loss. He had a previous history of transitional cell carcinoma of the bladder.

a What diagnoses would you consider?
b What further investigations would be indicated?

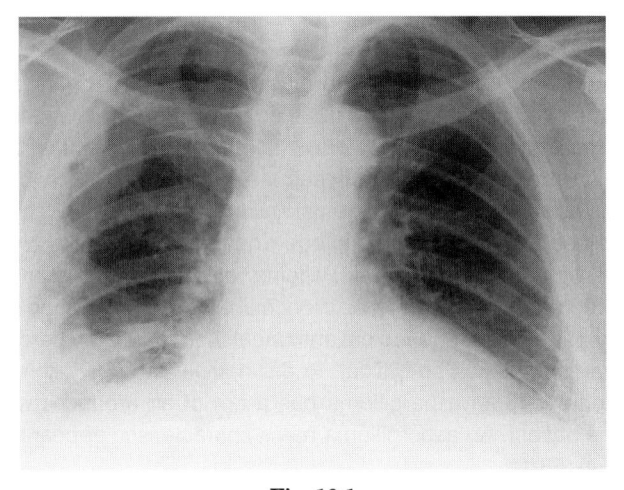

Fig. 19.1

ANSWER 19

a There is lobulated pleural thickening along the right lateral chest wall. The differential diagnosis for these appearances includes mesothelioma or metastatic carcinoma.

b CT scan of the thorax. A biopsy of the pleural mass may differentiate between the two conditions.

Discussion

Mesothelioma is associated with occupational exposure to asbestos in approximately 80% of cases, and is invariably unilateral. Unlike asbestosis, the development of a mesothelioma has no relation to the extent or duration of exposure to asbestos. It may appear up to 30 years after the initial exposure. Diagnosis depends on a positive occupational history, typical radiological features and a positive pleural biopsy. The latter can be performed as a percutaneous procedure under CT guidance or as a video-assisted thoracoscopic surgical (VATS) procedure. Unfortunately, the histological features of mesothelioma can mimic carcinoma or sarcoma, making distinction difficult. Furthermore, mesothelioma readily 'seeds' down the needle track, resulting in an open tumour-filled communication with the skin. Mesothelioma has no effective treatment and carries a dismal prognosis. A CT scan of the thorax (Fig. 19.2) demonstrates mesothelioma of the chest wall.

Primary tumours may metastasize to the pleura. They include:

- lung (40%);
- breast (20%);
- lymphoma (10%);
- ovary; uterus; gastrointestinal tract; pancreas; bladder.

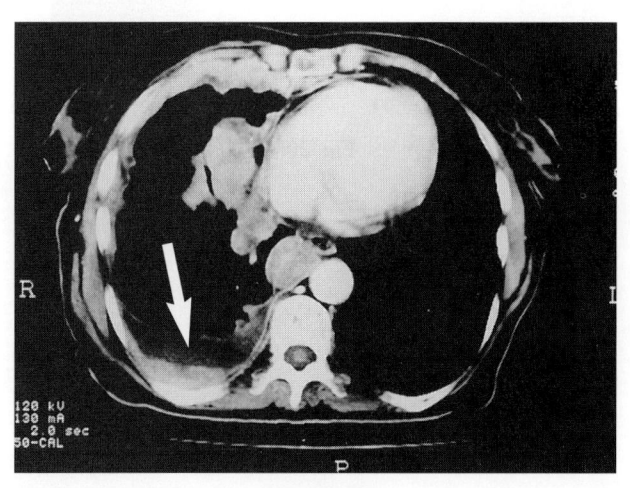

Fig. 19.2
CT thorax. Mesothelioma – a thick lobulated pleural mass encircles the right chest wall. Note the pleural effusion (arrow).

QUESTION 20

This 55-year-old man complains of epigastric pain.

a What are the two radiological signs?
b Suggest a condition which could explain both features.

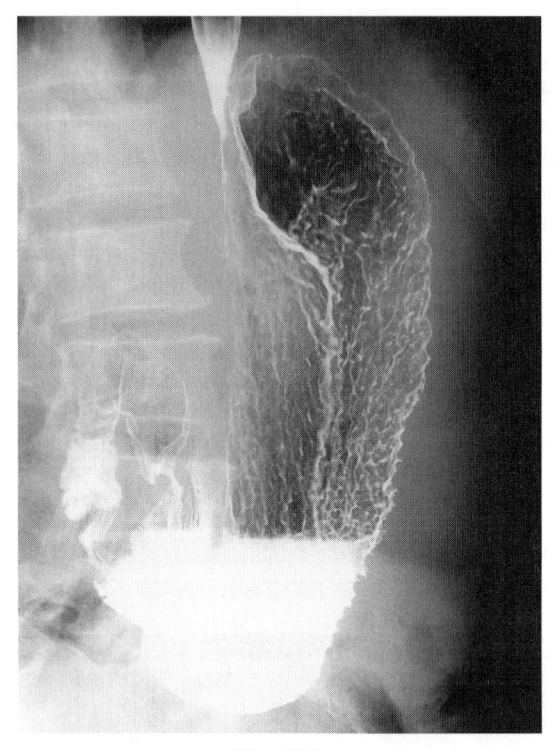

Fig. 20.1

ANSWER 20

a There is erosive (haemorrhagic) gastritis and marked splenomegaly.
b Chronic myeloid leukaemia is a cause of a huge spleen. It can cause gastric erosions either as a result of steroids or as a stress response.

Discussion

Erosive gastritis (Fig. 20.2) accounts for up to 20% of all cases of blood loss from the gastrointestinal tract. It may present with dyspeptic symptoms or haematemesis. An underlying cause is not found in up to 50% of cases.

Causes of erosive gastritis include the following:

- drugs – steroids; aspirin; non-steroidal anti-inflammatory agents; alcohol;
- infection in immunocompromised hosts – viral (herpes simplex, cytomegalovirus); candida.

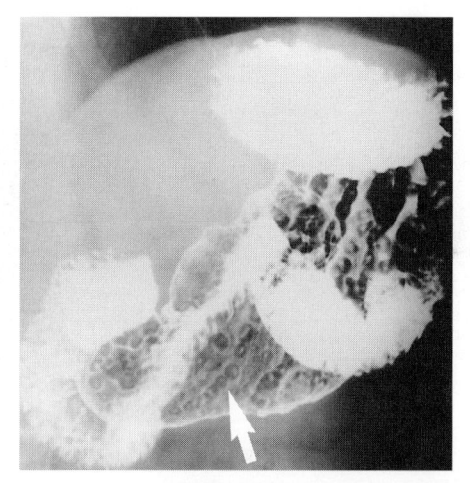

Fig. 20.2
Erosive gastritis in another patient. Note typical target lesions (arrow).

QUESTION 21

This 67-year-old man complains of progressive dyspnoea.

a Describe the radiological features.
b What is the diagnosis?

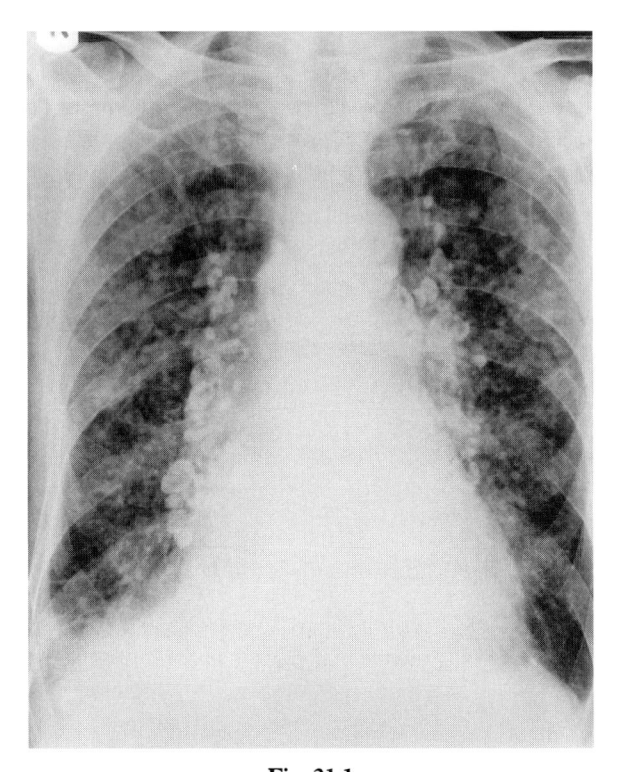

Fig. 21.1

ANSWER 21

a There are numerous nodular densities throughout both lungs with sparing of the bases. 'Eggshell' hilar lymph node calcification is present.
b The appearances are those of *silicosis*.

Discussion

Silicosis is a fibrosing pulmonary disease caused by chronic exposure to crystalline silica. Occupational exposure occurs in mining, tunnelling, quarrying and sandblasting. Small particles of silica are inhaled and engulfed by macrophages. Cell death results when the silica is expelled. Collagen is then formed, leaving 2–3 mm nodules with layers of hyalinized connective tissue.

There are three types of silicosis:

  i chronic – moderate exposure over 20–40 years;
  ii accelerated – increased particle load over 5–15 years;
  iii acute – heavy exposure over a period of less than 5 years.

The radiographic features are multiple soft tissue nodules, mainly in the upper zones. This distribution may be explained by lymphatic clearance of dust being more efficient at the bases. Some nodules show central calcification. Eggshell calcification of hilar lymph glands occurs in 5% of cases.

Complications of silicosis are as follows:

  i Progressive massive fibrosis (PMF), in which the coalescence of multiple silicotic nodules forms conglomerate masses. These start in the upper and mid zones and migrate towards the hila ('angel's wings'). They tend to be bilateral and symmetrical.
  ii Tuberculosis. This may present as cavitation within an area of PMF.
  iii Caplan's syndrome. This is the combination of pulmonary rheumatoid nodules and silicotic nodules.

QUESTION 22

A 25-year-old male had sustained a fracture of his right femur 48 hours earlier. He became acutely confused and restless. On examination he was tachypnoeic with crackles throughout his chest. At the time of admission his chest radiograph was normal.

a What is the diagnosis?

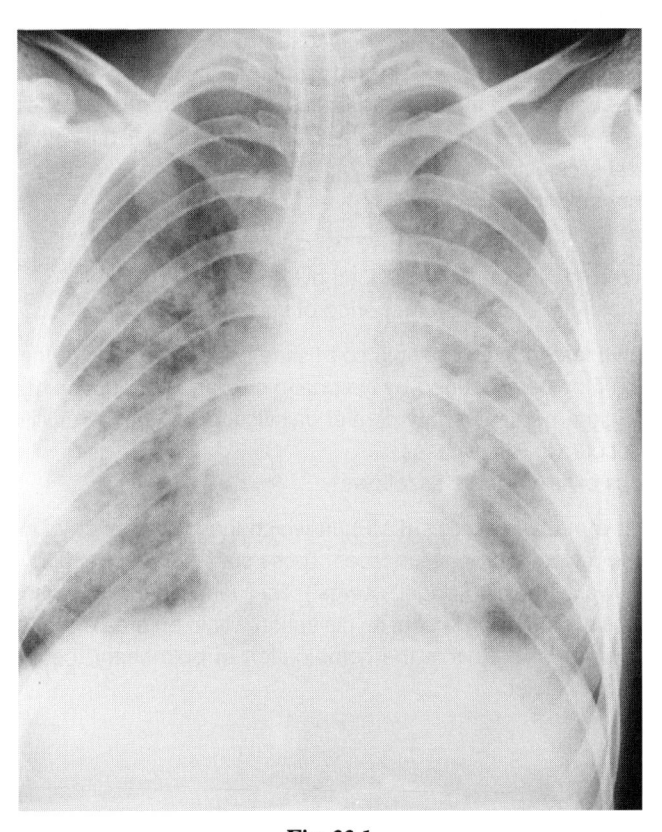

Fig. 22.1

Answer 22

a The patient has fat embolism.

Discussion

The chest radiograph shows an endotracheal tube just above the carina and bilateral air space shadowing (consolidation). This shadowing is more marked peripherally than centrally, which is the reverse of cardiogenic pulmonary oedema. An air bronchogram is present in the left mid zone.

Fat embolism usually occurs in young people who sustain leg fractures in road traffic accidents, and in elderly people with femoral neck fractures. It can also occur after hip replacement surgery. Fat released from the bone marrow at the time of the fracture lodges in peripheral pulmonary arteries. Symptoms appear approximately 40 hours after injury and include dyspnoea, cough, haemoptysis and pleuritic pain. Confusion, restlessness and coma herald involvement of the central nervous system. Petechiae are common, and occur in the conjunctiva, retina and anterior axillary skin folds. This distribution is said to occur because the fat globules 'float' to the uppermost vessels. Patients become hypoxaemic.

The abnormal chest radiograph appearances occur 24 to 48 hours after trauma. The pathological changes in the lungs are due to pulmonary oedema from increased permeability.

QUESTION 23

This child is febrile and breathless.

a What is the most likely diagnosis?

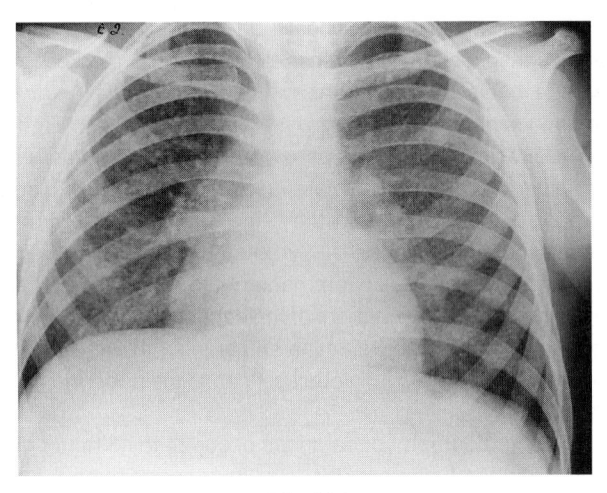

Fig. 23.1

ANSWER 23

a Miliary tuberculosis (TB).

Discussion

Miliary TB results from bloodborne spread of the tubercle bacilli throughout the body. Multiple granulomas, no larger than about 2 mm, are seen throughout both lungs. These nodules are so well defined that they resemble millet seeds – hence the term 'miliary' TB.

Miliary TB can occur as a complication of both primary and reactivation forms of the disease. In this patient there is hilar lymphadenopathy, indicating that miliary spread has complicated primary TB. When the patient is febrile and unwell, miliary TB is the first consideration. However, there are other causes of miliary shadowing on the chest radiograph:

- sarcoidosis;
- silicosis;
- acute extrinsic allergic alveolitis;
- fibrosing alveolitis;
- viral pneumonia, e.g. glandular fever.

The important points to remember are as follows:

    i The incidence of TB is increasing due to:
- immunosuppression (HIV disease, steroids, diabetics);
- homelessness.

    ii TB is a treatable but potentially fatal condition and should never be forgotten.

    iii A normal chest radiograph does not exclude the diagnosis of miliary TB.

Question 24

These two patients have the same disease.

a Describe one radiological feature in Fig. 24.1a.
b Describe two radiological features in Fig. 24.1b.
c What is the underlying diagnosis?
d What complication has occurred in the patient depicted in Fig. 24.1b?

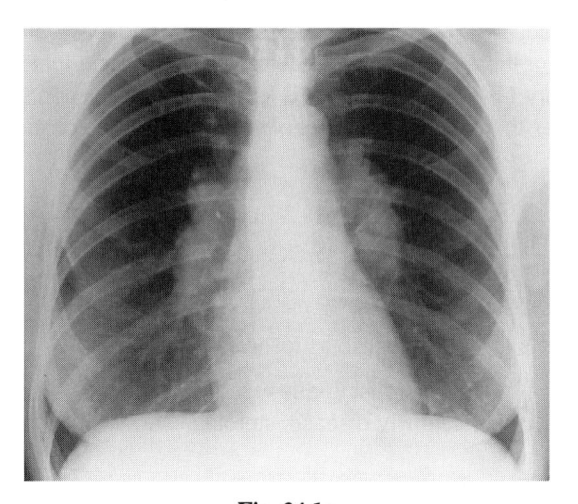

Fig. 24.1a

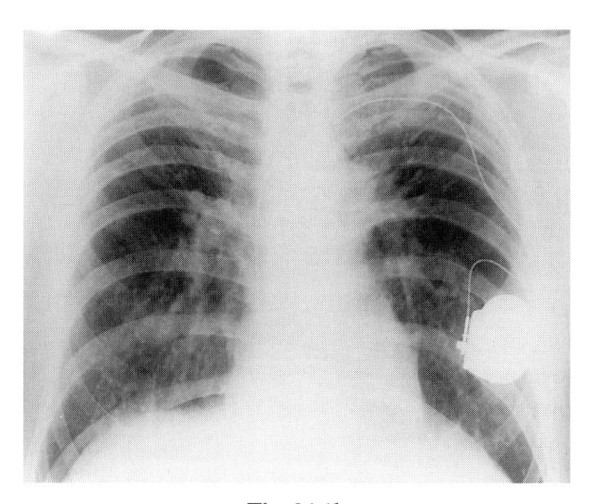

Fig. 24.1b

ANSWER 24

a Bilateral hilar lymphadenopathy.
b Bilateral upper zone fibrosis. Permanent single-chamber pacemaker.
c Sarcoidosis.
d Granulomatous involvement of the myocardium and conducting pathways causing complete heart block.

Discussion

Sarcoidosis is a granulomatous disorder of unknown aetiology, and can affect any system. The commonest clinical presentations are erythema nodosum (30%), abnormal chest radiograph in the absence of symptoms (25%), and respiratory symptoms (20%).

Intrathoracic sarcoidosis has the following four stages.

Stage 0   Normal chest radiograph
Stage I   Nodal enlargement (bilateral hilar and sometimes also paratracheal lymphadenopathy)
Stage II   Node enlargement and parenchymal shadowing
Stage III Parenchymal shadowing only (± fibrosis).

Symmetrical bilateral hilar lymphadenopathy (BHL) is the commonest manifestation of sarcoidosis seen on chest radiography. Lymph node enlargement, for practical purposes, *always* precedes the onset of parenchymal shadowing. The paratracheal lymph nodes do not enlarge to the same extent as the hilar glands. In lymphoma, hilar lymphadenopathy tends to be asymmetrical and paratracheal adenopathy usually predominates.

Causes of BHL include the following:

- sarcoidosis;
- lymphoma;
- metastases, e.g. from small-cell lung cancer. Tend to be unilateral or asymmetrical.
- TB;
- extrinsic allergic alveolitis;
- pneumoconiosis, e.g. silicosis;
- chronic lymphatic leukaemia;
- cystic fibrosis.

Stage III sarcoidosis incorporates those cases in which there are parenchymal infiltrates with or without fibrosis. The fibrosis in sarcoidosis tends to be upper and mid zone in distribution, as can be seen in Fig. 24.1b. The heart may be directly or indirectly involved in sarcoidosis. When granulomata directly involve the heart, patients develop arrythmias, heart block, congestive cardiac failure or cardiomyopathy, depending on the site and extent of the disease. Indirect involvement is the development of cor pulmonale secondary to lung disease and hypoxaemia.

QUESTION 25

This 60-year-old lady has acute on chronic dyspnoea.

a List three radiological abnormalities.
b What is the underlying diagnosis? What complication has occurred?

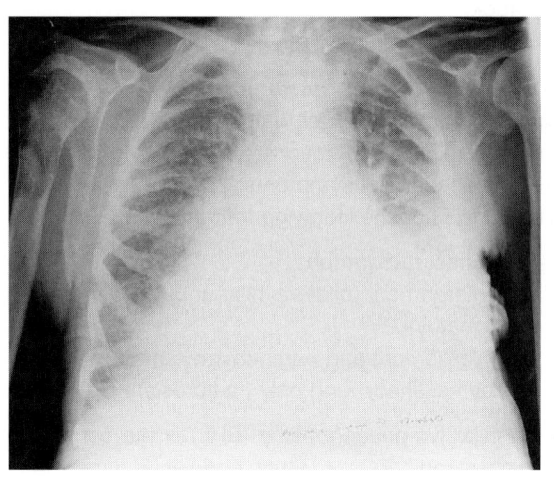

Fig. 25.1

Answer 25

a Brown tumour of right humerus.
Cardiomegaly.
Interstitial pulmonary oedema.
b Hyperparathyroidism due to chronic renal failure. Congestive heart failure.

Discussion

Renal osteodystrophy is the term applied to a range of skeletal changes in chronic renal failure. The combination of hyperparathyroidism and osteomalacia (rickets) is responsible for the skeletal manifestations. Deficiency of 1,25-dihydroxycholecalciferol (vitamin D) occurs because of ineffective 1-hydroxylation in the kidneys. This results in osteomalacia (in adults) and rickets (in children). The chronically low serum calcium causes secondary hyperparathyroidism. Both processes contribute to the osteopenia seen in renal bone disease.

The main feature of osteomalacia is defective mineralization of bone matrix. The quantity of bone matrix is unchanged. The radiological differences between rickets and adult osteomalacia are due to unfused epiphyses in children. At the ends of the long bones in rickets, the metaphyses become cupped and the growth plate is widened with unossified osteoid. In adults with osteomalacia, the hallmark is the presence of Looser's zones. Found in long bones, they are usually symmetrical in distribution and represent focal areas of unossified osteoid. Looser's zones are located perpendicular to the cortex of the bone along its concave border, unlike Paget's disease where stress fractures occur along the convexity. Looser's zones may also occur in the ribs, scapulae and pelvic bones. Histologically, seams of uncalcified osteoid are seen throughout affected bone.

In hyperparathyroidism, increased circulating levels of parathyroid hormone lead to excessive osteoclastic activity, increased quantity of osteoid and woven bone and marrow fibrosis. The main radiological hallmark is subperiosteal resorption of bone on the radial aspect of the phalanges. This sign may also be seen in the outer ends of the clavicles, the sacroiliac joints, symphysis pubis and along the proximal medial tibial metaphyses. Local areas of marked osteoclastic resorption occur in the long bones, jaw and ribs and are termed 'brown tumours' (osteitis fibrosa cystica). They are well-defined, expansile, lytic 'soap-bubble' lesions.

QUESTION 26

This 26-year-old woman has intermittent dizziness, syncope and visual disturbance.

a What is the investigation?
b What is the most likely diagnosis? Suggest an alternative diagnosis.

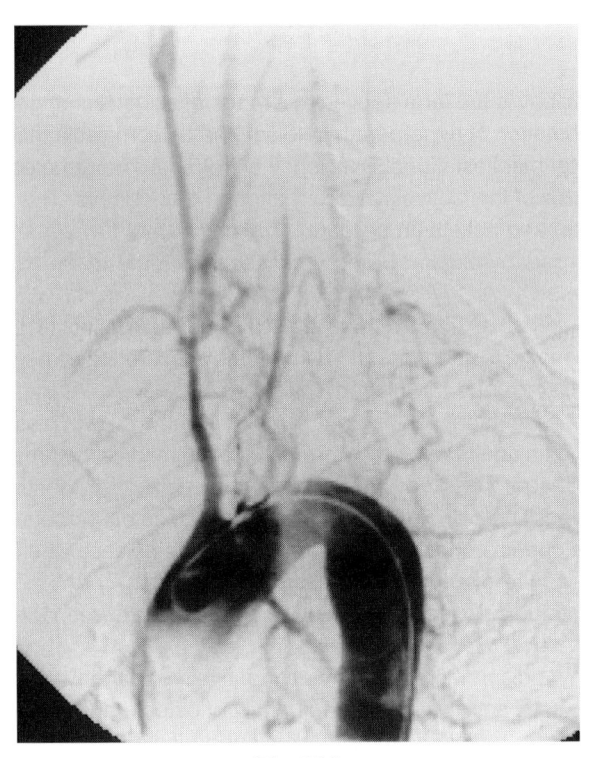

Fig. 26.1

Answer 26

a Arch aortography.
b Takayasu's arteritis. Behçet's disease.

Discussion

Takayasu's arteritis is a granulomatous disorder of unknown cause. It may affect any branch of the aorta, especially the great vessels. Females are affected eight times more often than males, and there is an increased incidence in the Far East. The typical patient is a young female between 20 and 40 years of age.

Other clinical features of this condition include convulsions, hemiplegia, amblyopia and optic atrophy.

Aortography typically shows narrowing of the great vessels and the adjacent aorta. Pulses in the arms are lost when the subclavian arteries are involved – hence the term 'pulseless' disease. Poor flow in the subclavian arteries may lead to reversed flow in the vertebral arteries – the subclavian 'steal' syndrome. Vertebrobasilar ischaemia with vertigo and blackouts may occur. Takayasu's arteritis can be treated with steroids, and reconstructive surgery is necessary when pulses are lost.

Behçet's disease more usually affects the venous system. When it affects arteries, Behçet's disease may produce either arterial occlusive disease similar to Takayasu's disease, or arterial dilatation.

QUESTION 27

This is an unenhanced CT scan of a 50-year-old man with recent onset of diabetes and arthralgia.

a What structures are labelled 1 and 2?
b What is the diagnosis?

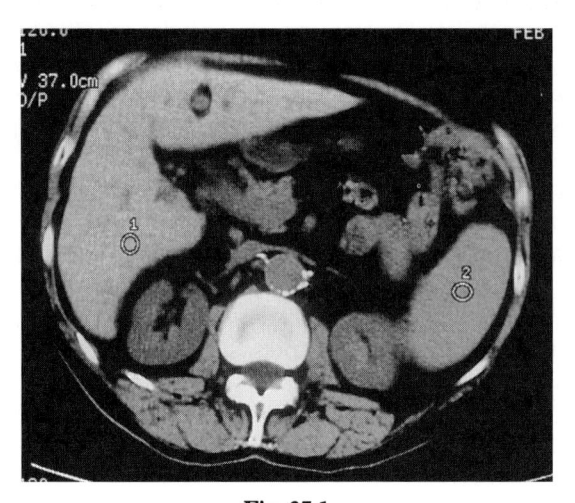

Fig. 27.1

Answer 27

a 1 = Liver. 2 = Spleen.
b Haemochromatosis.

Discussion

Haemochromatosis is an autosomal recessive condition characterized by increased iron absorption from the small intestine. It is rare before middle age. Excess iron deposited in the liver, pancreas, heart and joints gives rise to the typical clinical manifestations of cirrhosis, bronze skin pigmentation, diabetes, cardiomyopathy, loss of libido and testicular atrophy, arthralgia and chondrocalcinosis.

Iron deposition increases the attenuation of the liver, making it look 'whiter' than the spleen on CT. In normal subjects the liver and spleen have almost the same Hounsfield attenuation value, i.e. they have a similar greyness. On MRI, iron deposition in the liver causes a low signal on both T1 and T2 sequences, as shown in Fig. 27.2.

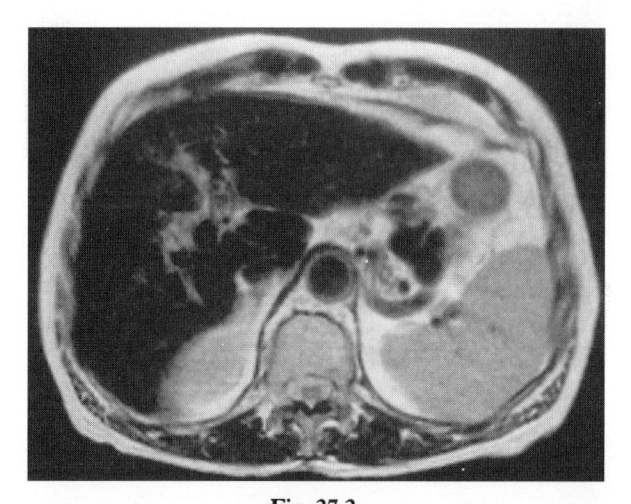

Fig. 27.2
T2-weighted MR scan through the liver and spleen showing low signal in the liver parenchyma.

Question 28

This 40-year-old man has loin pain and haematuria.

a What is the diagnosis?
b Name one extrarenal abnormality with which this condition is associated.

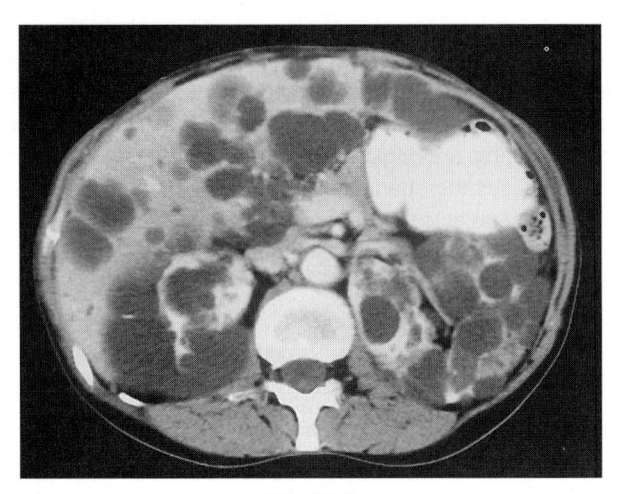

Fig. 28.1

Answer 28

a Adult polycystic kidney disease.
b Intracranial berry aneurysms.

Discussion

Adult polycystic kidney disease (APCKD) is an autosomal dominant condition characterized by the development of cysts in the kidneys, liver, pancreas and, rarely, the spleen. The kidneys are enlarged, but the quantity of functioning renal tissue is decreased.

Patients may present in adult life with haematuria, loin pain, hypertension, uraemia and abdominal masses. APCKD is increasingly detected during ultrasound screening of relatives of affected individuals. Intravenous urography typically shows 'spidery calyces' due to extrinsic pressure by intrarenal cysts on the calyx, and lobulated enlargement of *both* kidneys.

Intracranial berry aneurysms occur in 10% of patients with APCKD. Figure 28.2 shows a subarachnoid haemorrhage following rupture of an aneurysm.

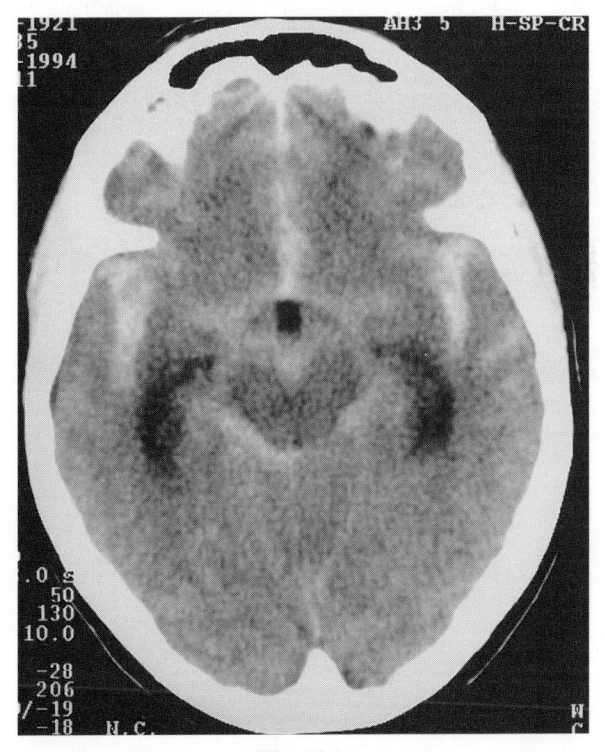

Fig. 28.2
CT brain. Subarachnoid haemorrhage. Fresh blood collects in the basal cisterns, Sylvian fissures and interhemispheric fissures.

QUESTION 29

This is the unenhanced CT scan of the brain in a 35-year-old man with headache.

a Name two radiological abnormalities.
b What is the diagnosis?

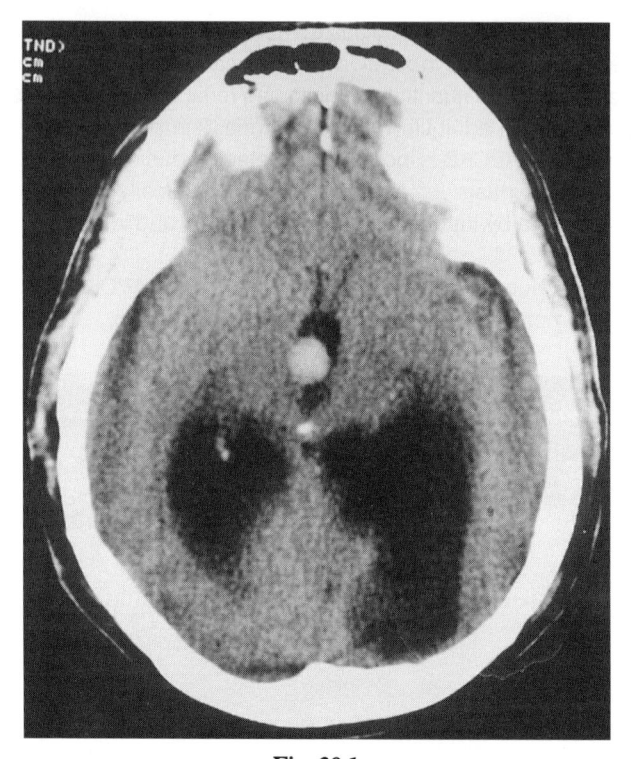

Fig. 29.1

Answer 29

a Hyperdense spherical lesion in the third ventricle. Hydrocephalus.
b Colloid cyst of the third ventricle.

Discussion

Colloid cysts are rare benign lesions affecting young adults. They are found in the anterior portion of the third ventricle and obstruct the foramina of Monro, giving rise to hydrocephalus. Patients may experience headache and intermittent loss of consciousness in addition to memory and cognitive changes. Classically, the headache worsens when leaning forward, due to anterior movement of the cyst acting as a ball-valve on the foramina. Patients are treated with a ventricular shunt when hydrocephalus is present. These lesions are very rarely excised because of the high incidence of total amnesia following surgery.

QUESTION 30

Enhanced CT of the abdomen in a 28-year-old man with mouth ulcers, weight loss and left hip pain.

a What is the radiological abnormality?
b What is the most likely underlying cause?
c What further management is necessary?

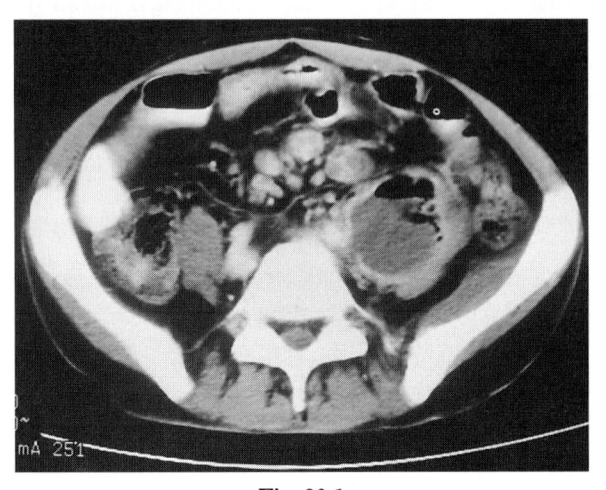

Fig. 30.1

Answer 30

a There is a thick-walled abscess in the left psoas muscle with an air-fluid level.
b Crohn's disease.
c Aspiration of pus for bacteriology and TB culture. Drainage procedure under CT guidance.

Discussion

Psoas abscess, as a complication of Crohn's disease, occurs when there is a localized perforation with fistula formation from bowel into the psoas muscle. It indicates active disease. A psoas abscess is best shown by CT and frequently contains air, as in this case. As the psoas is inserted into the lesser trochanter of the femur, any inflammation of this muscle will cause hip flexion and restriction of hip movement.

Other causes of psoas abscess include tuberculosis (Fig. 30.2), carcinoma of the colon and penetrating trauma. Post-tuberculous psoas abscesses will calcify during resolution.

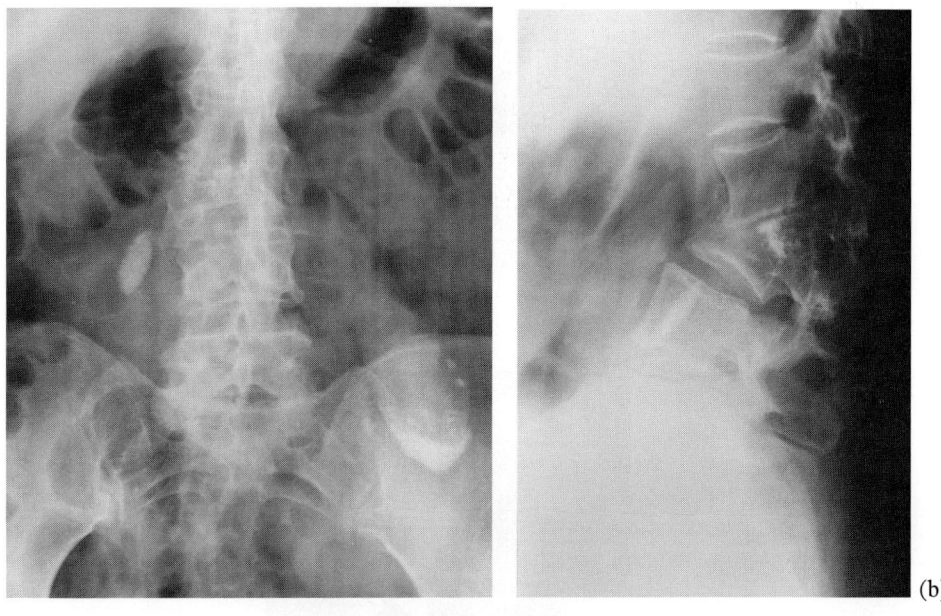

Fig. 30.2a and b
Lumbar spine. Healed paravertebral tuberculous abscess with calcified psoas muscles, calcified paravertebral region and a gibbus.

QUESTION 31

A 60-year-old hypertensive male presents with chest pain and collapse. Figure 31.1 shows a sagittal T1-weighted cardiac-gated MRI.

a What feature has been shown?
b What is the diagnosis?
c What treatment is necessary?

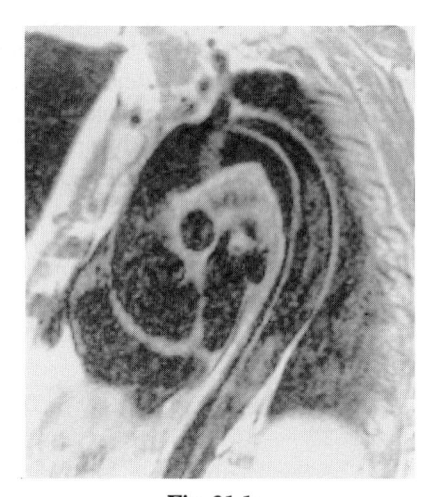

Fig. 31.1a

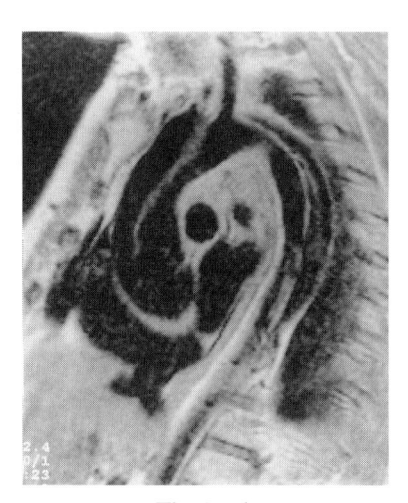

Fig. 31.1b

ANSWER 31

a Intimal flap starting in the ascending aorta, involving the arch and descending aorta.
b Acute aortic dissection of the ascending and descending aorta (Stanford type A).
c Surgical treatment.

Discussion

Spontaneous aortic dissection usually results from weakening of the intima due to repeated hypertensive 'trauma' to the intima. Eventually a tear develops and blood tracks between the intima and media, creating a false lumen. An established dissection can extend in an antegrade or retrograde direction, and can 'spiral' its way around the artery. The great vessels may be occluded and patients may present with ischaemia in the head and neck. The renal and mesenteric vessels can also be involved. A complete dissection, which has both an entry and exit site, occurs in the majority of cases (90%), but occasionally the dissection is incomplete.

Aortic dissection is most usefully classified using the Stanford classification, which also indicates the type of treatment required.

Type A – dissection involving the ascending aorta (with or without extension into the arch and descending aorta).
Type B – dissection at or below the ligamentum arteriosum only.

Surgery and aortic grafting is necessary for Type A dissections. Type B dissections can be treated medically with hypotensive agents.

Figure 31.2 shows a Type A dissection on CT.

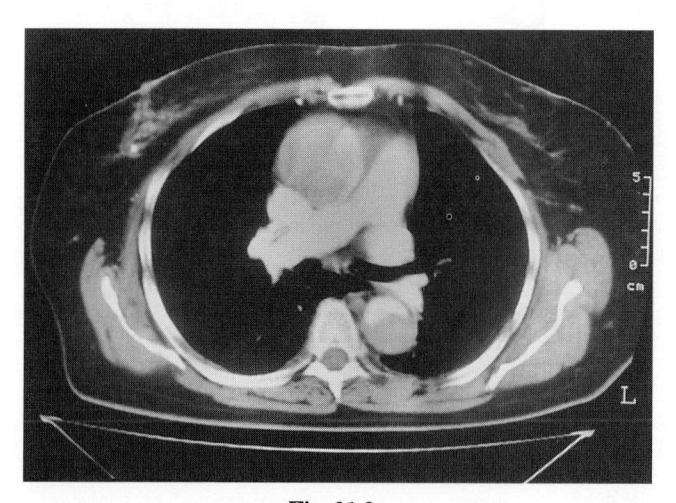

Fig. 31.2
Contrast-enhanced CT thorax. Type A dissection. A false lumen (grey part of vessel) is demonstrated in an ectatic ascending aorta. It extends into the descending aorta.

QUESTION 32

A 50-year-old jaundiced man has pruritus and intermittent abdominal pain.

a What is the investigation?
b What is the diagnosis?
c With which disease is it associated?

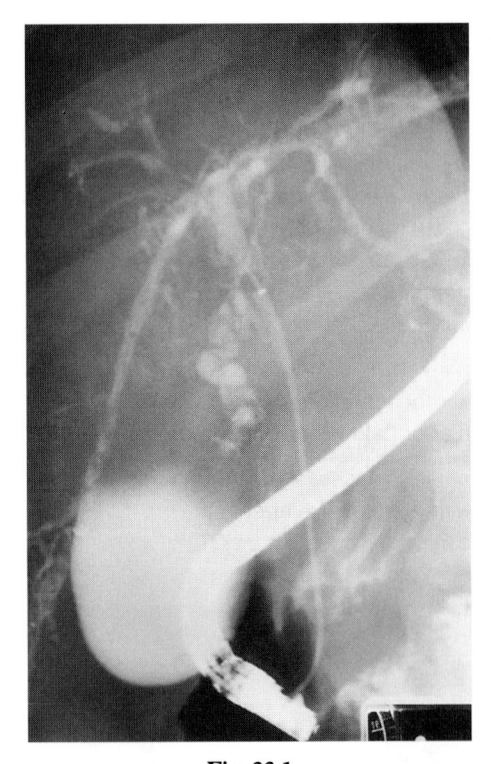

Fig. 32.1

Answer 32

a Endoscopic retrograde cholangiopancreatography (ERCP).
b Sclerosing cholangitis.
c Inflammatory bowel disease (ulcerative colitis).

Discussion

Sclerosing cholangitis is a chronic inflammatory process affecting both the intra- and extra-hepatic bile ducts. It is classified into primary and secondary types. Secondary sclerosing cholangitis results from chronic obstruction of the extra-hepatic duct. Primary sclerosing cholangitis (PSC) has no known cause, but is associated with inflammatory bowel disease in about 50% of patients. It is more common in association with ulcerative colitis than Crohn's disease. Some patients with ulcerative colitis have only minimal symptoms of PSC, which may only be evident as persistent elevation of serum alkaline phosphatase.

PSC has a characteristic cholangiographic appearance. There are multifocal intra- and extra-hepatic strictures. Diffuse cholangiocarcinoma is a complication of long-standing PSC, and the two conditions may be radiologically indistinguishable. In such cases, brush cytology or core biopsies are required to establish the diagnosis.

QUESTION 33

This middle-aged man has intermittent vertigo and nystagmus.

a What is the investigation?
b What is the diagnosis?

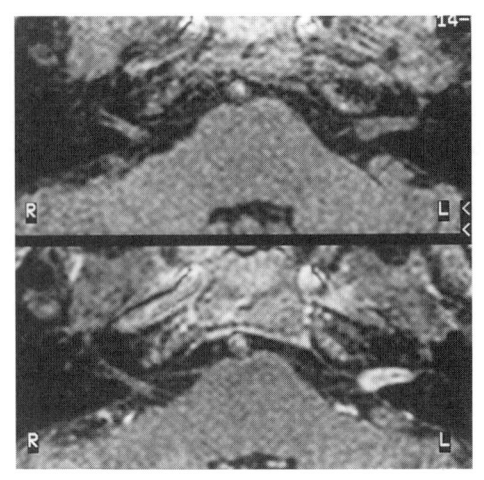

Fig. 33.1

Answer 33

a Pre- and post-gadolinium-enhanced T1-weighted MRI of the internal auditory meati.
b Left acoustic neuroma (intracanalicular).

Discussion

Acoustic neuromas arise from Schwann cells of the eighth cranial nerve. About 60% of them arise from the vestibular division of the nerve. They may develop entirely within the internal auditory meatus, as in this case, or they may extend intracranially (Fig. 33.2). MRI is the most accurate imaging method. The sensitivity for detection is further increased by the administration of gadolinium, which is avidly taken up by the tumour.

Bilateral acoustic neuromas are rare, but when present are invariably associated with neurofibromatosis.

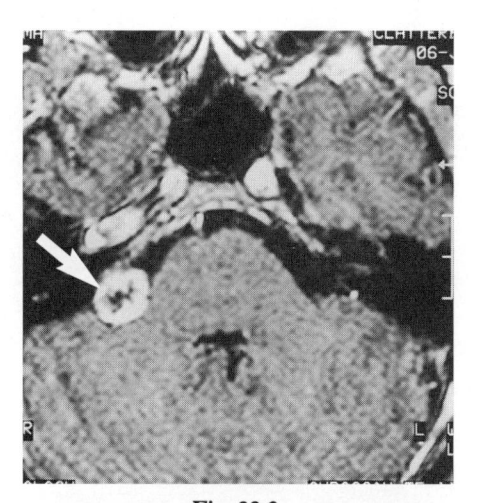

Fig. 33.2
MRI of both IAMs with i.v. gadolinium showing an enhancing rounded tumour (arrow) arising from the right eighth nerve and extending to lie adjacent to the brainstem.

QUESTION 34

This 31-year-old man complains of severe abdominal pain, vomiting and arthralgia.

a Describe three radiological features.
b What is the diagnosis?
c How do you explain the abdominal pain?

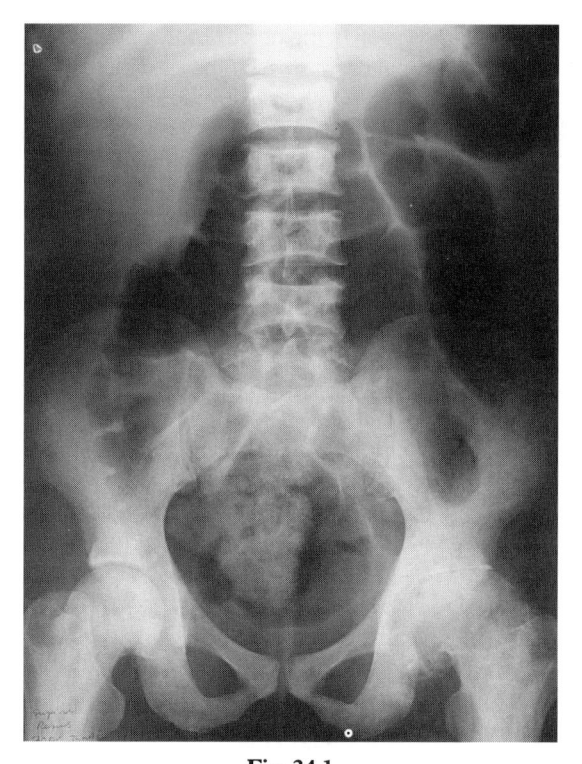

Fig. 34.1

Answer 34

a Generalized osteosclerosis. Central vertebral body end-plate depression. Avascular necrosis in the left femoral head.
b Sickle cell disease.
c Painful crisis caused by thrombosis of small mesenteric vessels.

Discussion

Sickle cell disease is a severe haemolytic anaemia that occurs predominantly in blacks. Affected individuals are homozygous for a gene which controls production of HbS. Polymerization of abnormal haemoglobin occurs when oxygen tensions are low. Red cells containing HbS 'sickle', thereby blocking small arteries. The sickled cells are fragile, and haemolysis readily occurs when these cells come into contact with the damaged vessel wall.

Sickle cell disease is an important cause of avascular necrosis. This occurs not only in the femoral head but also in the humeral head, giving the classical 'snow-cap' sign. In the vertebral body, the end-plate is supplied by small end arterioles, with a well-developed network of arteries in the periphery of the end-plate. In sickle cell disease, thrombosis of the end arterioles results in osteonecrosis of the vertebral body with a classical central depression. In extreme cases, the vertebral body resembles an 'H'-shape.

The spleen may be slightly enlarged in childhood, but by adulthood the spleen shrinks due to repeated infarction. This predisposes patients to pneumococcal infection. Patients are also prone to developing *Salmonella* infections. Dactylitis, due to either ischaemia or infection, may occur in the phalanges of hands and feet. Sickle cell disease is an important cause of renal papillary necrosis, which is due to thrombosis of the arteries supplying the renal papillae. Pulmonary infarction may also occur – the so-called 'sickle lung'. It may be difficult to distinguish radiologically between infection and infarction, and the two conditions often coexist.

QUESTION 35

A 14-year-old boy is short in stature.

a What radiological feature is present?
b What are the two possible diagnoses?
c How would you distinguish between them?

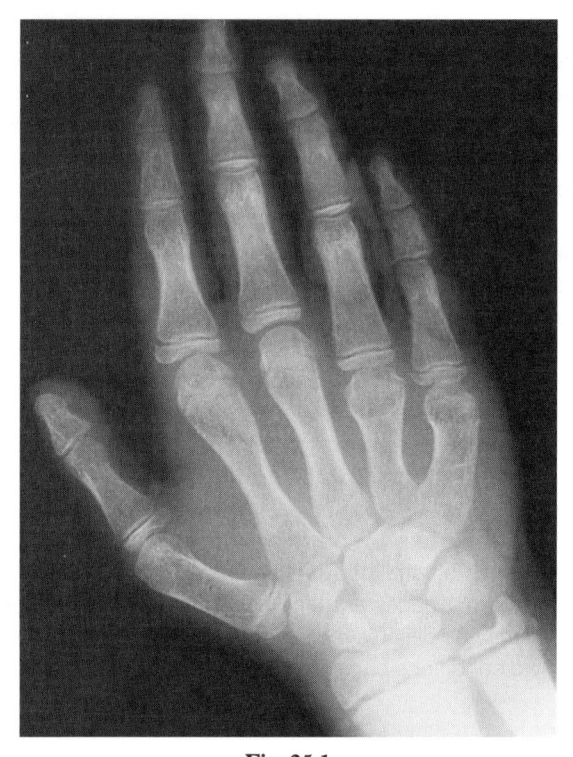

Fig. 35.1

ANSWER 35

a Short fourth and fifth metacarpals.
b Pseudohypoparathyroidism. Pseudopseudohypoparathyroidism.
c Plasma calcium.

Discussion

Pseudohypoparathyroidism (PsH) is an inherited condition resulting from failure of target organs to respond to parathyroid hormone (PTH). This results in hypocalcaemia and, by negative feedback, elevation in PTH (Table 35.1). There are characteristic somatic features in PsH: short fourth and fifth metacarpals and metatarsals; small stature; low IQ and round face. Pseudopseudohypoparathyroidism (PsPsH) has identical somatic features to PsH, but with normal biochemistry.

Symptoms of hypocalcaemia include tetany, circumoral paraesthesia, depression, carpopedal spasm (Trousseau's sign) and facial twitching on facial nerve tapping (Chvostek's sign). There is prolongation of the QT-interval on the ECG.

Primary hypoparathyroidism (PrH) occurs when secretion of PTH is absent or reduced. This may be a complication of neck surgery, or it may be due to autoimmune failure of the parathyroid gland.

Table 35.1 Biochemical features of primary hypoparathyroidism, pseudohypoparathyroidism and pseudopseudohypoparathyroidism

Condition	Calcium	Phosphate	PTH	Alkaline phosphatase
PrH	Reduced	Normal or increased	Decreased	Normal
PsH	Reduced	Increased	Normal or increased	Normal or increased
PsPsH	Normal	Normal	Normal	Normal

QUESTION 36

This is a transverse ultrasound scan through the left lobe of the liver to show the heart.

a What is the diagnosis?

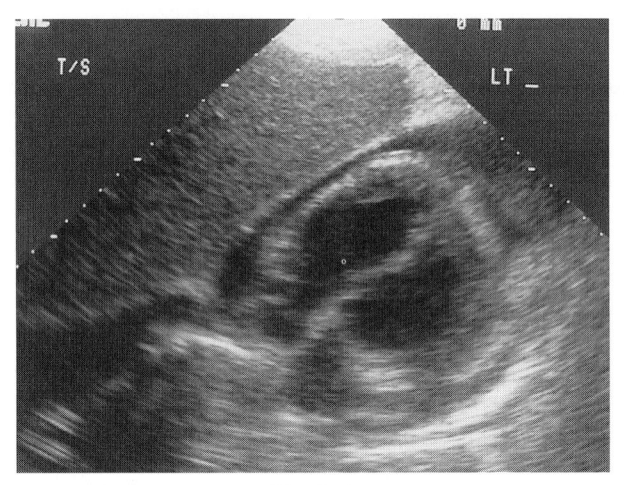

Fig. 36.1

Answer 36

a Pericardial effusion.

Discussion

There is an echo-free zone between the myocardium and pericardium. This is the characteristic ultrasound (and echocardiographic) appearance of a pericardial effusion. There are characteristic appearances of a pericardial effusion on CT (Fig. 36.2).

See Question 3 for further discussion.

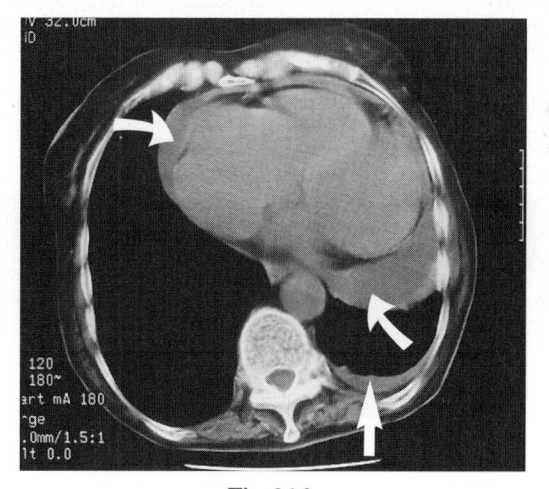

Fig. 36.2

CT thorax. Pericardial effusion. There are crescents of water density between the pericardium and myocardium on both sides of the heart (curved arrows). An associated left pleural effusion is present (arrow).

Question 37

This 27-year-old man has a long history of painful joints.

a What is the most likely diagnosis?
b Can you give an alternative diagnosis?

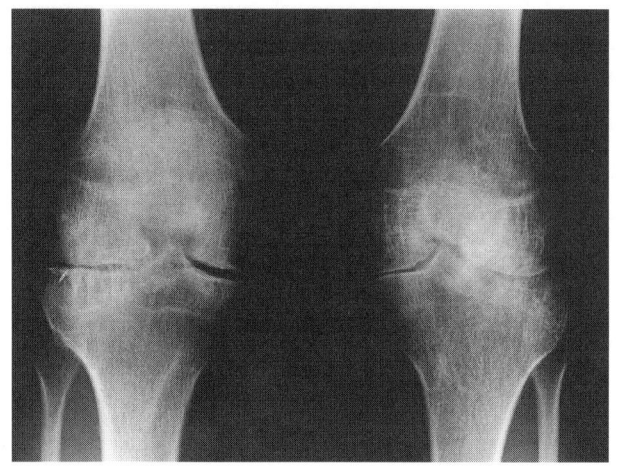

Fig. 37.1

ANSWER 37

a Haemophiliac arthropathy.
b Juvenile chronic arthritis.

Discussion

Haemophilia A or classical haemophilia is an X-linked recessive disorder characterized by deficiency of factor VIII. Haemarthroses are a common complication and most frequently occur in childhood. Intra-articular bleeding produces a red, swollen and tender joint. Radiography may show an increase in density within the soft tissues of the joint. Following repeated bleeds, not all of the blood is resorbed. Synovial hyperaemia and thickening then occur. The bone becomes osteopenic. Synovial inflammatory tissue or pannus develops at the articular margin, eroding cartilage and bone. Continuing damage leads to enlarging cysts and bone expansion (femoral condyles in this example). Loss of cartilage leads to an irregular narrowed joint space. In the knee joint, a squared intercondylar notch classically occurs. Other causes of this appearance include juvenile chronic arthritis, rheumatoid arthritis and TB. All of these conditions cause pannus formation, although changes are more likely to be unilateral in the case of TB.

Away from the joint, haematomas of soft tissue can elevate the periosteum and cause extensive bony erosion – the so-called haemophiliac pseudotumour – in approximately 2% of cases (Fig. 37.2).

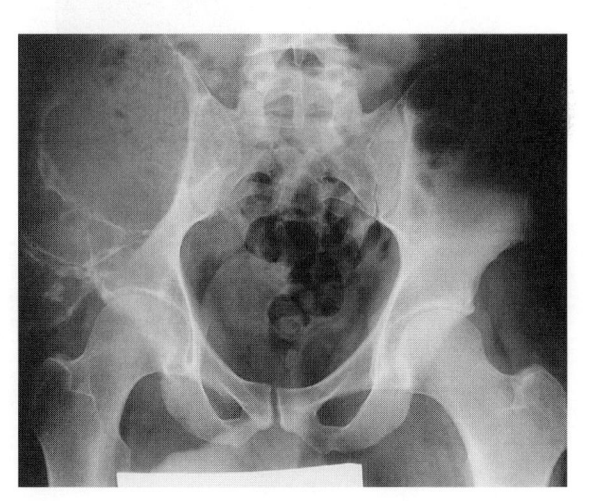

Fig. 37.2
Pelvis. Haemophiliac pseudotumour. There is a huge well-defined lytic mass replacing and expanding the right iliac bone.

Question 38

This is the barium swallow examination of a 50-year-old man with dysphagia.

a What two radiological abnormalities are present?
b Which one of these abnormalities has an association? What is that association?

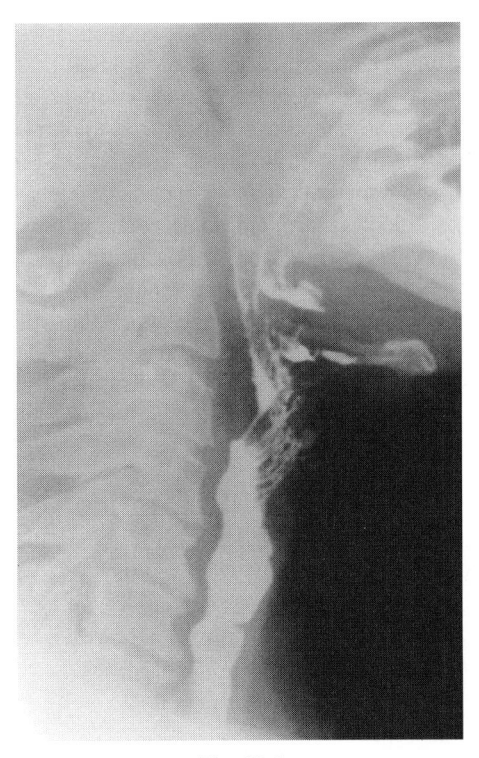

Fig. 38.1

ANSWER 38

a Post-cricoid pharyngeal web. Extrinsic impressions on the posterior oesophagus by osteophytes.
b Post-cricoid pharyngeal web. Webs are associated with iron deficiency anaemia. There is an increased risk of post-cricoid carcinoma.

Discussion

A pharyngeal web is a thin shelf of mucosa projecting from the anterior pharyngeal wall. It is more common in females, and can occasionally cause severe dysphagia for solids. It may disappear with treatment of the anaemia, but there is an increased risk of developing carcinoma.

Question 39

This is a CT scan of the thorax in a 49-year-old woman with cough.

a What is the radiological diagnosis?
b What is the next most useful investigation?

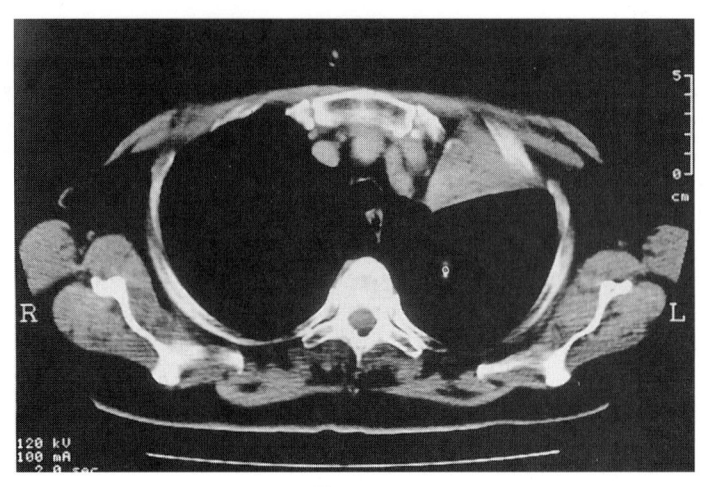

Fig. 39.1

Answer 39

a Left upper lobe collapse.
b Bronchoscopy.

Discussion

There are many causes of large airway obstruction, but the most important is carcinoma of the bronchus. The causes of airway obstruction can be classified into those occurring in the lumen, in the wall and outside the wall.

Luminal causes include:

- tumour (carcinoma, adenoma);
- foreign body;
- mucous plug (asthma/postoperative).

Mural causes include:

- stricture – granulomatous (TB or sarcoid);
- trauma/surgery;
- vasculitis, e.g Wegener's granulomatosis.

Extrinsic causes include:

- lymphadenopathy;
- mediastinal masses;
- aortic aneurysm.

When the left upper lobe collapses, the oblique or major fissure moves anteriorly and medially. On CT viewed with soft tissue windows, the deflated lobe appears grey and wedge shaped because it no longer contains air. It therefore assumes the same attenuation as soft tissue. However, the left lower lobe and right lung appear black because they contain air.

Occasionally, CT may show a hilar mass or an endobronchial lesion in association with a collapsed lobe. Unless there is a known extrapulmonary primary cancer, bronchoscopy is the most useful further investigation in adults. In routine practice, CT scans of the thorax include the adrenal glands and liver to search for distant metastatic spread. Figure 39.2 shows the classic appearances of left upper lobe collapse on a chest radiograph.

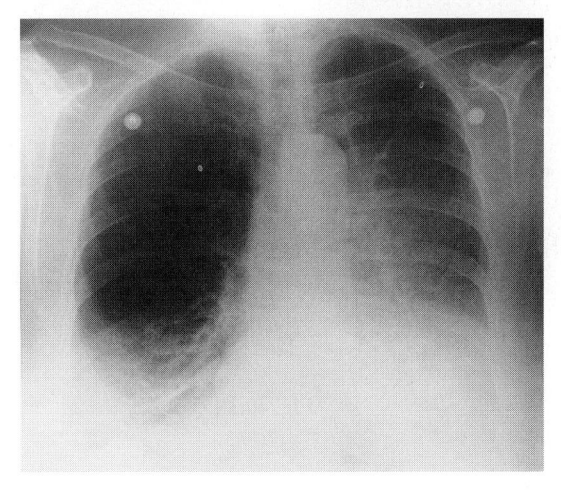

Fig. 39.2
Chest radiograph. Left upper lobe collapse. There is a hazy 'veil' over the left lung field due to collapse of the upper lobe towards the anterior chest wall.

QUESTION 40

This is a chest radiograph in a 38-year-old man.

a What are the two radiological abnormalities?
b What is the most likely diagnosis?
c What two physical signs may be present in this condition?

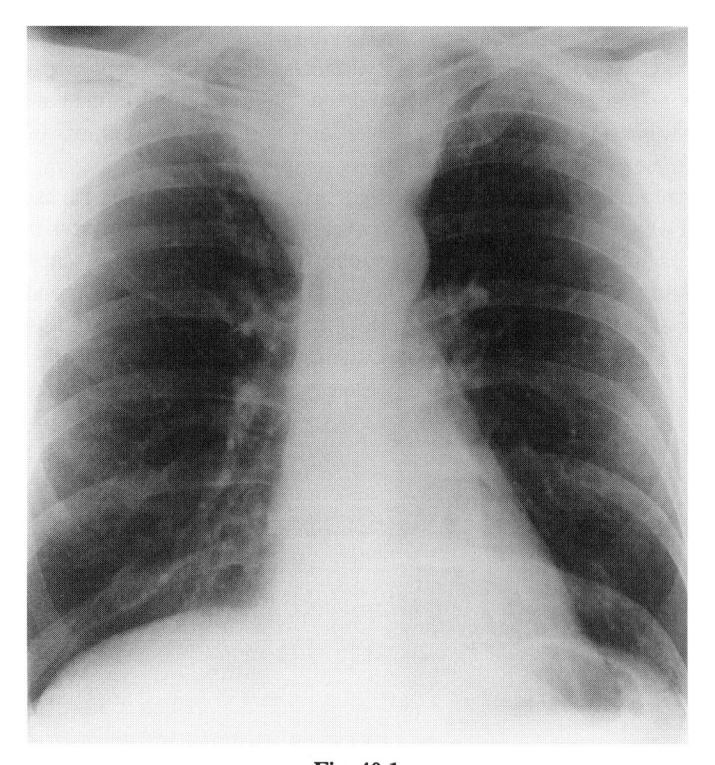

Fig. 40.1

Answer 40

a Superior mediastinal mass extending above and below the clavicles. Tracheal deviation.
b Retrosternal or intrathoracic goitre.
c Stridor. Pemberton's sign.

Discussion

An intrathoracic goitre originates in the neck and grows into the superior mediastinum. This continuity can be shown as an extension of the superior mediastinal mass above the clavicles on chest radiography, CT and MRI. It is usually due to benign multinodular goitre or adenoma, but may rarely be due to carcinoma. Tracheal deviation is common and, when narrowed, can give rise to stridor and sometimes dyspnoea. Elevation of the arms can result in compression of the brachiocephalic veins by the mediastinal mass. This may cause Pemberton's sign (facial plethora and venous engorgement). Occasionally, in longstanding cases, the superior vena cava (SVC) may become permanently obstructed by the goitre, resulting in the SVC syndrome.

Intrathoracic goitres can be imaged with isotope studies, CT or MRI. The latter is particularly useful when defining the anatomical relationship of the intrathoracic goitre to the great vessels prior to surgery. Figure 40.2a shows heterogenous tracer uptake in a different patient with an enlarged multinodular goitre. The dense circular area of increased tracer marks the suprasternal notch and indicates that functioning thyroid tissue is confined to the neck. In an intrathoracic goitre, there would be tracer activity seen below the suprasternal marker. Figure 40.2b shows a retrosternal goitre on CT.

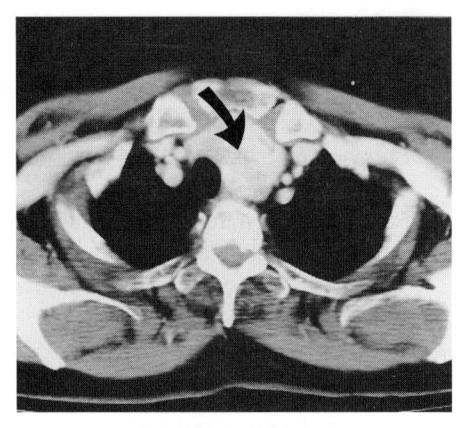

Fig. 40.2b
CT thorax. Retrosternal goitre (curved arrow). Note deviation of the trachea to the right.

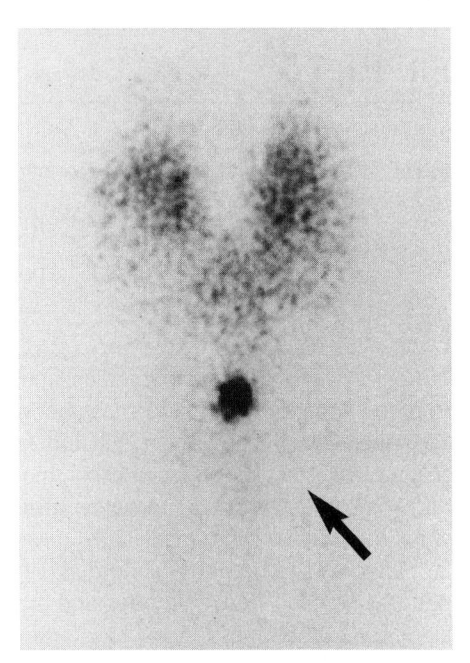

Fig. 40.2a
Isotope thyroid scan. Multinodular goitre. The suprasternal notch (arrow) confirms that functioning thyroid tissue is confined to the neck.

QUESTION 41

This is the hand radiograph of a sick 7-year-old boy with gum hypertrophy.

a What is the exact diagnosis?
b List three possible mechanisms by which this appearance may otherwise occur.

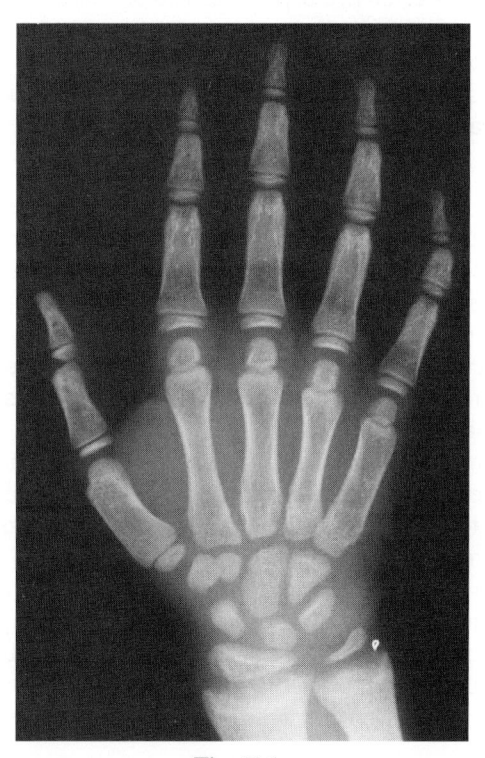

Fig. 41.1

ANSWER 41

a Anticonvulsant rickets.

b Possible mechanisms include:

- *Vitamin deficiency* – poor diet; lack of sunlight; malabsorption;
- *Defective production of 25-hydroxycholecalciferol* – liver disease; anticonvulsant therapy;
- *Ineffective 1-hydroxylation in the kidneys* – renal failure;
- *Resistance to vitamin D* – X-linked dominant condition due to proximal tubular insensitivity to vitamin D.

Discussion

The radiological features of rickets in the wrist are classical. There is deficiency of vitamin D resulting in defective mineralization of bone. This is seen radiographically as osteopenia. The epiphyseal growth plates widen due to hypertrophy of cartilage which is laid down without ossification. An irregular epiphyseal line is present with accompanying metaphyseal cupping. Other radiological features of rickets are bow legs, defective cranial bones (craniotabes) and frontal bossing, kyphoscoliosis and costochondral beading ('rickety rosary').

Rickets and osteomalacia have an identical pathological basis and are both metabolic bone diseases due to vitamin D deficiency. Rickets is osteomalacia of the growing skeleton. The commonest causes of rickets in the UK are renal osteodystrophy and malabsorption. Dietary rickets is now rare in this country.

The mechanism of vitamin D deficiency due to anticonvulsants is thought to be multifactorial and associated with dose of drug, sunlight exposure and physical activity of the child. Drugs particularly implicated are phenytoin and phenobarbitone, which cause a decrease in serum 25-hydroxycholecalciferol levels. There is increased hepatic microsomal hydroxylase activity, resulting in increased levels of inactive vitamin D metabolites.

QUESTION 42

This 50-year-old woman has a painful red knee.

a What radiological abnormality is shown?
b What is the diagnosis?
c Name three associated conditions.

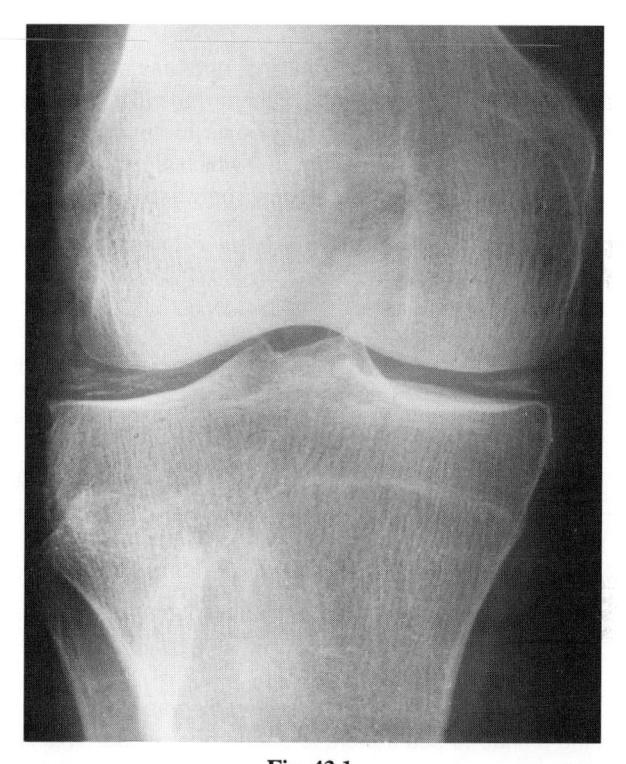

Fig. 42.1

ANSWER 42

a Chondrocalcinosis.
b Pseudogout or calcium pyrophosphate dihydrate deposition disease (CPPD).
c Degenerative joint disease; hyperparathyroidism; haemochromatosis; Wilson's disease; acromegaly.

Discussion

Chondrocalcinosis is calcification of joint cartilage, and may affect hyaline or fibrocartilage. In this case, there is calcification of both the articular (hyaline) cartilage and menisci (fibrocartilage). Chondrocalcinosis may be asymptomatic or can be associated with episodes of intermittent arthritis (pseudogout) which are similar in character, but not in distribution to gout. The important differences between gout and pseudogout are shown in Table 42.1.

Table 42.1 Important differences between gout and pseudogout

	Crystals	Birefringence	Distribution
Pseudogout	Calcium pyrophosphate dihydrate	Weakly positive	Large joints
Gout	Sodium urate	Negative	Joints of feet and hands

Chondrocalcinosis due to CPPD has other important associations which are listed above. It affects both sexes equally and its incidence increases with age.

In the examination, if you are shown a lateral skull radiograph in an acromegalic, do not forget to look at the pinnae to see if there is chondrocalcinosis. This finding is sure to impress your examiner!

QUESTION 43

This is an oblique lateral chest radiograph in a 43-year-old man with ascites.

a What is the diagnosis?
b Give three possible causes.
c List four physical signs which may be present.

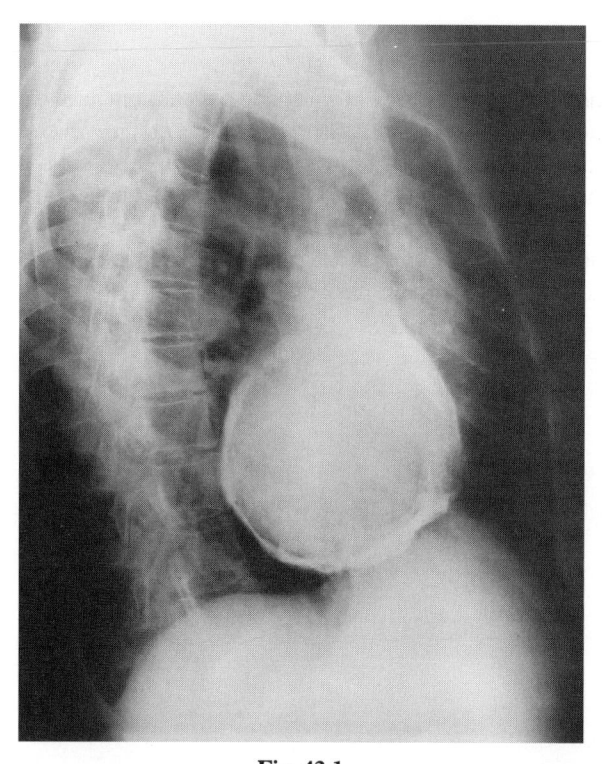

Fig. 43.1

Answer 43

a Calcific constrictive pericarditis.
b Tuberculous pericarditis; haemopericardium; pericarditis of rheumatic, viral or bacterial origin.
c Kussmaul's sign; pulsus paradoxus; Friedreich's sign; hepatomegaly; raised jugular venous pressure; atrial fibrillation (in 30%) and third heart sound.

Discussion

Constrictive pericarditis is a condition in which the pericardium fails to stretch. The main effect is impairment of systemic venous filling of the right atrium, which is responsible for the plethora of physical signs listed above. The third heart sound is due to rapid ventricular filling, and a pericardial 'knock' may occasionally be heard on cardiac auscultation. The heart is small on the chest radiograph, which usually, but not always, shows pericardial calcification. However, a calcified pericardium does not necessarily imply constrictive pericarditis, which is a clinical diagnosis.

QUESTION 44

a What is the diagnosis?

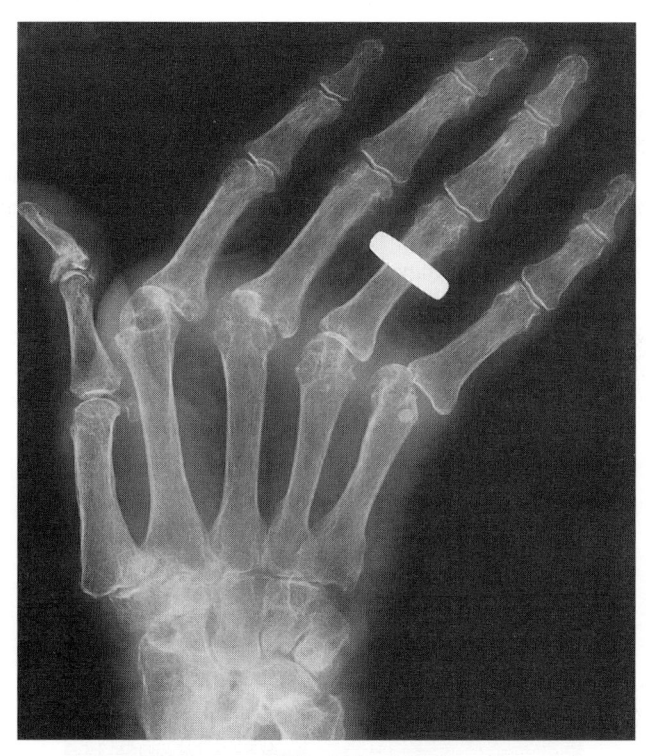

Fig. 44.1

Answer 44

a Rheumatoid arthritis.

Discussion

The bones are osteopenic and there are marked marginal erosive changes in the metacarpophalangeal (MCP) joints and carpal bones. There is ankylosis of the scaphoid and radius. There is joint space narrowing in the carpal and radiocarpal joints. The MCP joints are subluxed and there is ulnar deviation of the phalanges. Identical changes were seen in the opposite hand. These are classical radiological features in severe rheumatoid disease.

Similar changes of ulnar deviation and subluxation, without erosion and ankylosis, may be seen in systemic lupus erythematosus.

Figure 44.2 shows arthritis mutilans, a complication of severe rheumatoid disease. There is marked osteopenia, the phalanges have a tapered appearance and there is marked subluxation of joints. Severe psoriatic arthropathy can also cause this appearance.

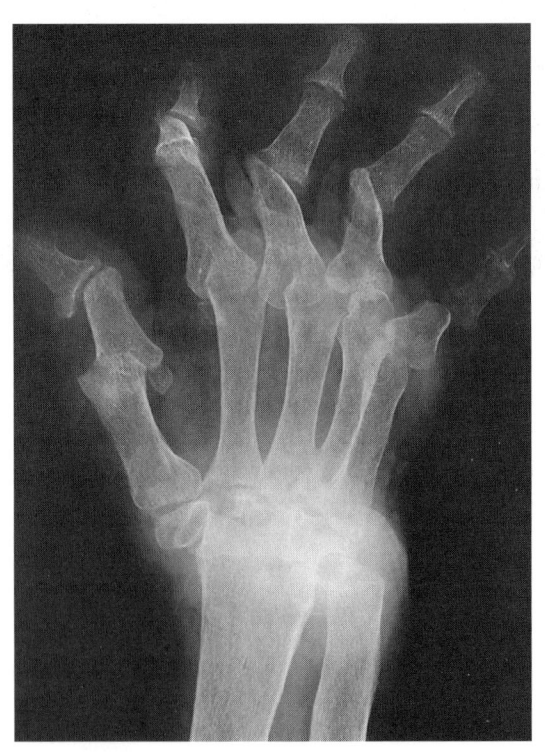

Fig. 44.2
Hand radiograph. Arthritis mutilans.

QUESTION 45

a Name five causes of the abnormality shown in Fig. 45.1.

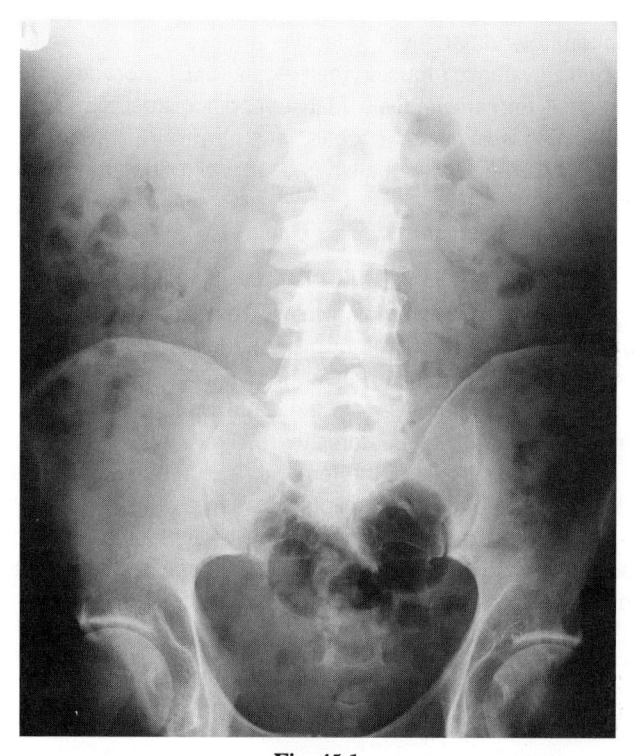

Fig. 45.1

Answer 45

a There is mild/moderate splenic enlargement.

The possible causes are portal hypertension, lymphoma, leukaemia, haemolytic anaemia, infection (glandular fever, infective endocarditis and reaction to sepsis), rheumatoid arthritis, systemic lupus erythematosis (SLE), storage diseases (Gaucher's disease), sarcoidosis and amyloidosis. Malaria and schistosomiasis should be considered in those returning from endemic areas.

Massive splenic enlargement in the UK is usually due to chronic myeloid leukaemia and myelofibrosis.

Discussion

Splenic enlargement is detected radiologically by depression of the splenic flexure and 'ground glass' opacification in the left upper quadrant. The cause of splenic enlargement in this patient was non-Hodgkin's lymphoma.

When splenic enlargement is seen on the abdominal radiograph, it is important to inspect the film for any associated features that will give a clue to the underlying cause. For example, avascular necrosis of the femoral head may suggest SLE or Gaucher's disease. Sickle cell disease may cause splenic enlargement in childhood, but by adult life the spleen has diminished in size due to infarction. Increased bony density (osteosclerosis) may suggest myelofibrosis. Always look carefully for the presence of gallstones which may be a feature suggestive of haemolytic anaemia.

QUESTION 46

This is a 60-minute film from a small bowel meal examination in a 50-year-old woman with dysphagia, malabsorption and hypertension.

a List two radiological abnormalities that are present.
b What is the diagnosis?

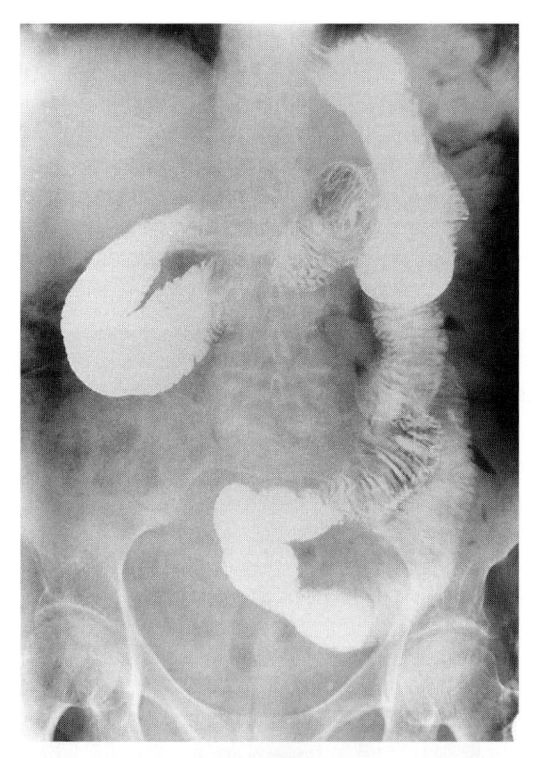

Fig. 46.1

ANSWER 46

a 'Coiled-spring' small bowel dilatation with normal fold thickness. Soft tissue calcification adjacent to the left femoral neck.
b Systemic sclerosis or scleroderma.

Discussion

Scleroderma, a disease that is four times more frequent in women, is characterized by diffuse fibrosis and vasculitis. It may be localized and affect the skin alone, or it may affect multiple organs (skin, joints, oesophagus, kidney, lung, heart, small and large bowel). The skin becomes taut and shiny, especially in the extremities and face. Scleroderma may sometimes have features which resemble rheumatoid disease or systemic lupus erythematosus, and can be grouped into a mixed connective tissue disease overlap syndrome.

In its pure form, scleroderma causes sclerodactyly. This is due to soft tissue atrophic change and occurs in the fingers and toes. Telangiectasia occurs in the digits and

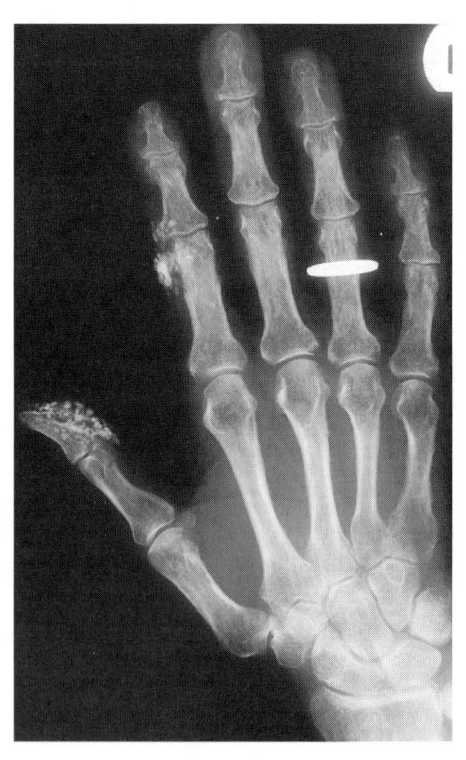

Fig. 46.2
Hand radiograph. Scleroderma. There is dense punctate calcification in the subcutaneous tissue over the phalanges.

around the face, lips and tongue. Subcutaneous calcification occurs in the fingertips and over bony prominences (see Fig. 46.2). Bony erosion occurs in the tips of the terminal phalanges. Vasospasm of the digital arteries leads to Raynaud's phenomenon.

The most common abnormality in the gastrointestinal tract is oesophageal dysmotility, which manifests as dysphagia and reflux. Fibrosis occurs in the submucosa of the gastro-oesophageal junction, impairing the sphincter and allowing gastric contents to enter the oesophagus. The bowel becomes hypomotile, slowing down the transit of food (and barium), resulting in small bowel dilatation. Classically, this resembles a 'coiled spring' on barium studies. Malabsorption occurs, due to bacterial overgrowth within stagnant dilated bowel. Advanced disease leads to degeneration of the muscularis mucosa, causing air to enter the submucosa (pneumatosis cystoides intestinalis). Smooth muscle atrophy allows wide-necked pseudosacculations to develop in both the small and large bowel.

Scleroderma is associated with basal interstitial pulmonary fibrosis. This is thought to be primarily an immunological phenomenon, but chronic aspiration pneumonitis may also play a part. Vasculitis of small renal arteries leads to nephrosclerosis, hypertension and renal failure.

The so-called CREST syndrome occurs when the patient exhibits the following: **c**alcinosis; **R**aynaud's phenomenon; **o**esophageal dysmotility; **s**clerodactyly and **t**elangiectasia.

Question 47

This is an unenhanced pelvic CT in a 43-year-old male patient from the Middle East presenting with haematuria.

a What two abnormalities are present?
b What is the diagnosis?
c What recognized complication may occur?

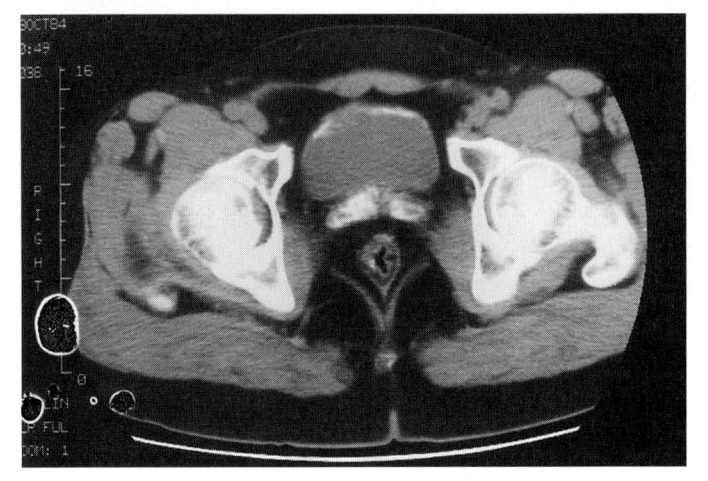

Fig. 47.1

Answer 47

a Calcified bladder wall. Calcified seminal vesicles.
b Schistosomiasis.
c Squamous cell carcinoma of the bladder.

Discussion

Schistosoma haematobium is a fluke found in fresh water and carried by intermediate snail hosts, which is endemic in Africa and the Middle East. Human infection results from contact with *Bulinus* snails during bathing. Fork-tailed cercariae develop in the snail and penetrate human skin, usually the sole of the foot. After passing into the portal venous circulation, the cercariae mature over the next 3 months and pass into the vessels of the bladder (or in the case of *S. japonicum* and *S. mansoni* into the vessels of the intestines). The life cycle is complete when the infested human host passes eggs in the urine and/or faeces.

Symptoms depend on the stage of disease. A pruritic papular rash develops at the site of entry of cercariae, and when adult worms are formed in the liver the patient may be febrile (Katayama fever) with eosinophilia, urticaria and hepatosplenomegaly. Haematuria, dysuria and frequency occur in established bladder infection. Advanced disease causes hydroureteronephrosis secondary to ureteric fibrosis and stricture. Bladder wall fibrosis occurs. Calcification may encircle the bladder completely, appearing as a concentric calcified ring when the bladder is full. The bladder remains distensible, unlike the extremely rare tuberculous calcification of the bladder.

S. haematobium may also cause seminal vesicle (Fig. 47.1) and distal ureteric calcification (Fig. 47.2a). Bladder stones are not infrequent. There is an increased incidence of squamous cell carcinoma of the bladder.

S. japonicum is endemic in the Far East. Chronic infection primarily affects the liver. The life cycle is similar to that of *S. haematobium*, but in addition to snails, domestic and farm animals may be intermediate hosts. Cercariae are trapped in the small portal venules in the liver or mesenteric vessels of the intestines. Granulomatous reactions lead to periportal fibrosis and intestinal wall fibrosis. The liver and intestinal wall may calcify (Fig. 47.2b).

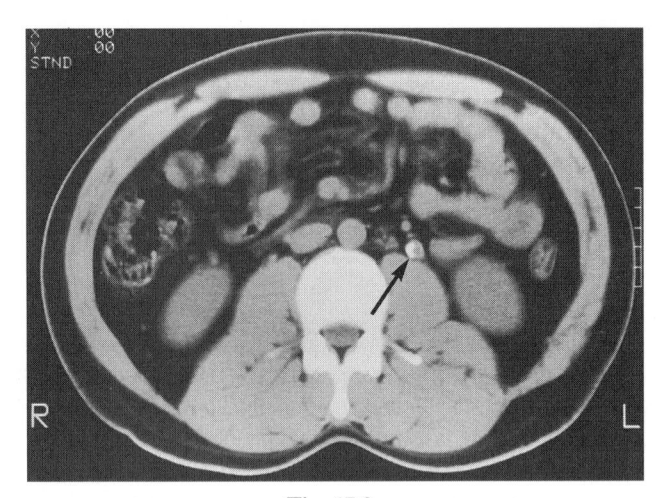

Fig. 47.2a
CT abdomen. *Schistosoma haematobium* infection. Calcification of left ureter (arrow).

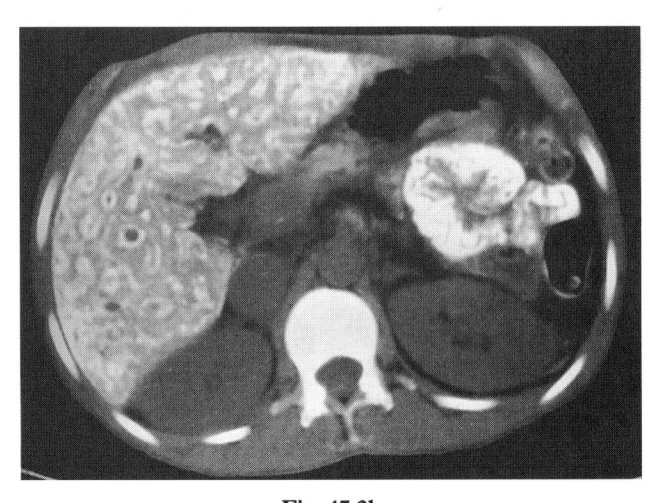

Fig. 47.2b
CT abdomen. *Schistosoma japonicum* infection. There is calcification of small bowel in the left flank. Note the characteristic 'tortoise shell' calcification in the liver.

QUESTION 48

This is a CT scan of the thorax in a 60-year-old female.

a Name three radiological abnormalities.
b What is the diagnosis?

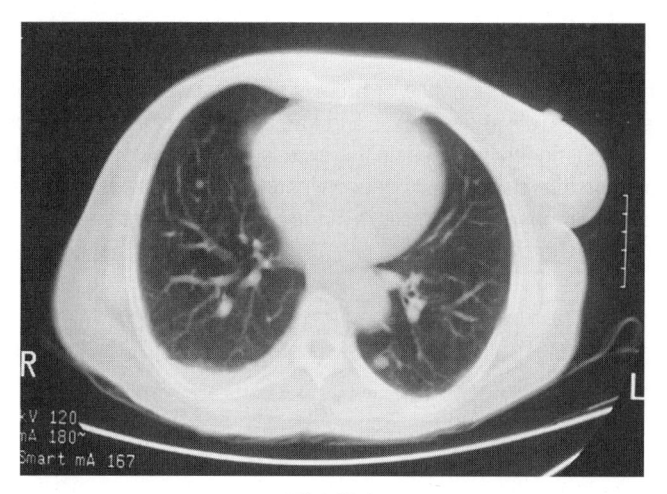

Fig. 48.1

ANSWER 48

a Right mastectomy.
   Multiple pulmonary nodules.
   Right pleural effusion.
b Breast carcinoma with pulmonary and pleural metastases.

Discussion

In females, the presence or absence of breasts should always be assessed before any other observation. This rule applies to CT and MRI as well as chest radiography. There are at least three intrapulmonary nodules on this slice, and an associated pleural effusion. It is of great importance that inspection is not confined to the lung fields alone, since the correct diagnosis of pulmonary metastases is made by noting the mastectomy.

QUESTION 49

This is a CT of the brain in a 40-year-old man.

a What is the diagnosis?
b What further management is indicated?

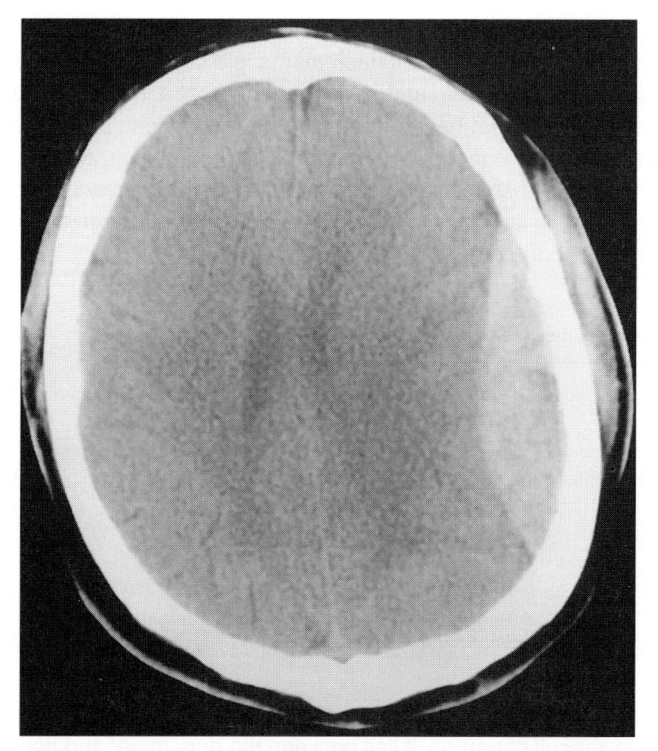

Fig. 49.1

Answer 49

a Acute extradural haematoma with mass effect in the left parietal region.
b Urgent evacuation of the extradural haematoma.

Discussion

It is clinically important to differentiate between acute subdural and extradural haematomas (Table 49.1). A subdural haematoma is a collection of blood between the dura mater and arachnoid mater, and is due to slow blood loss from a bridging dural vein (see Fig. 49.2). Subdural haematoma may be traumatic in origin. It is more common in alcoholics with concomitant cerebral atrophy or in patients with blood dyscrasias. The crescent-shaped haematoma 'follows' the convexity of the brain with gyri interdigitating along its concave medial border. A subdural haematoma can cross a suture but not the falx or tentorium.

Table 49.1 Differences between subdural and extradural haematomas

	Shape	Crosses sutures?	Mechanism	Associated fracture?
Extradural haematoma	Lentiform Smooth	No	Disruption of meningeal vessel	Very common
Subdural haematoma	Crescent Ragged	Yes	Disruption of bridging vein	35%

An extradural haematoma occurs after bleeding from the middle meningeal artery (or vein), usually as a result of trauma. It lies between the dura mater and periosteum of the inner table of the skull, and has a characteristic lentiform shape due to dissection of the dura from the skull. As the dura is tightly bound to the skull sutures, extradural collections do not cross suture lines but may cross the attachment of the tentorium and falx. In Fig. 49.1 the anterior tip of the haematoma demarcates the position of the coronal suture and the posterior tip demarcates the position of the lambdoid suture.

Both subdural and extradural haematomas can exert a significant mass effect. This causes compression of normal structures and a rise in intracranial pressure, which is particularly common in extradural collections. Such mass effect is an early complication necessitating urgent surgical evacuation. Classically a 'lucid' interval occurs in up to 40% of patients with extradural haematomas. Although the development of mass effect tends to be slower and more sustained with a subdural collection, a rise in intracranial pressure can be a dangerous complication requiring decompression. It is important to remember that whilst both types of haematoma are associated with trauma, either can occur in the absence of vault fracture. A normal skull radiograph therefore does not exclude serious intracranial injury.

An acute subdural haematoma can be differentiated from a chronic haematoma by the attenuation characteristics within the collection. An acute bleed raises the attenuation value, rendering the collection white on CT. This change may persist for approximately 2 weeks. There is a 2-week period when haemoglobin is removed – a collection can sometimes be very difficult to see as it becomes isodense with brain. From then on, the collection can become hypodense with respect to brain, thus appearing dark grey or black.

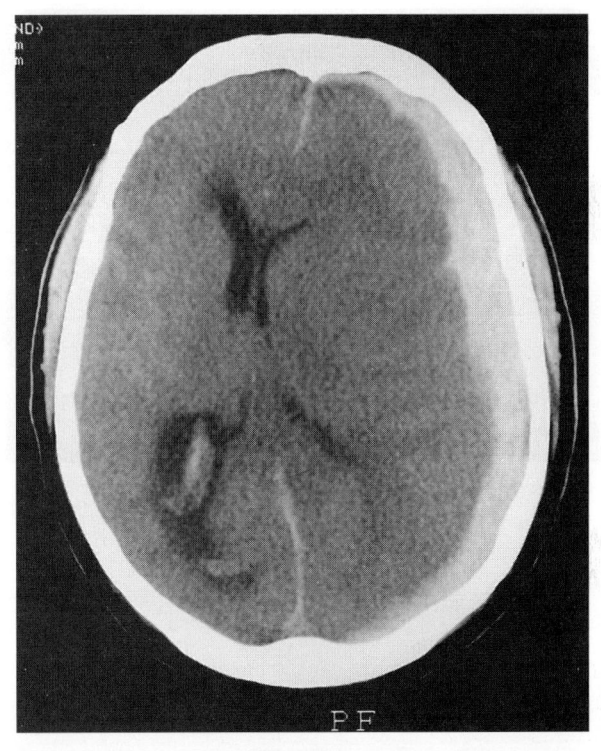

Fig. 49.2
CT Brain. Acute subdural haematoma with midline shift.

QUESTION 50

This 45-year-old Asian man has low back pain.

a What is the investigation?
b What two abnormalities are present?
c What is the most likely diagnosis?

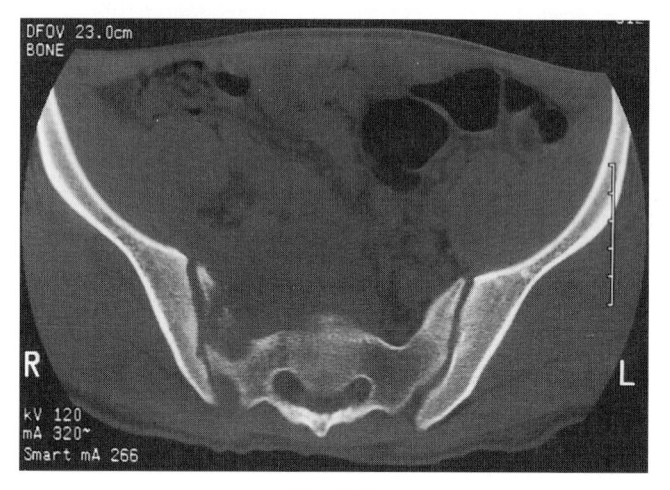

Fig. 50.1

Answer 50

a CT of the sacroiliac joints.
b Presacral soft tissue mass. Destruction of both sides of the right sacroiliac joint.
c Tuberculous sacroiliitis.

Discussion

The sacroiliac joints may become infected by haematogenous spread, local spread from pelvic sepsis or following surgery. Radiologically, early infection is suggested by blurring of the subchondral bone on both sides of the joint which is narrowed. The contralateral joint is normal, which is a strong pointer to an infectious aetiology. Tuberculous infection is suggested by the patient's racial origin and the presence of a soft tissue mass in the presacral area. Direct needle puncture for acid-fast bacilli and culture will confirm the diagnosis.

While infective sacroiliitis is unilateral, sacroiliitis in individuals with the HLA B27 genotype (associated with ankylosing spondylitis, inflammatory bowel disease, Reiter's disease or psoriasis) usually shows bilaterally symmetrical involvement of the sacroiliac joints.

QUESTION 51

This 56-year-old woman has right-sided weakness.

a What three abnormalities are shown in Fig. 51.1a?
b Figure 51.1b is the CT brain on the same patient. What is the exact diagnosis?

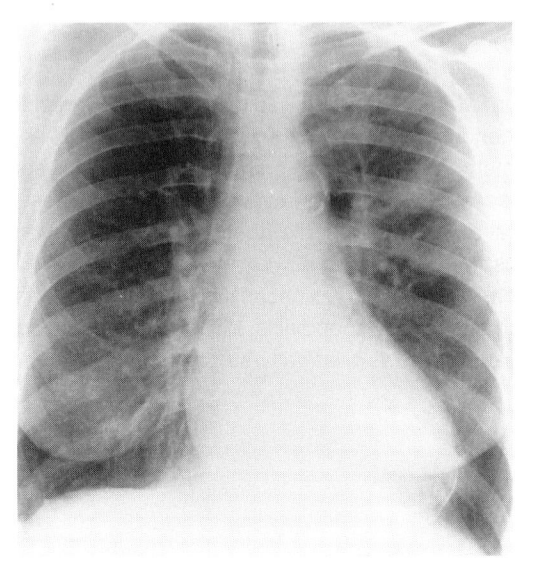

Fig. 51.1a

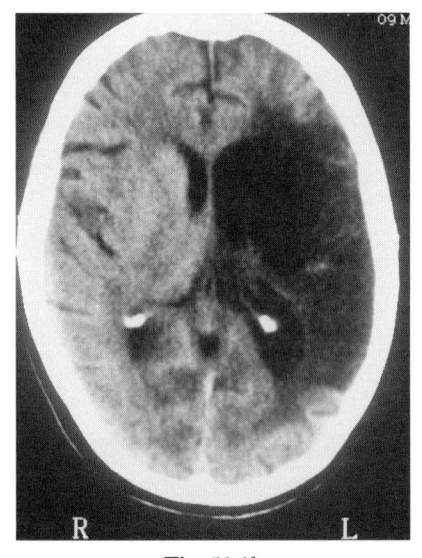

Fig. 51.1b

Answer 51

a Cardiomegaly. Calcified left ventricular aneurysm. Ill-defined pulmonary shadowing in mid-zone of left lung.
b Acute cerebral infarction caused by a left middle cerebral artery embolus secondary to a left ventricular aneurysm.

Discussion

A ventricular aneurysm occurs when a large transmural anterior infarct is surrounded by viable myocardium. It is particularly associated with occlusion of the left anterior descending coronary artery. An aneurysm very rarely ruptures, but is a source of systemic embolization when mural thrombi become detached. Ventricular aneurysms often cause arrhythmias, and patients frequently present with left heart failure. The ECG classically shows fixed ST elevation in the anterior leads.

Figure 51.1b shows a wedge-shaped non-haemorrhagic infarct in the left parietal area. It is of low attenuation and its borders precisely demarcate the boundaries of the middle cerebral arterial territory. It is due to an embolus lodged in the left middle cerebral artery. There are no areas of high attenuation and no significant mass effect.

QUESTION 52

This 50-year-old man has weakness and wasting of both arm muscles.

a What is the diagnosis?
b What other physical signs may be elicited?

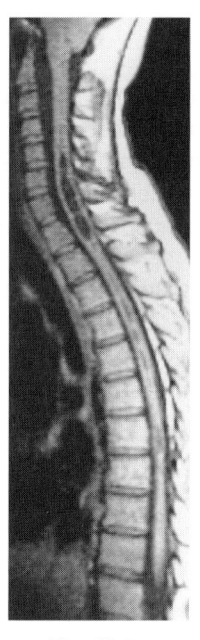

Fig. 52.1a

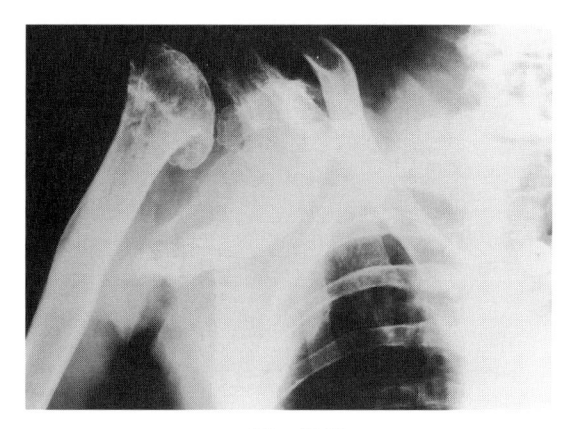

Fig. 52.1b

Answer 52

a Syringomyelia causing Charcot's neuropathy of the shoulder.
b Pain and temperature sensory loss over the upper trunk in a 'cape' distribution, joint deformities, Horner's syndrome, upper motor neurone signs in the legs.

Discussion

Syringomyelia is due to a fluid-filled cavity within the spinal cord. It is usually located in the cervical cord, but may involve the cord at any point along its length. The brainstem may be involved and it is then termed syringobulbia. The syrinx is lateral and posterior to the central canal which explains the asymmetry of sensory signs. It is associated with acquired conditions: intramedullary tumours and trauma and with developmental anomalies (Arnold–Chiari malformations and spinal dysraphism).

The syrinx interrupts pain and temperature fibres as they decussate in the cord. The patient will first notice burns or cuts in the fingers. An area of paraesthesia then extends proximally to envelop the shoulders in a cape-like distribution. Involvement of the pyramidal tracts causes upper motor neurone signs in the legs. Occasionally, anterior horn cells may be involved producing fasciculation and muscle wasting at the level of the syrinx. Horner's syndrome occurs in involvement of the cervical sympathetic plexus.

In longstanding syringomyelia, the shoulder and elbow joints (Fig. 52.2) become anaesthetic and are prone to repeated trauma. A Charcot's or neuropathic joint will result. This is usually unilateral due to the lateral position of the syrinx. However, large syringes may give rise to bilateral arthropathy.

Radiologically, a Charcot's joint can be diagnosed when the joint is **d**eformed, **d**isorganized, **d**istended (effusion), **d**islocated, **d**ense (sclerotic) and containing **d**ebris. Remember all the 'd's'!

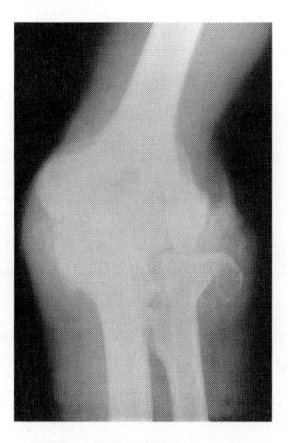

Fig. 52.2
Elbow joint. Charcot's joint. There is deformity, disorganization, sclerosis and debris within the joint.

QUESTION 53

This 40-year-old alcoholic presents with cough and weight loss.

a What are the two radiological abnormalities?
b What is the most likely diagnosis?
c Name two other clinical conditions which predispose to its development.

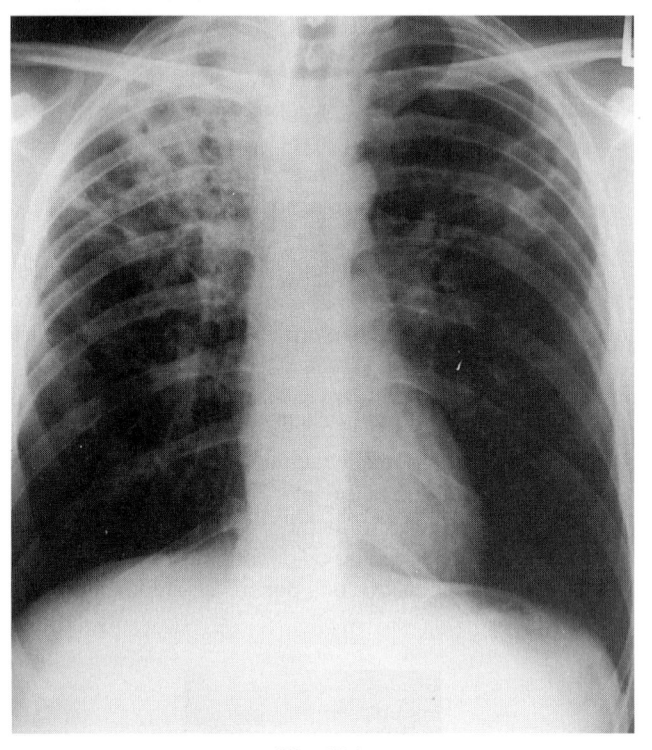

Fig. 53.1

ANSWER 53

a Consolidation and cavitation in the right upper lobe and left mid-zone.
b Reactivation or post primary tuberculosis (TB).
c Diabetes mellitus; malnutrition; uraemia; cancer; silicosis; immunosuppression; homelessness.

Discussion

Reactivation, or post primary TB classically involves the apical and posterior segments of the upper lobes and the apical segments of the lower lobes. Formerly, this distribution was thought to occur because aerobic tubercle bacilli thrive in areas of high oxygen concentration. It is now thought that poor lymphatic clearance in these areas is primarily responsible for this distribution. In advanced disease, any segment may be affected but an upper zone distribution predominates. Lymph node enlargement and pleural effusion are unusual in reactivation TB. When the infection has resolved, calcified fibro-nodular infiltrates are seen, usually in one of the upper lobes. However, this appearance on its own does not imply inactivity, which must always be confirmed bacteriologically and by observing no change on an interval radiograph (usually 6 months later).

Primary TB has three main radiographic findings. One of these alone or in combination may be present: parenchymal consolidation (most frequently in the periphery of the lower lobes); hilar and mediastinal lymphadenopathy; pleural effusion (more common in adults).

Both primary and reactivation TB can be complicated by miliary spread. Figure 23.1 shows miliary seeding in a child with hilar lymphadenopathy due to primary TB.

Unusual radiographic manifestations of TB may occur in a variety of situations: pneumothorax in cavitary disease; atelectasis secondary to endobronchial disease; tuberculoma in primary or reactivation TB; bronchopleural fistula as a complication of a chronic tuberculous pleural effusion. Primary TB in immunosuppressed individuals can lead to spread to one or both lungs without cavitation. TB may be a presenting feature of cancer, and carcinoma can occasionally develop in a TB scar.

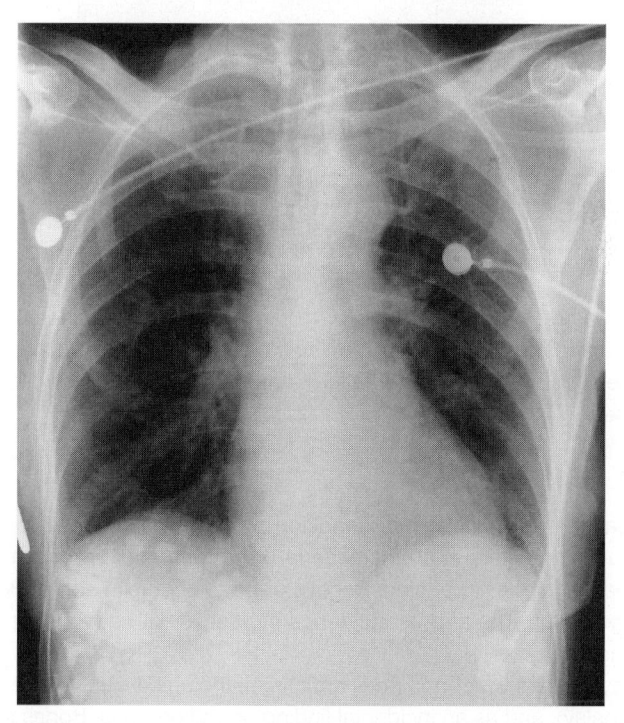

Fig. 53.2
Chest radiograph. Calcified tuberculous granulomata in the liver and spleen.

QUESTION 54

a What is the diagnosis?
b Name five complications.

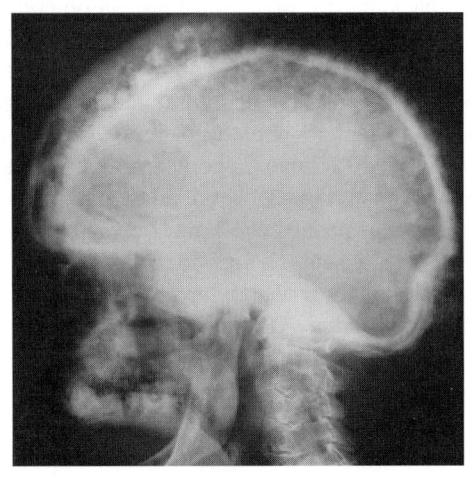

Fig. 54.1

ANSWER 54

a Paget's disease.
b Pathological fracture; bone overgrowth causing cranial nerve palsies (especially VIIIth nerve); high output cardiac failure; immobilization hypercalcaemia and sarcomatous change.

Discussion

Paget's disease is an idiopathic condition in which increased osteoclastic and osteoblastic activity results in an increase in bone resorption and formation. The end result is haphazard bone expansion. Paget's disease occurs in about 4% of the population over 40 years of age, and its incidence increases with advancing age. It is more common in men.

Patients may present with bone pain, arthritis, pathological fracture, deafness (or other cranial nerve palsy), and as an incidental finding on radiographs. Bones such as the tibia and skull may enlarge, giving symptoms of bowing and increasing hat size, respectively. The commonest sites for Paget's disease are the spine and pelvis (Fig. 54.2).

Paget's disease has a classic radiographic appearance. In long bones, the disease begins in a subarticular position extending down the diaphysis as a flame-like area of lysis due to excessive osteoclastic activity. In the skull, osteoclastic lysis appears well demarcated. This is known as osteoporosis circumscripta. Osteoblastic activity intervenes giving a mixed pattern on the radiograph – the so-called 'cotton wool' appearance (Fig. 54.1). Note the thickening of the outer table of the vault.

Paget's disease has a characteristic appearance on a technetium-MDP bone scan (Fig. 54.2). There is intense confluent and uniform increased tracer activity in expanded bone, reflecting marked osteoblastic activity. Serum alkaline phosphatase and urinary hydroxyproline levels are elevated.

Deafness is due to a combination of Paget's disease of the ossicles and VIIIth nerve compression. Compression of the cord may complicate spinal involvement, and obstructive hydrocephalus may result in cases of severe basilar invagination. Paget's disease softens bone and predisposes to pathological fracture. Stress fractures tend to occur along the convex cortex of a bowed bone. Sarcomatous change is said to affect 1% of patients and may be of any cell type. The onset of sarcoma is heralded by increased pain.

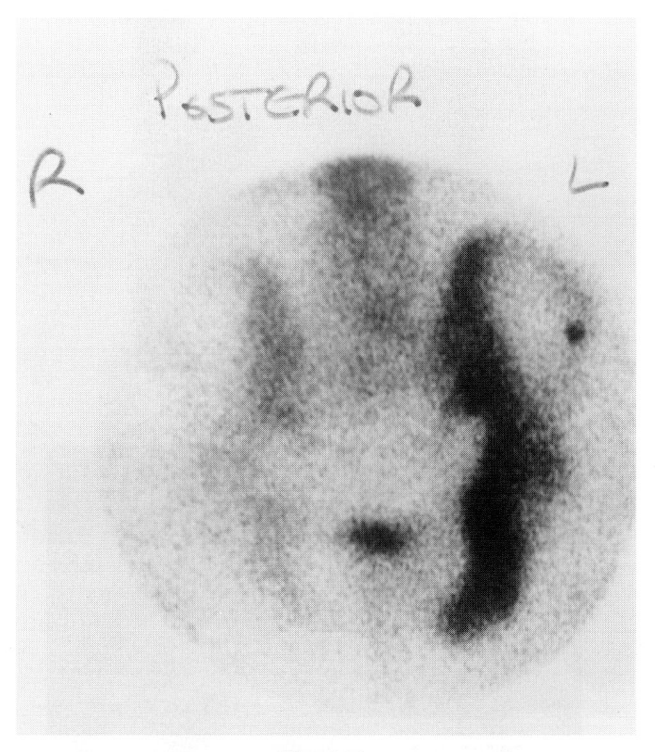

Fig. 54.2
Isotope bone scan. Paget's disease of the pelvis. There is intense tracer uptake in an expanded ilium, ischium and inferior pubic ramus.

QUESTION 55

This 60-year-old woman presents with jaundice.

a What abnormalities are shown on **i** ERCP
ii liver ultrasound?
b What is the most likely underlying diagnosis?

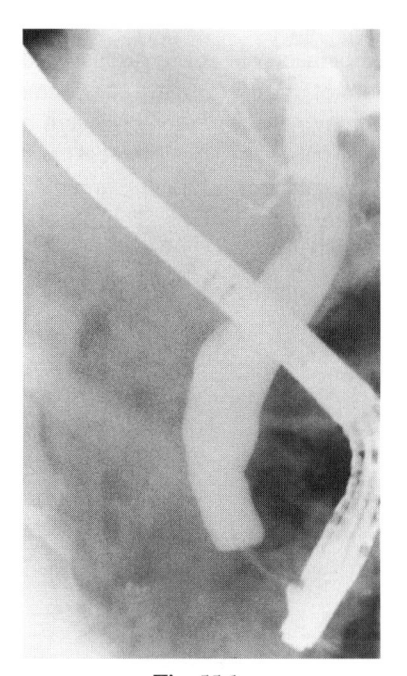

Fig. 55.1a

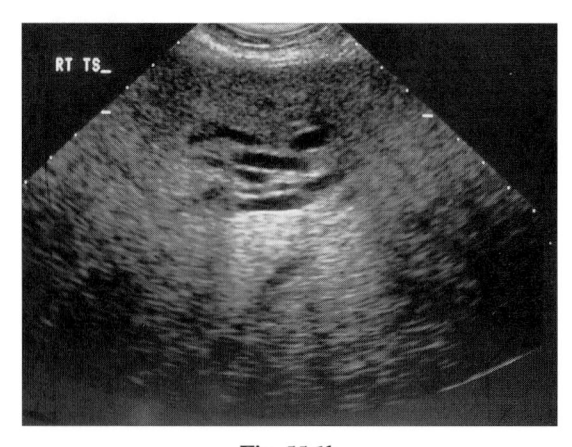

Fig. 55.1b

Answer 55

a i Dilatation of the common bile duct (CBD) and intrahepatic ducts. Shouldered stricture of the distal CBD.
  ii Dilatation of the intrahepatic ducts.
b Carcinoma of the ampulla of Vater.

Discussion

Ampullary carcinomas are slow-growing neoplasms. At presentation, they are usually small although local lymph node involvement and distant metastases have been reported in up to 20% of cases. Overall, they have a more favourable prognosis than the more diffuse and infiltrative neoplasms of the pancreas. Although bile duct dilatation is readily demonstrated on CT and ultrasound, the tumour itself is not often seen on these studies. ERCP is the preferred imaging method as it enables direct inspection and biopsy of the lesion. If no distant disease is detected, these lesions are resected using a Whipple's procedure.

Question 56

This is an enhanced abdominal CT scan in a 14-year-old girl.

a What is the diagnosis?
b What two main complications may arise in this condition?

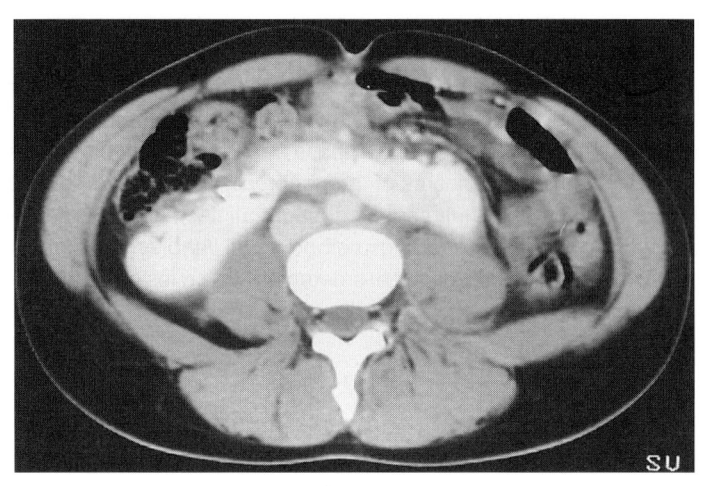

Fig. 56.1

Answer 56

a Horseshoe kidney.
b Upper ureteric obstruction, urinary stasis and stone formation.
Increased predisposition to trauma.

Discussion

Horseshoe kidney is the commonest of the renal fusion anomalies. Both lower poles are joined in the midline by an isthmus of functioning renal tissue. Occasionally the isthmus is a non-functioning fibrotic bridge. Both ureters course anterior and medial to the lower poles, and it is at this point that ureteric obstruction occurs. Urinary stasis predisposes to stone formation and, in cases of chronic irritation, to the development of transitional cell carcinoma.

The isthmus of the kidney is at risk of direct injury when it becomes trapped between the lumbar spine and the traumatic force.

QUESTION 57

This is a contrast-enhanced CT of the brain in a 45-year-old man with epilepsy.

a What is the diagnosis?
b What major complication may occur?

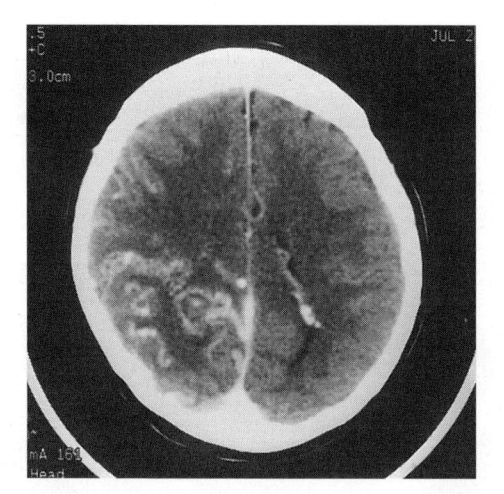

Fig. 57.1

ANSWER 57

a Arteriovenous malformation of the brain.
b Subarachnoid haemorrhage.

Discussion

An arteriovenous malformation (AVM) of the brain may present with headache, epilepsy or progressive neurological deficit. The CT appearances are characteristic – serpiginous feeding arteries and draining veins readily delineated by contrast medium (Fig. 57.1). AVMs may calcify and this is best shown on unenhanced CT. There may, in addition, be areas of reduced attenuation around the lesions due to ischaemia. When the blood–brain barrier is breached a diffuse contrast blush may be seen.

AVMs are responsible for 10% of cases of subarachnoid haemorrhage. Presentation is then similar to subarachnoid haemorrhage of any other cause. Obstructive hydrocephalus may complicate.

QUESTION 58

This is a CT scan of the thorax in an elderly male with a brisk haemoptysis.

a   How has the scan been performed?
b   What is the diagnosis and with which underlying disease process is it associated?
c   Name two methods of treating this patient.

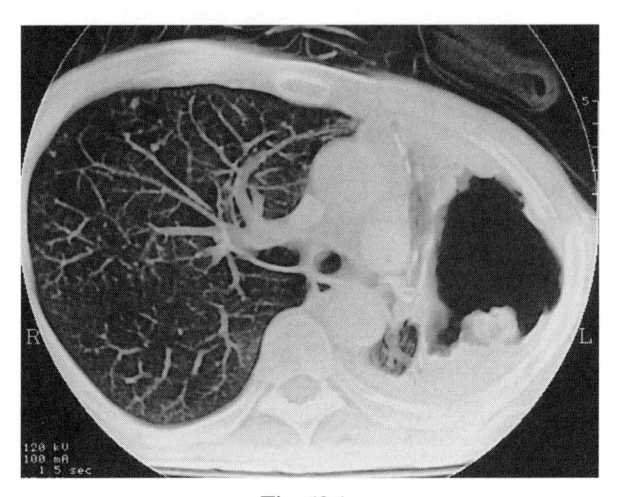

Fig. 58.1a

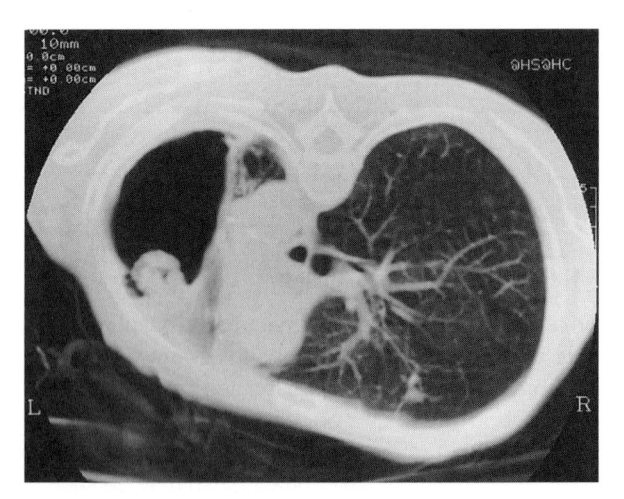

Fig. 58.1b

Answer 58

a Prone and supine CT.
b Aspergilloma (mycetoma) in a tuberculous cavity.
c Left upper lobectomy. Bronchial artery embolization.

Discussion

An aspergilloma can be easily demonstrated on CT. In this example, there is volume loss and medial pleural calcification, highly suggestive of previous TB. The finding of a discreet, mobile fungus ball within a cavity represents the end of a spectrum of changes seen in this condition. It represents the condensation of fungal hyphae and fibrinous material (see also Fig. 18.2). The cavity wall has a rich supply from branches in the bronchial circulation.

Cough is the commonest symptom. Haemoptysis has been reported in up to 95% of cases and can be life threatening. In the emergency situation, the patient should be turned into the decubitus position on the same side as the lesion to prevent aspiration of blood into the contralateral main bronchus. Bronchial artery embolization or lobectomy may be necessary in severe cases. A typical radiographic appearance (see Fig. 18.1) and a strongly positive precipitin test confirm the diagnosis. About 10% of cases undergo spontaneous resolution.

QUESTION 59

This 50-year-old man has recently developed diabetes mellitus and hypertension.

a What is the diagnosis?
b Name four additional features in this condition.

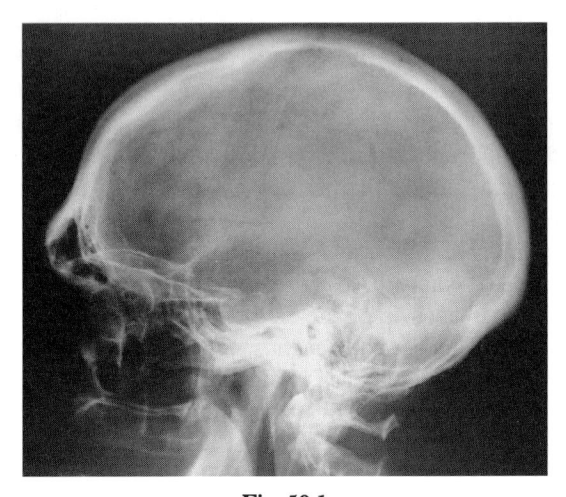

Fig. 59.1

ANSWER 59

a Acromegaly.

b Cardiomyopathy and hypertension; deep voice (due to laryngeal cartilage hypertrophy); thick, greasy skin; arthralgia (and chondrocalcinosis); proximal myopathy; peripheral neuropathy (carpal tunnel syndrome); visual field defects in suprasellar extension (bitemporal hemianopia); macroglossia; prominent supra-orbital ridge; prognathism; spade-like hands; terminal phalangeal tufting and widely spaced teeth.

Discussion

Acromegaly is a condition due to excessive secretion of growth hormone (GH) after epiphyseal fusion. It is usually caused by a chromophobe adenoma of the pituitary and occurs between the third and fifth decades. If there is excess GH prior to epiphyseal fusion, gigantism will result.

The earliest manifestation in acromegaly is coarsening of facial features and swelling of the hands and feet. Impaired glucose tolerance is present in about 50% of cases, although clinically significant diabetes occurs in only 10% of cases.

The radiological features of acromegaly are classical. Skull radiograph shows cortical vault thickening, enlarged frontal sinuses, enlarged sella turcica with erosion of the dorsum, enlarged mandible, and chondrocalcinosis in the pinna.

Hand radiograph shows increased joint spaces due to hypertrophy of articular cartilage, spade-like hands, enlargement of the terminal phalangeal tufts, and prominent flanges along the phalangeal shafts at the site of muscle insertion.

Lateral heel radiograph shows increased heel pad thickness (more than 23 mm).

The pituitary adenoma can be imaged with MRI which demonstrates the tumour in every orthogonal plane. MRI is excellent at showing its relationship to the optic chiasm. Characteristically, pituitary adenomas do not enhance with i.v. gadolinium.

QUESTION 60

This young patient presents with cardiovascular collapse.

a What investigation is this?
b What is the diagnosis?
c What treatment is indicated?

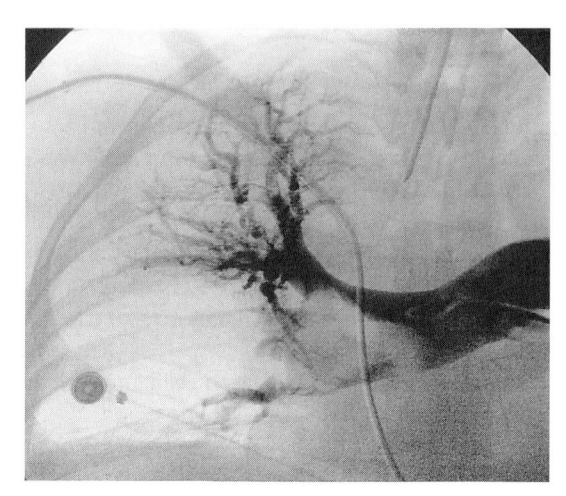

Fig. 60.1

ANSWER 60

a Pulmonary angiography.
b Large right main pulmonary artery embolus with emboli in the right basal and upper lobe pulmonary arteries.
c Systemic thrombolysis or thrombectomy (via catheter or thoracotomy).

Discussion

A massive pulmonary embolus requires immediate investigation and management. A clot of this magnitude may be lysed with systemic thrombolysis using streptokinase or tissue plasminogen activator. In some centres suction thrombectomy may be achieved with specialized catheters and with specialized expertise. It is very rare for patients to survive a journey to a cardiothoracic surgical unit for consideration of a thoracotomy and manual thrombectomy.

QUESTION 61

This is an ultrasound image of the liver in a 46-year-old man, 24 hours after an alcoholic drinking binge.

a What abnormality is shown?
b What is the most likely explanation?
c What investigation would confirm the diagnosis?

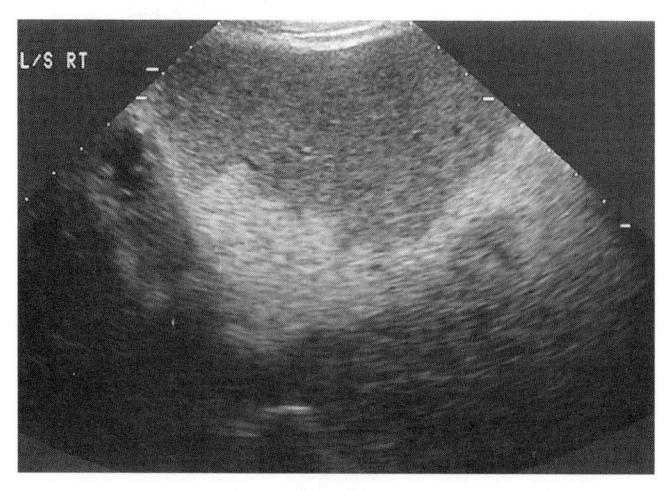

Fig. 61.1

ANSWER 61

a Geographical area of increased echogenicity within the liver.
b Focal fatty infiltration.
c CT of the liver.

Discussion

Fatty infiltration of the liver is normally diffuse. Occasionally it may be focal as illustrated in Fig. 61.1. Fat causes a high echogenicity on ultrasound. CT of the liver will show the fatty infiltration as low attenuation (see Fig. 86.1). Furthermore, fatty infiltration does not alter the architectural integrity of the liver, enabling this condition to be distinguished confidently from neoplasia.

QUESTION 62

A 59-year-old man has weight loss and iron deficiency anaemia.

a What investigation is this?
b What is the most likely diagnosis?
c Suggest a possible alternative diagnosis.

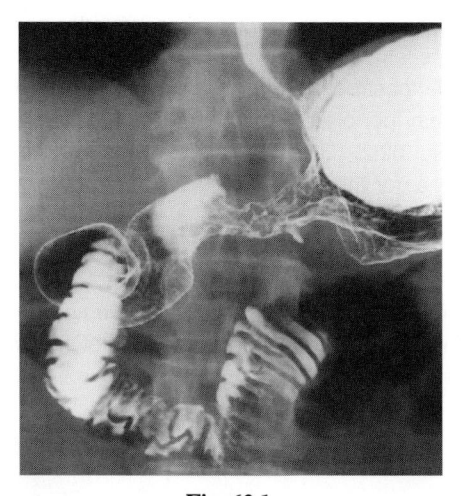

Fig. 62.1

Answer 62

a Barium meal.
b Carcinoma of the stomach.
c Crohn's disease.

Discussion

Advanced gastric cancer may appear as a large irregular gastric mass or, as in this example, a more diffuse lesion infiltrating and narrowing the stomach. Gastric cancers may cause gastric outlet obstruction when they involve the antrum.

Localized cancers may perforate the stomach wall. A fistula may develop between stomach and colon (Fig. 62.2). Other causes of a gastro-colic fistula are Crohn's disease, diverticular disease of the large bowel, carcinoma of the large bowel and gastrointestinal lymphoma.

Gastric involvement is a rare manifestation of Crohn's disease, usually associated with involvement elsewhere in the gastro-intestinal tract. Radiologically, there is rugal thickening and aphthoid ulceration, but severe involvement may mimic gastric carcinoma. The distal stomach is involved, causing tapering of the pyloric region and usually extending into the duodenum.

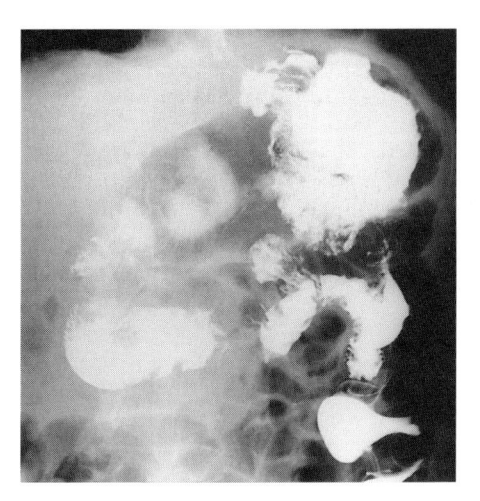

Fig. 62.2
Barium meal. Gastro-colic fistula secondary to gastric cancer. There is a communication between the fundus of the stomach and the descending colon.

QUESTION 63

This is a contrast-enhanced CT of the brain in a 60-year-old man with cerebellar signs.

a What abnormality is shown?
b What are the two most likely causes?

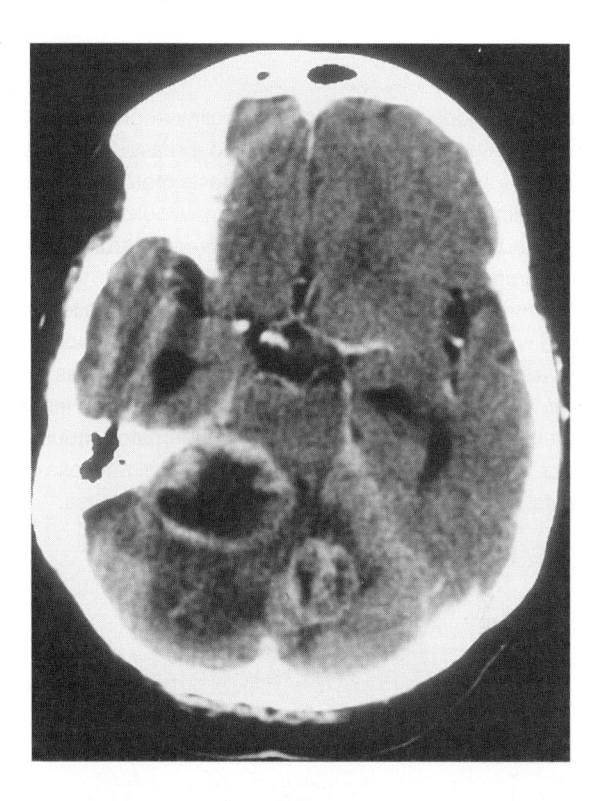

Fig. 63.1

Answer 63

a Two rim-enhancing space-occupying lesions with surrounding oedema in the cerebellum.
b Metastases.
 Abscesses.

Discussion

Metastases are the commonest brain tumours in clinical practice. The most common primary sites are carcinoma of the bronchus and breast. The presence of multiple intracranial space-occupying lesions strongly suggests metastases, especially if there is a known history of malignancy. On CT, metastases may look identical to abscesses, and the latter are suggested if the patient is febrile or has endocarditis, a right-to-left cardiac shunt or is immunosuppressed.

Both metastases and abscesses tend to occur at the grey–white matter junction, and both are associated with surrounding oedema which appears black on CT. A thick irregular wall suggests a metastasis and a thinner, more regular wall is more suggestive of abscess. However, it may be difficult to distinguish the two lesions on CT. Brain abscesses are often streptococcal and arise from haematogenous spread in 50% of cases and by direct local spread in the remainder. A fungal abscess occurs in immunosuppressed patients, but appears identical to a pyogenic abscess.

QUESTION 64

a What is the radiological diagnosis?
b What investigation would you request next and why?
c Name five other associated conditions.

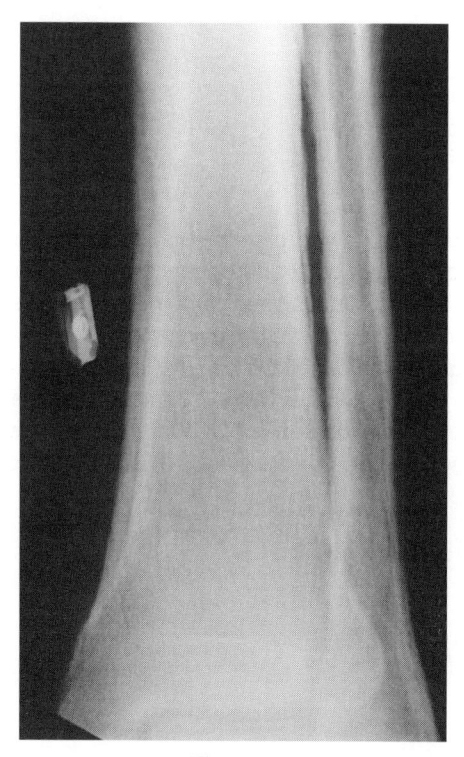

Fig. 64.1

Answer 64

a Hypertrophic pulmonary osteoarthropathy (HPOA).
b Chest radiograph, to exclude carcinoma of the bronchus or other thoracic disease.
c Bronchiectasis.
  Mesothelioma.
  Cyanotic congenital heart disease.
  Cirrhosis.
  Inflammatory bowel disease.
  Benign pleural fibroma.

Discussion

Clubbing of the fingers and toes was once thought to be the result of thoracic disease alone – hypertrophic pulmonary osteoarthropathy (HPOA). It is now known to be associated with a host of other conditions. When clubbing is associated with a bronchial neoplasm, it may be accompanied by hyperhidrosis. Arthralgia similar to that of rheumatoid disease is present in up to 30% of patients.

Radiologically there is periosteal new bone extending from the diaphysis to the metaphysis, sparing the epiphysis. The bones of the forearm and lower legs are most commonly involved, but metacarpals, metatarsals and occasionally phalanges may also be affected.

QUESTION 65

This ERCP is from a 65-year-old man with maturity-onset diabetes mellitus.

a What are the radiological findings?
b What is the diagnosis?
c List two other possible symptoms in this patient.

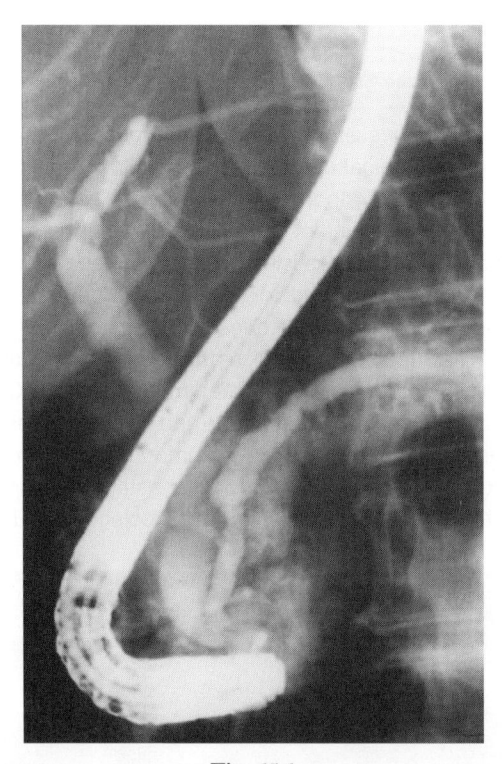

Fig. 65.1

Answer 65

a The main pancreatic duct is dilated and has an irregular calibre. The acinae are delineated by contrast medium.
b Chronic pancreatitis.
c Pain (epigastric radiating to the back).
Weight loss.
Steatorrhoea.

Discussion

Chronic pancreatitis is a progressive inflammatory process of the pancreas characterized by irreversible morphological changes. This results in pain and loss of endocrine and exocrine function. Clinically, the diagnosis may take the form of recurrent acute attacks of pancreatitis or of a persistent, chronic pain. The most common cause is alcohol excess. Other causes include gallstones, hyperlipidaemia, hypercalcaemia, congenital anomalies of the pancreatic and biliary ducts and trauma.

Ultrasound helps to demonstrate gallstones or other causes of duct obstruction in a patient suspected of having chronic pancreatitis. CT of the pancreas is useful for demonstrating the calcification or any associated mass lesion. ERCP findings of chronic pancreatitis are dilatation of the pancreatic duct and side branches and areas of calcification. The distal pancreatic segment of the common bile duct may also be narrowed. Figure 65.1 shows chronic pancreatitis due to longstanding obstruction in the duct. Figure 65.2 shows chronic calcific pancreatitis in association with hyperparathyroidism.

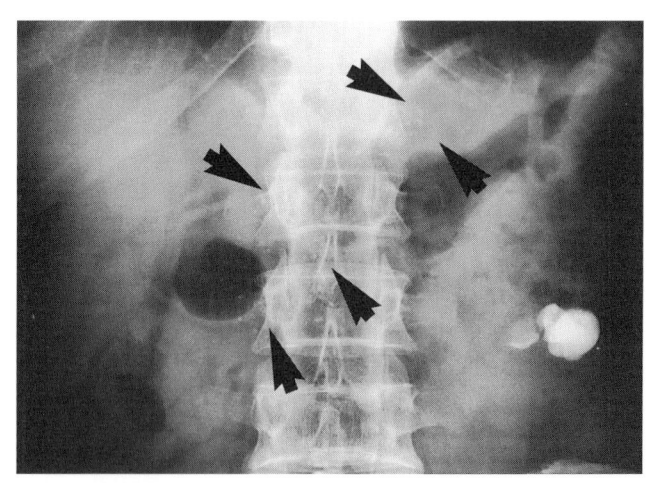

Fig. 65.2
Hyperparathyroidism. Chronic calcific pancreatitis and left renal calculi. Note the spotty, irregular distribution of calcification crossing the midline towards the left upper quadrant (arrows).

QUESTION 66

This was an incidental finding during a liver ultrasound in an asymptomatic 50-year-old New Zealander.

a Describe the abnormality.
b What diagnosis should be excluded?
c How would you confirm it?

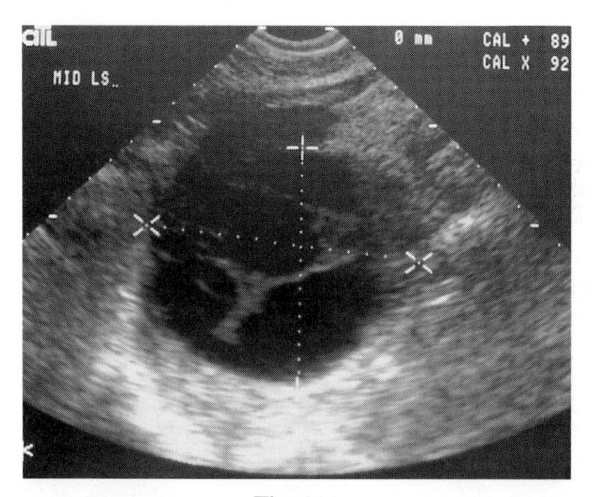

Fig. 66.1

Answer 66

a There is a 9-cm-diameter septated cyst within the liver parenchyma.
b Hydatid disease.
c Skin test (Casoni test).

Discussion

Hydatid disease is caused by *Echinococcus granulosus*. The adult worm lives in the intestines of dogs and other canines. The worm releases eggs into the stool. These eggs are then ingested by an intermediate host (humans and sheep). The embryos penetrate the intestinal wall of the host and are carried to the liver by the portal circulation. Some embryos will reach the lungs, kidneys and bones. The larvae develop into hydatid cysts which develop pressure symptoms as they slowly enlarge. The fluid-filled cyst contains scolices, brood capsules and daughter cysts.

Hydatid disease is common in sheep-rearing areas including Australia, New Zealand, Wales and South Africa. The cysts may be unilocular or multilocular and septated. CT shows the cyst and its frequently calcified wall to advantage. The daughter cysts are located in the periphery of the lesion.

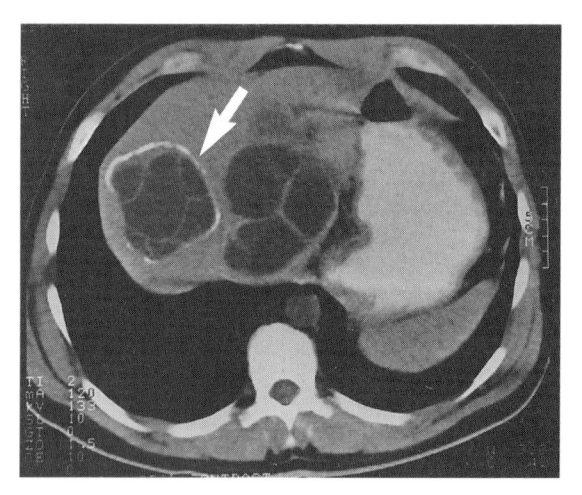

Fig 66.2
CT Liver without i.v. contrast medium. Note rim calcification of a septated hydatid cyst (arrow).

Question 67

This is a static renal scan in a patient with hypertension.

a What radiopharmaceutical has been used?
b What is the abnormality?
c Suggest a possible cause for this abnormality.

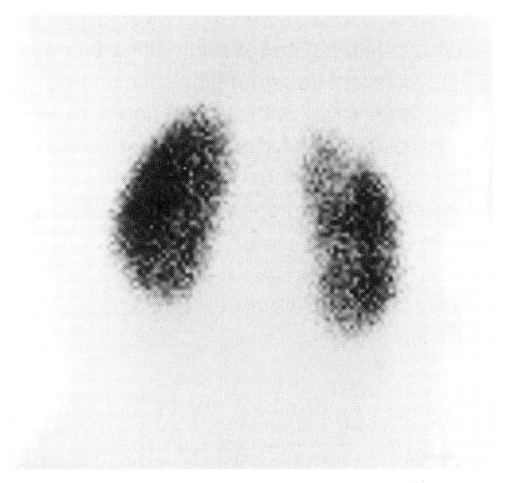

Fig. 67.1

Answer 67

a Tc99m dimercaptosuccinic acid (DMSA).
b There is an area of photopenia in the upper pole of the right kidney. This is due to a cortical scar.
c Reflux.

Discussion

Tc99m DMSA is taken up by the renal cortex and retained for a prolonged time in a stable state. This makes it an excellent tracer for high-resolution imaging of the cortex. The maximum uptake of tracer is achieved within 3 to 6 hours. A dynamic radiopharmaceutical such as Tc99m DTPA or Tc99m MAG3 would not be suitable for cortex imaging because it is rapidly cleared from the kidney.

An area of poor tracer uptake, or photopenia, is the result of a scar or space-occupying lesion. The scar results in hypertension.

QUESTION 68

This 65-year-old woman has developed respiratory failure. She is on long-term immunosuppression for Wegener's granulomatosis.

a What complication has occurred as a result of immunosuppression?
b What additional complication has occurred and how has it been treated?

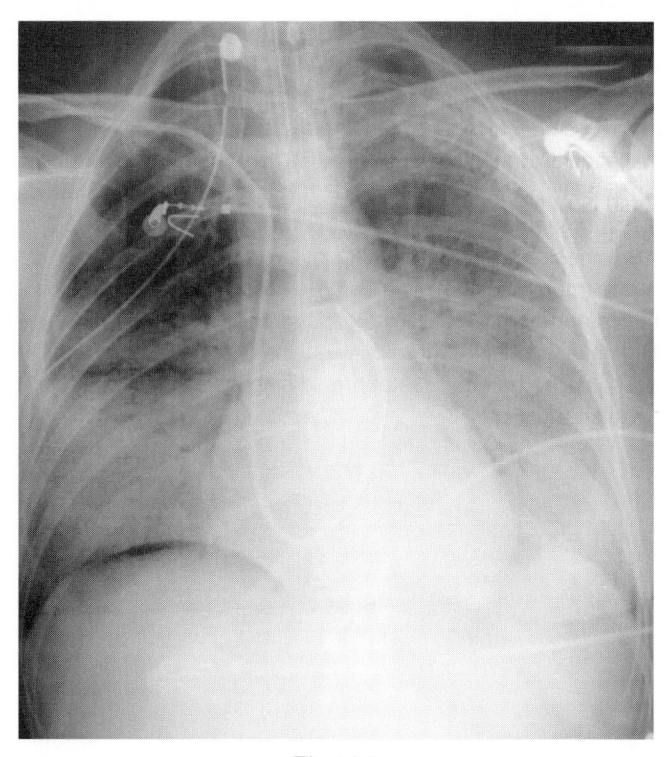

Fig. 68.1

ANSWER 68

a Bilateral perihilar consolidation due to *Pneumocystis carinii* pneumonia (PCP).
b Right-sided pneumothorax. An intercostal drain has been placed in the right side.

Discussion

PCP affects immunocompromised individuals and starts insidiously with a dry cough and breathlessness. Later, hypoxaemia and fever occur, but there are seldom any significant auscultatory signs. *Pneumocystis carinii* is a fungus. PCP has a predilection for the perihilar regions without zonal predominance (Fig. 68.1). The chest radiograph is normal in 10% of cases, and in early cases the subtle perihilar shadowing may be overlooked. Pleural effusions and hilar or mediastinal lymphadenopathy are unusual in PCP.

Pneumothorax can complicate PCP when pneumatoceles are present. Pneumatoceles represent air cysts which develop in areas of consolidation and are due to a check-valve mechanism. Intermittent positive pressure ventilation can cause and exacerbate a pneumothorax in this condition. The lucent crescent below the silhouette of the right hemidiaphragm (Fig. 68.1) on this supine chest radiograph is the only sign that the patient has a pneumothorax. Air in the pleural space collects in the least dependent part, i.e. the anterior costophrenic sulcus, and it is vital that it is promptly treated in a ventilated patient.

QUESTION 69

This child has abdominal pain, ataxia and a hypochromic microcytic anaemia.

a What abnormality is shown?
b What is the diagnosis?

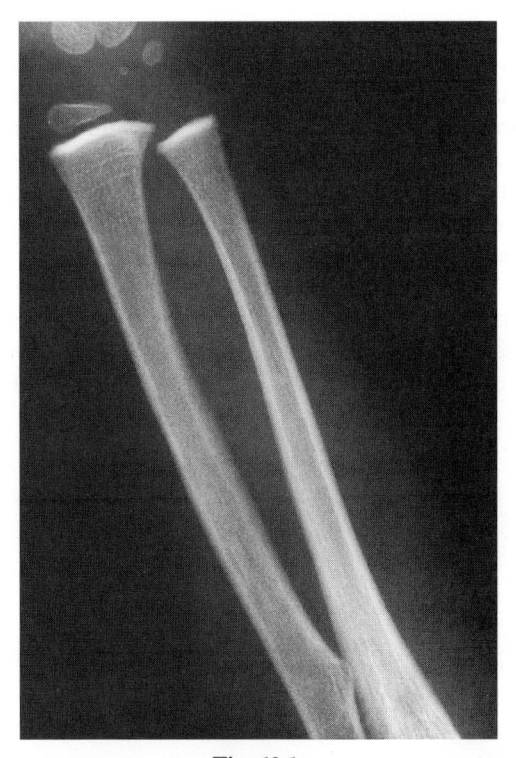

Fig. 69.1.

Answer 69

a Dense metaphyseal bands in the distal radius and ulna.
b Lead poisoning.

Discussion

Lead poisoning occurs mainly in children, and is most commonly due to lead paint ingestion. The dense metaphyseal bands seen in lead poisoning are a result of calcium deposition in the cartilaginous matrix. There is radiographic evidence of raised intracranial pressure (widened sutures) in 10% of patients with chronic lead poisoning. Opaque lead particles may be seen in the bowel lumen on abdominal radiographs. However, dense metaphyseal bands can be seen in normal subjects, and a diagnosis of lead poisoning should therefore not be made on the basis of the radiographic appearances alone. In children, acute poisoning presents over a few days with persistent and forceful vomiting, ataxia, seizures and altered consciousness due to encephalopathy. These symptoms cease spontaneously if exposure is interrupted. Long-term lead intoxication causes a hypochromic, microcytic anaemia with stippled red blood cells. A definitive diagnosis can be made by measuring the blood lead concentration.

QUESTION 70

This 50-year-old man has a left hemiplegia.

a What abnormality is shown?
b What is the diagnosis?
c What facial features would you expect to find?

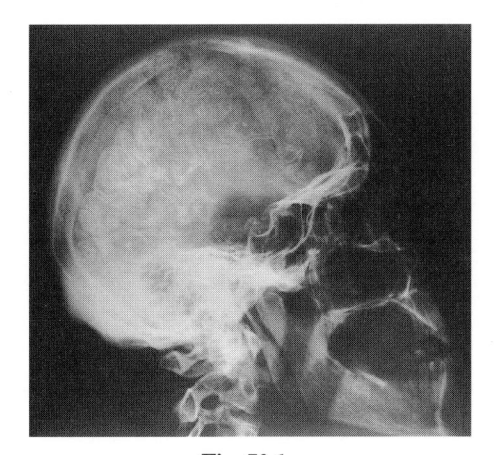

Fig. 70.1a

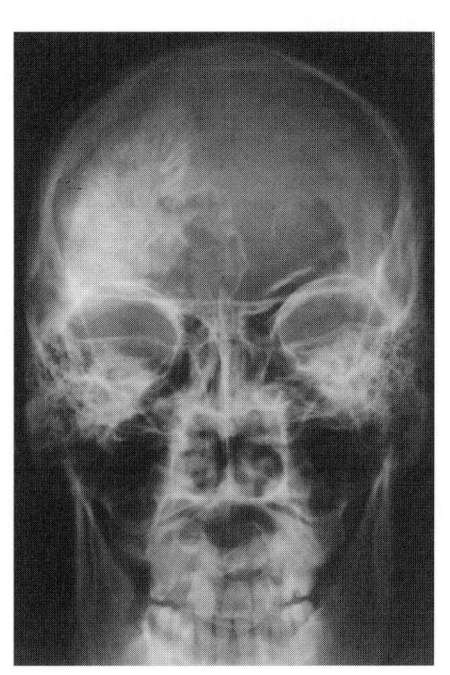

Fig. 70.1b

Answer 70

a 'Tramline' calcification of the parieto-occipital cortex of the right cerebral hemisphere.
b Sturge-Weber syndrome.
c Cutaneous angioma in a distribution above the palpebral fissure which is usually ipsilateral to the cortical calcification.

Discussion

The Sturge-Weber syndrome is a neuroectodermal disorder characterized by a leptomeningeal angiodysplasia with atrophy of the underlying cerebrum. About 50% of patients have the classical 'tramline' calcification in the surface of the cortex of the parieto-occipital lobes. A port-wine stain or cutaneous angioma is associated with the brain abnormality and is located above the palpebral fissure.

Patients with this condition have epilepsy and contralateral pyramidal signs.

QUESTION 71

A 58-year-old man has right pleuritic pain, fever and a productive cough.

a What is the cause of the pleuritic pain?
b What disease must be excluded?

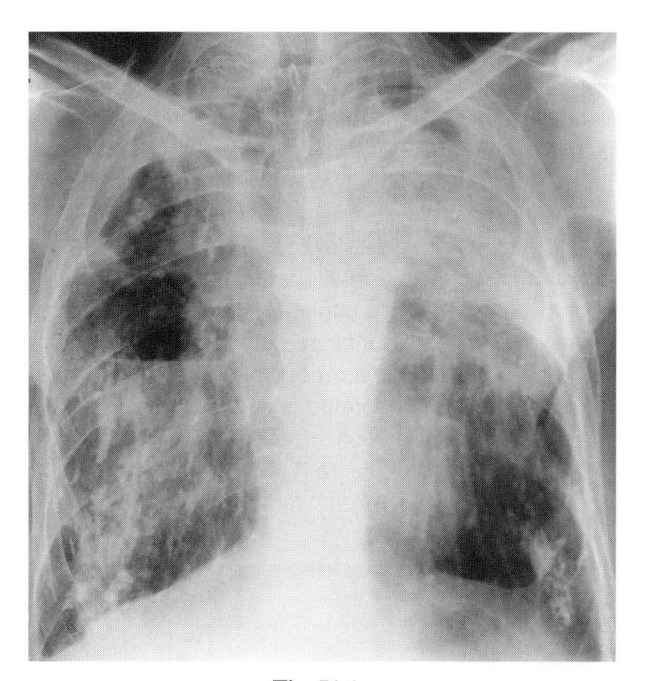

Fig. 71.1a

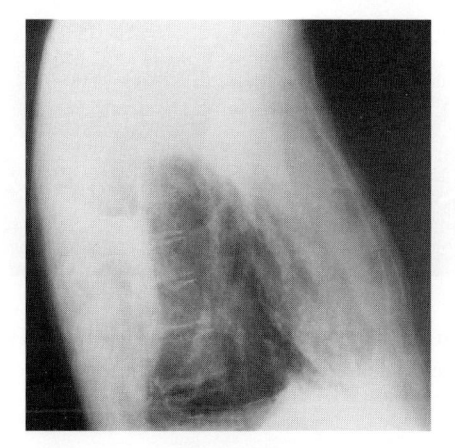

Fig. 71.1b

Answer 71

a Right-sided empyema.
b Tuberculosis (TB).

Discussion

The frontal and lateral chest radiographs show an encysted hydropneumothorax in the right posterior pleural cavity. The history suggests an empyema. There are changes of previous TB – bilateral mid- and upper-zone fibrous and calcified plaques. The presence of an empyema raises the possibility of active TB, which must be excluded. The empyema should be drained with an intercostal tube and samples should be sent for both routine and TB staining and culture.

An empyema is a collection of pleural fluid containing a white blood cell count higher than 15×10^3 cells/mm^3 and protein level higher than 3 g/dl or positive cultures for the same organisms on two consecutive samples. Most empyemas are due to associated pneumonia but some occur after trauma, surgery and subdiaphragmatic sepsis. The usual organisms implicated are anaerobes, pneumococcus and *Staphylococcus aureus*. Tuberculous empyemas are formed from breakdown of localized tuberculous pleurisy. The empyema cavity may breach the visceral pleura and form a bronchopleural fistula or break through the parietal pleura and ulcerate on to the skin. The subcutaneous abscess that results is known as empyema necessitans (Fig. 71.2).

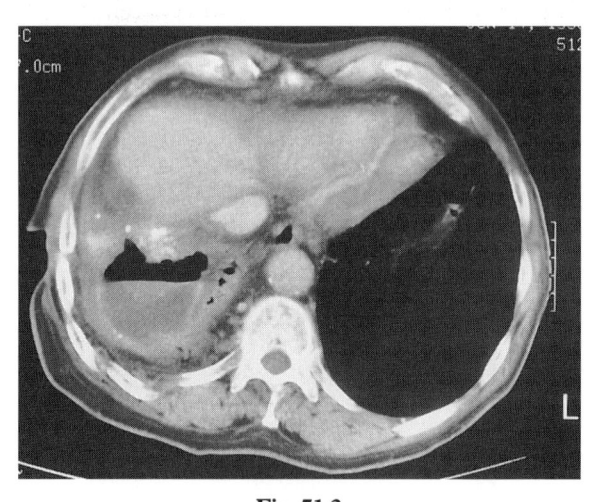

Fig. 71.2
CT. Empyema necessitans. Note the calcified, thickened visceral and parietal pleura and the subcutaneous depression on the right chest wall due to ulceration.

QUESTION 72

This is a contrast-enhanced abdominal CT in a 72-year-old Chinese man with abdominal pain, hepatomegaly and fever.

a What abnormalities are shown?
b What is the likely diagnosis?
c Which three investigations would you undertake?

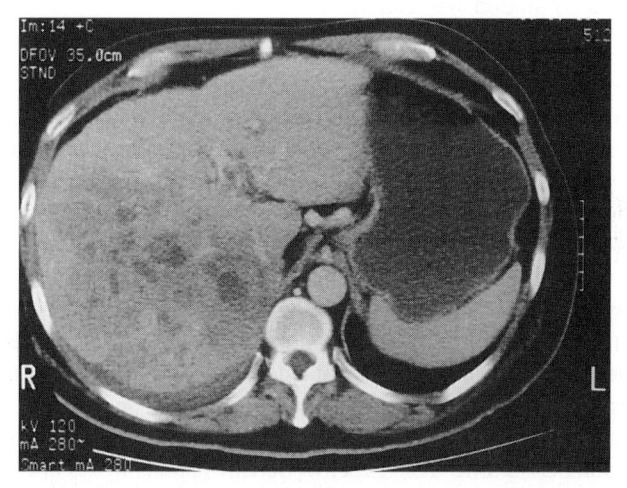

Fig. 72.1

Answer 72

a Multifocal non-enhancing expansile tumour in the right lobe of the liver.
Non-opacification of the inferior vena cava (IVC).
Right pleural effusion.
b Hepatocellular carcinoma (HCC).
c Serum alpha-fetoprotein.
Serum HBsAg.
Percutaneous CT-guided liver biopsy.

Discussion

Hepatocellular carcinoma (HCC) is much less common than metastatic disease of the liver, but it is the most common primary malignancy and an important cause of death in Southern Africa and South-Eastern Asia. In endemic areas, chronic hepatitis B virus (HBV) infection is responsible for a several hundredfold increase in the incidence of HCC compared to non-endemic areas. In carriers of HBV, viral DNA becomes incorporated into the genome and, by an unknown mechanism, hepatocytes undergo malignant transformation. Environmental factors are also implicated, with fungal aflatoxin, contaminating food such as nuts and corn, contributing to the high incidence of HCC in Africa. In developed countries, many patients with HCC have pre-existing cirrhosis which is known to have a high risk of malignant change.

Serum alpha-fetoprotein is a useful biochemical marker and is elevated in HCC and germ cell tumours. CT shows multifocal low-density lesions in the liver with or without surrounding cirrhosis. In this case, the IVC is not opacified because of tumour invasion, making the hepatoma non-resectable. Percutaneous biopsy will confirm the diagnosis, but there is a slightly higher risk of bleeding due to the increased vascularity of the tumour.

QUESTION 73

This is a T2-weighted MRI of the brain in a 26-year-old woman with unilateral blurred vision.

a What abnormalities are present?
b What is the diagnosis?
c How do you explain the blurred vision?

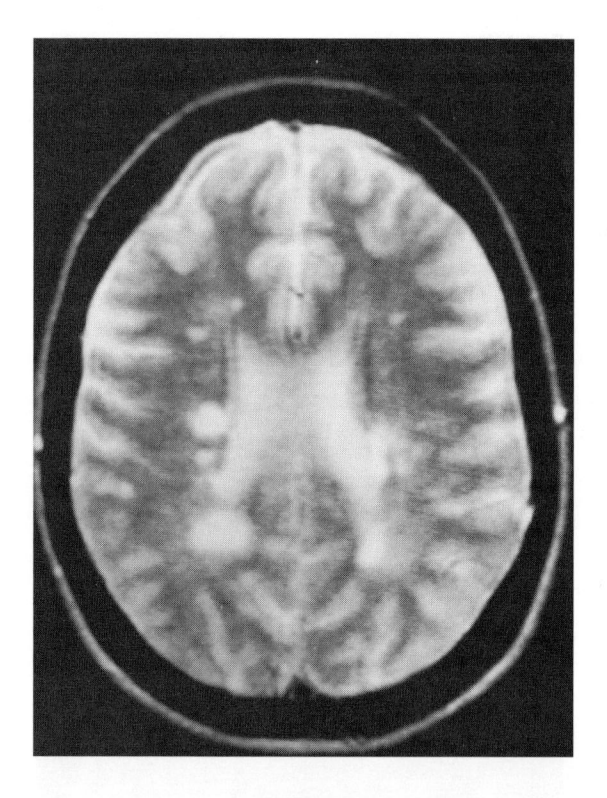

Fig. 73.1.

ANSWER 73

a High-signal lesions in the periventricular white matter of both cerebral hemispheres.
b Multiple sclerosis (MS).
c Optic neuritis.

Discussion

Multiple sclerosis (MS), a disease of unknown aetiology, is one of the commonest disorders of the central nervous system (CNS) in young people. The clinical diagnosis relies on demonstrating signs in at least two places in the CNS separated by time. Modern imaging has enabled the diagnosis to be made more readily. MRI is the first-line investigation in suspected MS. Multiple plaques of demyelination, with a high signal on T2-weighted images due to their high water content, occur in the periventricular white matter, cerebellum, brain stem, optic nerve and spinal cord (Fig. 73.2). Acute plaques enhance with gadolinium and may be confused with tumour except for the absence of mass effect. The plaques may disappear or persist with time, losing their contrast enhancement. CSF and 'free water' within brain lesions appear as high-signal (white) on T2-weighted images.

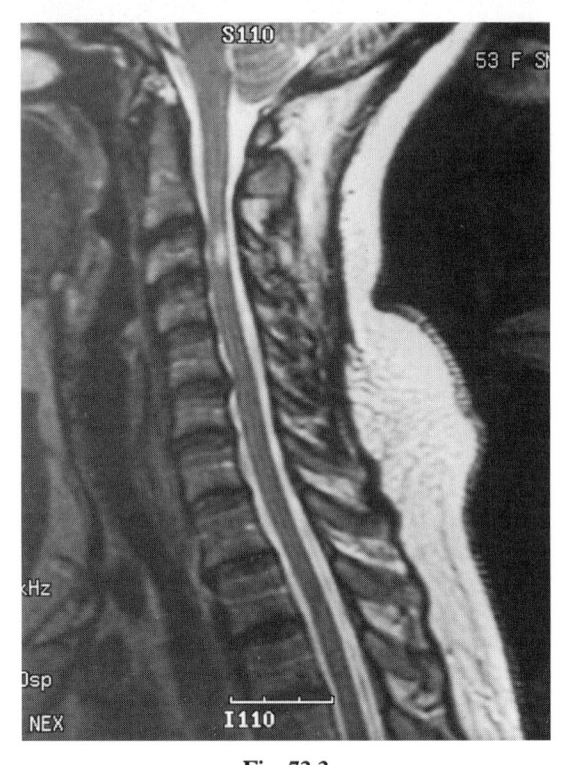

Fig. 73.2
Multiple sclerosis. T2-weighted MRI spinal cord demonstrating a high signal lesion within the cord at C3.

QUESTION 74

This is a chest radiograph of a 66-year-old woman who recently noticed a lump in her neck.
a What are the two radiological abnormalities?
b What is the most likely diagnosis?
c What investigation would you perform next?

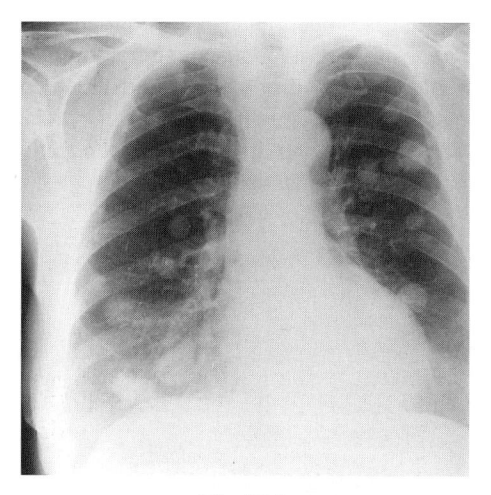

Fig. 74.1

ANSWER 74

a Multiple well-defined pulmonary nodules. Superior mediastinal mass (goitre).
b (Follicular) thyroid carcinoma with pulmonary metastases.
c Isotope thyroid scan.

Discussion

Thyroid cancer usually presents as an otherwise symptomless lump in the neck. Uncommonly it may present with metastases in the lungs, bones or lymph nodes. Papillary carcinoma is the commonest variant, comprising up to 70% of all thyroid cancers. It occurs more commonly in young females. It may also occur in the elderly, in whom there is a worse prognosis, spreading via the lymphatic system. Follicular carcinoma represents 15% of thyroid cancer, tends to occur in the elderly and has a more malignant course than papillary carcinoma with haematogenous spread. Both types are associated with prior neck irradiation.

An isotope thyroid scan classically demonstrates a cold defect in thyroid cancer. Only 4% of malignant tumours take up tracer. Up to 25% of 'cold' lesions are due to carcinoma, the remainder being cysts.

Pulmonary metastases appear as multiple well-defined nodules of varying size on a chest radiograph. In a young male the presence of well-defined pulmonary metastases strongly suggests a testicular carcinoma. Furthermore, the primary growth in the testis may be impalpable and may only be shown on testicular ultrasound. Other primary cancers that may present with pulmonary metastases include melanoma, ovarian carcinoma, breast carcinoma and stomach carcinoma. Primary bone tumours often have lung metastases at diagnosis. Spontaneous pneumothorax in association with pulmonary nodules is virtually diagnostic of metastatic osteosarcoma, although this has been described in Wilms' tumour. Miliary metastases can look identical to miliary TB on a chest radiograph (see Fig. 23.1), and are usually associated with thyroid, renal and bone malignancies, trophoblastic disease and melanoma.

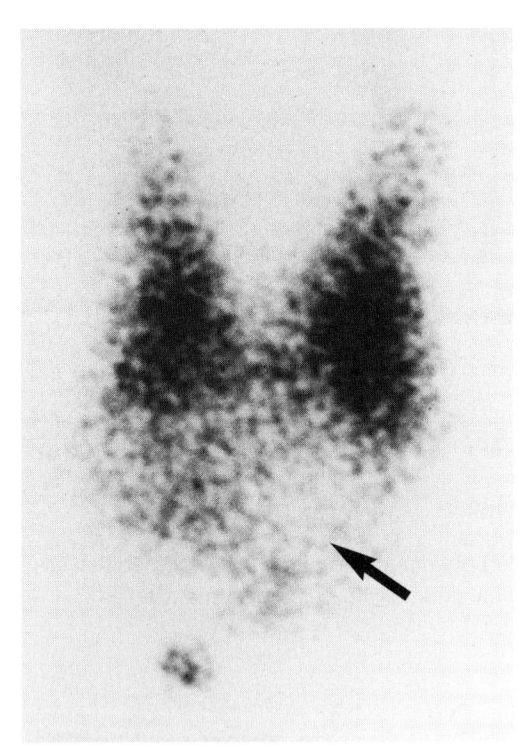

Fig. 74.2
Thyroid scan. Thyroid cancer. Large cold defect inferior left lobe (arrow).

QUESTION 75

This is a barium enema examination in a 65-year-old lady with profuse watery diarrhoea, muscle weakness and cramps.

a What abnormality is shown?
b What is the diagnosis?
c What other symptoms may be present?

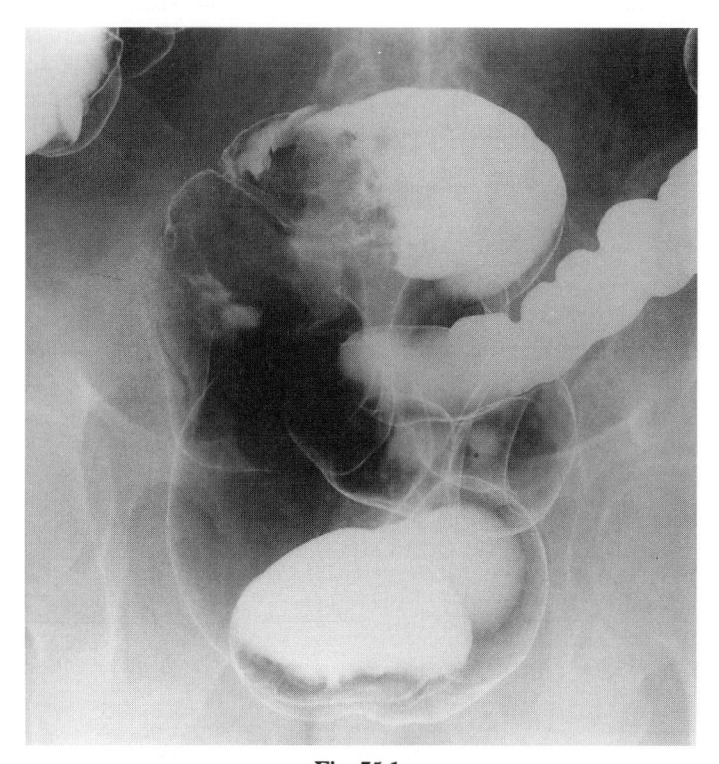

Fig. 75.1

ANSWER 75

a Large filling defect in the proximal rectum.
b Villous adenoma of the rectum.
c Rectal bleeding. Tenesmus.

Discussion

Villous adenomas of the rectum are sessile, frond-like masses. They produce excess mucus which characteristically leads to poor coating with barium. There is a tendency to malignant change. Local recurrence after excision occurs in about 10% of cases. Villous adenomas may present with profuse, watery diarrhoea which leads to hypokalaemia. Symptoms of hypokalaemia include:

- muscle weakness;
- hypotonia;
- arrhythmias;
- tetany;
- cramps.

Other symptoms associated with a villous adenoma include rectal bleeding and tenesmus.

QUESTION 76

This is a contrast enhanced abdominal CT in a 65-year-old woman with pyrexia of unknown origin.

a What abnormality is present?
b Which adjacent structures must be carefully examined on the CT study?
c Name three alternative modes of presentation.

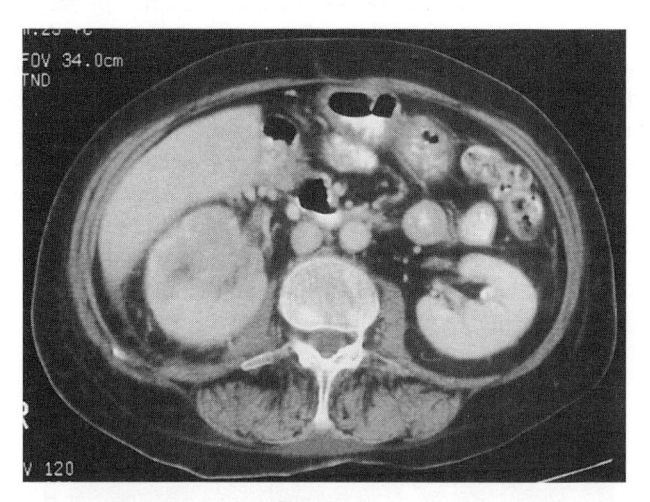

Fig. 76.1

ANSWER 76

a Mixed attenuation mass in the midpole of the right kidney due to hypernephroma.
b Renal vein and inferior vena cava (IVC).
c Haematuria, flank mass, pain, polycythaemia or hypertension.

Discussion

A hypernephroma or renal cell carcinoma is the most common primary malignant renal neoplasm. It is usually large at the time of symptomatic presentation but, with their increasing use, ultrasound (Fig. 76.2) and CT will often detect these tumours before symptoms arise. CT will provide information on its size, location and local extension. Both ultrasound and CT will detect venous invasion. CT is more sensitive for detecting nodal involvement. A chest radiograph is mandatory in patients with hypernephroma to exclude pulmonary metastases. Renal arteriography is occasionally employed to define the arterial anatomy prior to resection.

Haematuria and sometimes hypertension result when there is local extension of tumour into the calyx. A hypernephroma may occasionally produce erythropoietin, resulting in polycythaemia.

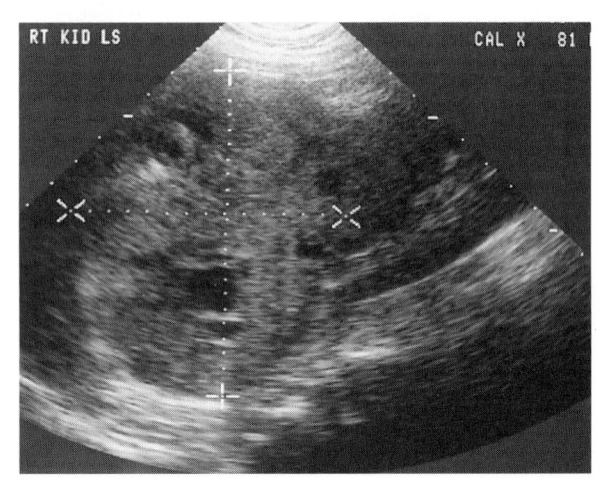

Fig. 76.2
Hypernephroma. Ultrasound right kidney shows a large mass of mixed echogenicity occupying the upper pole.

QUESTION 77

This 54-year-old man has headaches and breathlessness, which are worse in the supine position.

a What investigation is shown?
b What is the diagnosis? Give two possible causes.
c What other symptoms and signs may be present in this condition?

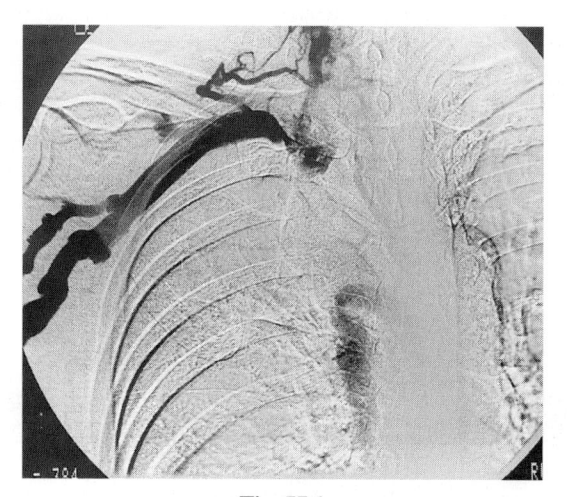

Fig. 77.1

ANSWER 77

a Superior venacavogram.
b Superior vena caval obstruction (SVCO). Lung cancer. Lymphoma.
c Dilated veins in the neck, face and upper chest. Plethora and oedema of the face, neck and upper chest.
Visual disturbance.
Stridor.
Syncope.

Discussion

The commonest cause of SVCO is compression and/or invasion of the SVC by tumour from a bronchogenic carcinoma. This may be primary invasion in the case of a squamous carcinoma, or lymph node metastases in the case of a small-cell carcinoma. Malignant lymphoma and metastases from testicular and breast cancer comprise the remainder of the malignant causes. SVCO may rarely be caused by benign disease – retrosternal goitre, aortic aneurysm, mediastinal fibrosis (secondary to TB or histoplasmosis) or thrombosis *in situ* (secondary to long-term indwelling catheters).

A contrast-enhanced CT must always be obtained in patients with SVCO in order to determine its cause. In most cases a tissue diagnosis will be required prior to treatment. Squamous carcinoma is radiosensitive, small-cell carcinoma is chemosensitive, and lymphomas may respond to both. Figure 77.2a shows obliteration of SVC by lymphoma. Note the contrast-filled collaterals around the right shoulder region. A metallic stent (Fig. 77.2b) can be placed in the superior vena cava in those patients who are refractory to treatment.

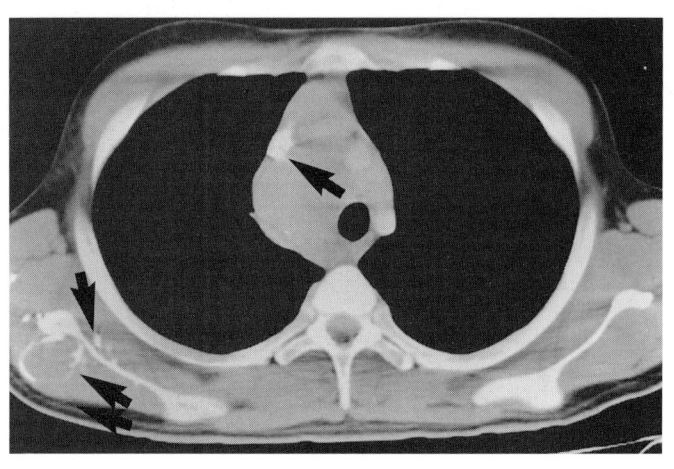

Fig. 77.2a
Non-Hodgkins lymphoma complicated by SVCO. CT scan. Note SVC (upper arrow) and the dilated contrast-filled venous collaterals around the right shoulder (lower arrows).

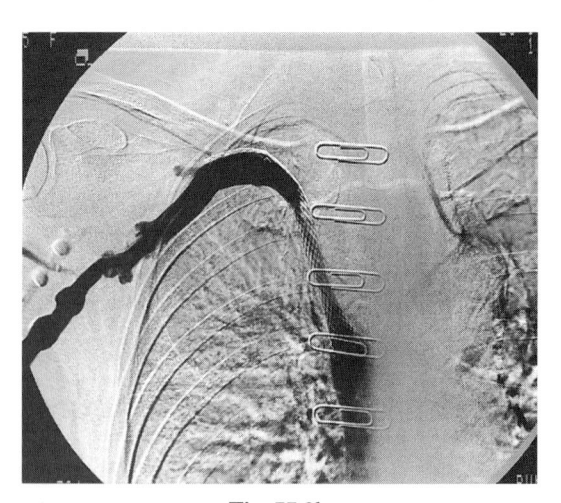

Fig. 77.2b
SVCO relieved with metallic stent. The flow is restored and there is now no flow into the neck veins.

QUESTION 78

a What investigation is this?
b What is the diagnosis?
c Name three modes of presentation.

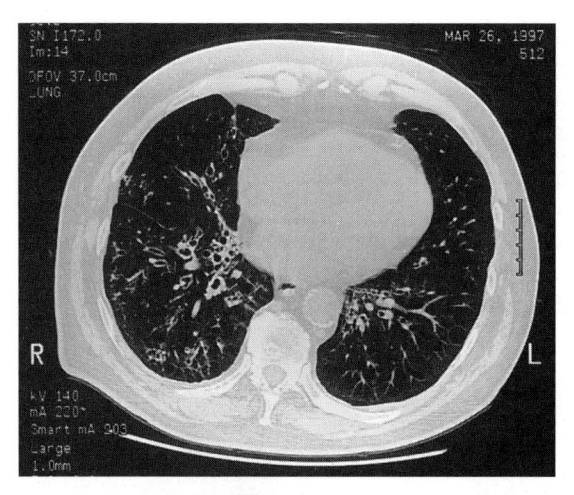

Fig. 78.1

ANSWER 78

a High-resolution CT (HRCT) of the chest.
b Bronchiectasis.
c Haemoptysis.
   Copious purulent sputum.
   Asthma.
   Clubbing.

Discussion

Bronchiectasis is irreversible dilatation of one or more bronchi and is invariably associated with inflammation. Bronchiectasis may be focal or generalized, and obstructive or non-obstructive. The main bronchi up to and including the fourth-order bronchi possess cartilaginous rings. Bronchiectasis only affects bronchi distal to this point. Three varieties of bronchiectasis, based on pathological and radiological findings, have been described:

- cylindrical bronchiectasis (mildest form);
- varicose bronchiectasis (greater dilatation with localized narrowing; associated with small airways disease);
- cystic (saccular) bronchiectasis (severest form, progressive dilatation distally).

The diagnosis of bronchiectasis is established on HRCT by demonstrating one enlarged bronchus adjacent to a smaller accompanying pulmonary artery.

In transverse section this resembles a signet ring (Fig. 78.2). HRCT has now replaced bronchography as the radiological investigation of choice in bronchiectasis.

Bronchiectasis has a number of causes. So far as examinations are concerned, the most important of these is Kartaganer's syndrome. You will not overlook this diagnosis if you carefully note the side markers on the chest radiograph.

The main causes of bronchiectasis are:

- childhood respiratory infection (whooping cough, measles, TB);
- cystic fibrosis;
- bronchial obstruction (endobronchial tumour or foreign body);
- agammaglobulinaemia (Bruton's disease);
- allergic bronchopulmonary aspergillosis.

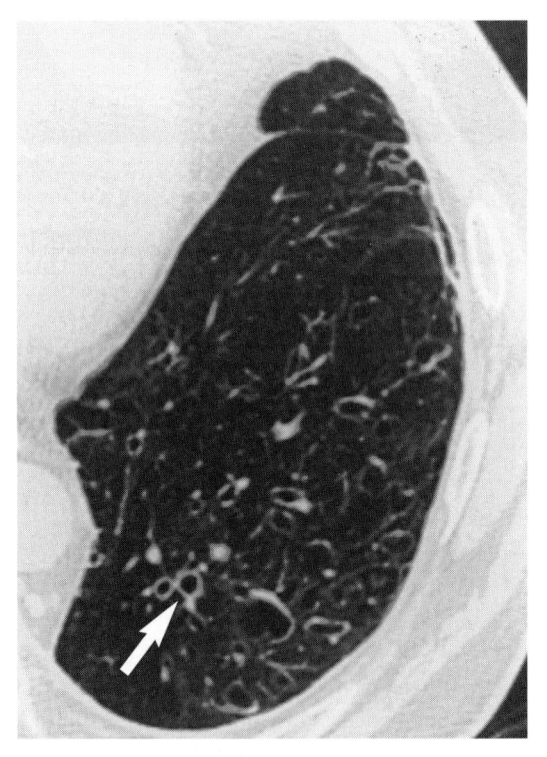

Fig. 78.2
HRCT. Bronchiectasis. Signet ring sign (arrow).

QUESTION 79

This is the chest radiograph of a 28-year-old breathless woman with known ovarian carcinoma.

a What is the most likely radiological diagnosis?
b With what other neoplasms is this condition associated?

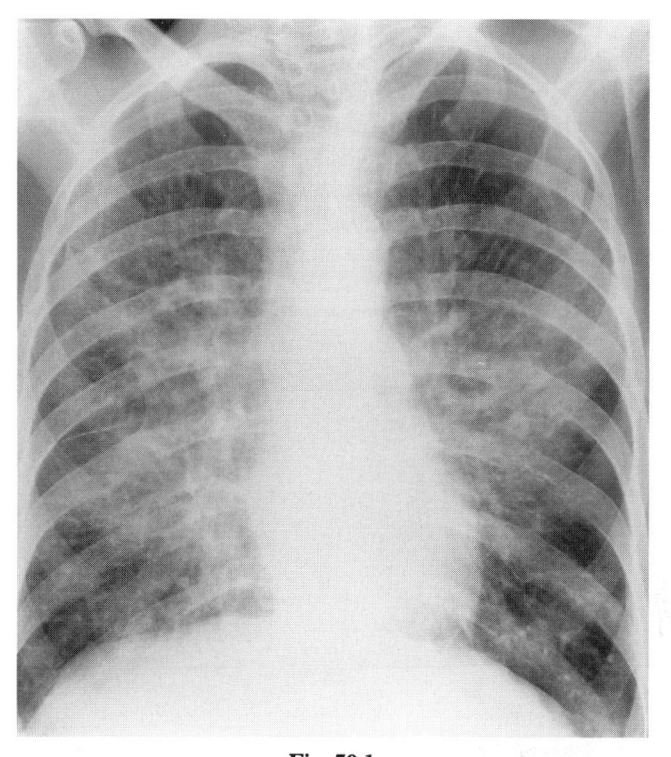

Fig. 79.1

ANSWER 79

a Lymphangitis carcinomatosa.
b Carcinoma of bronchus, breast, pancreas, stomach, uterus, prostate and colon. Lymphoma.

Discussion

Lymphangitis carcinomatosa is due to pulmonary lymphatic permeation by carcinoma cells. This results in centrally predominant reticulonodular shadows, thickening of septal lines and fissures and sometimes small pleural effusions. Hilar lymph node enlargement (not seen in this case) is present in up to 50% of cases. Patients are usually breathless, and quite often are considered to have pulmonary oedema unless there is a known history of primary malignancy. Figure 79.2 demonstrates unilateral lymphangitis in a patient with carcinoma of the bronchus. Lymphangitis may be widespread or focal and, when unilateral, it may be segmental or lobar in distribution.

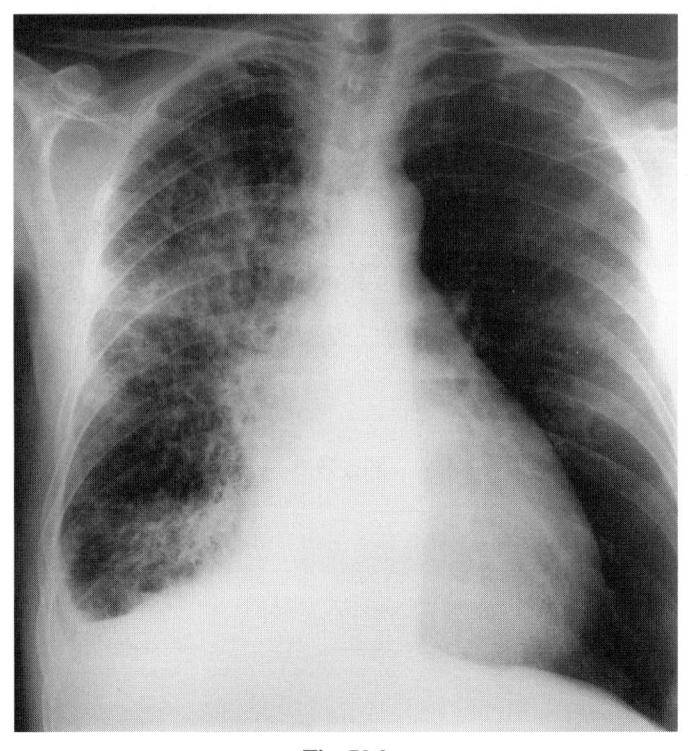

Fig. 79.2
Chest radiograph. Unilateral lymphangitis carcinomatosa from bronchial carcinoma. There is a right pleural effusion, thickening of the horizontal fissure and septae and central reticulonodular shadowing. Note enlargement of the right hilum.

Question 80

This is an intravenous urogram on a 65-year-old man who has backache.

a Name two radiological abnormalities
b What two diagnoses would you consider?
c What single blood test would you order?

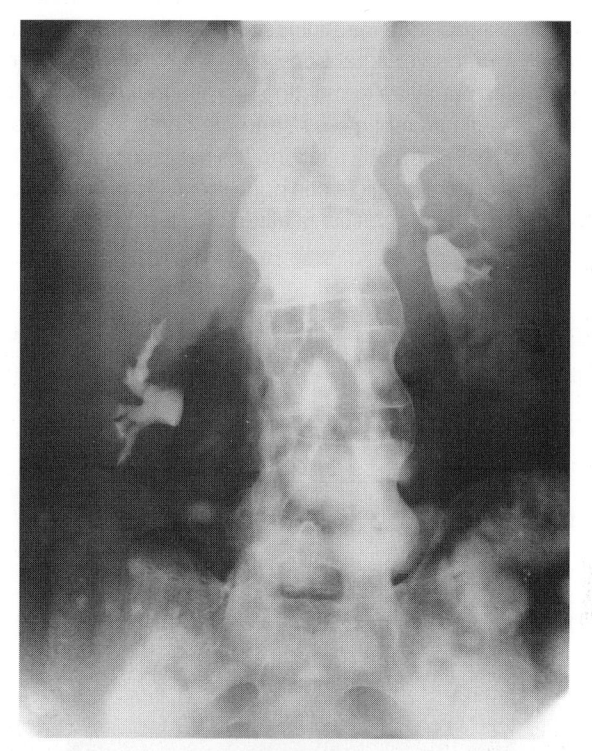

Fig. 80.1

Answer 80

a Bamboo spine associated with ankylosed sacro-iliac joints. Multiple sclerotic deposits in the spine and pelvis.
b Ankylosing spondylitis.
Prostatic carcinoma metastasizing to bone.
c Serum prostate-specific antigen (PSA).

Discussion

Ankylosing spondylitis (AS) is a seronegative disorder characterized by the presence of bilateral symmetrical sacro-iliitis. It is two to three times more common in men. Ninety per cent of affected individuals are HLA-B27 positive. Clinical features suggestive of the diagnosis include an insidious onset of low back pain, spinal stiffness and improvement with exercise. Patients are usually young at presentation and symptoms tend to persist longer than 3 months.

Radiologically, the earliest and most consistent sign of AS is bilateral symmetrical sacro-iliitis. Early changes in the lumbar spine are caused by an enthesopathy at the site of insertion of the outer fibres of the annulus fibrosus. This results in loss of the upper and lower anterior lips of the vertebral body and 'squaring' of the vertebral body, the Romanus lesion. Syndesmophytes form in the discal annulus fibrosus and calcification in the spinal longitudinal ligaments gives rise to the bamboo spine appearance. AS is also associated with an enthesopathy affecting the pelvis, os calcis and patella.

In addition to AS, this patient has sclerotic bone metastases from prostatic carcinoma. Approximately 80% of all bone metastases affect the axial skeleton – vertebrae, pelvis, ribs and skull.

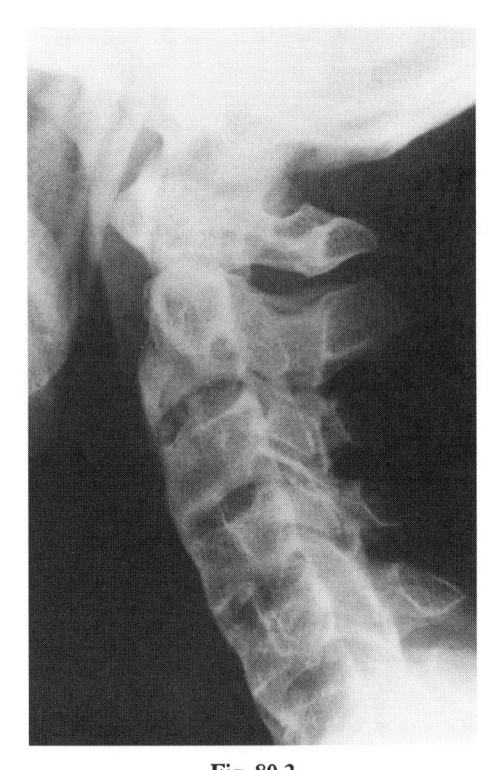

Fig. 80.2
Lateral cervical spine. Ankylosing spondylitis. There is calcification of the anterior longitudinal ligament. The vertebral bodies are 'squared' in appearance.

QUESTION 81

This is the lateral skull radiograph in a 40-year-old man with cardiomyopathy and bilateral ptosis.

a Name two radiological abnormalities.
b What is the diagnosis?
c Name three other features in this condition.

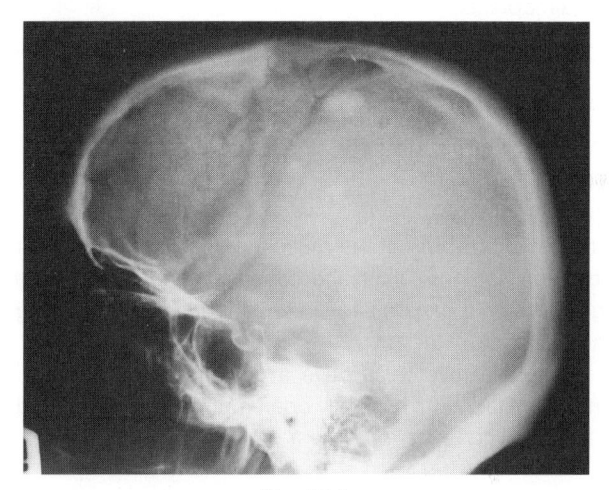

Fig. 81.1

ANSWER 81

a Small pituitary fossa.
  Hyperostosis of the skull vault.
  Thickening of the vault (occipital bone in Fig. 81.1).
b Dystrophia myotonica (myotonic dystrophy).
c Long, haggard face. Frontal balding. Difficulty relaxing muscle after strong contraction (i.e. delayed relaxation during shaking of the hand).
  External ophthalmoplegia.
  Wasting of masseters, temporal muscles.
  Cataracts.
  Reduced vital capacity.
  Small testes.

Discussion

Myotonia is increased excitability of the muscle membranes. The patient has difficulty relaxing muscles. For instance, when the patient's hand is shaken, there is a delay before 'letting go'. Myotonia can be seen in childhood (myotonia congenita) or middle age (dystrophia myotonica).

Patients with dystrophia myotonica have a characteristic appearance. Typically the patient has a long gaunt face with a slightly open mouth, thin neck and drooping eyelids.

QUESTION 82

a What is the diagnosis?
b How would you confirm it?

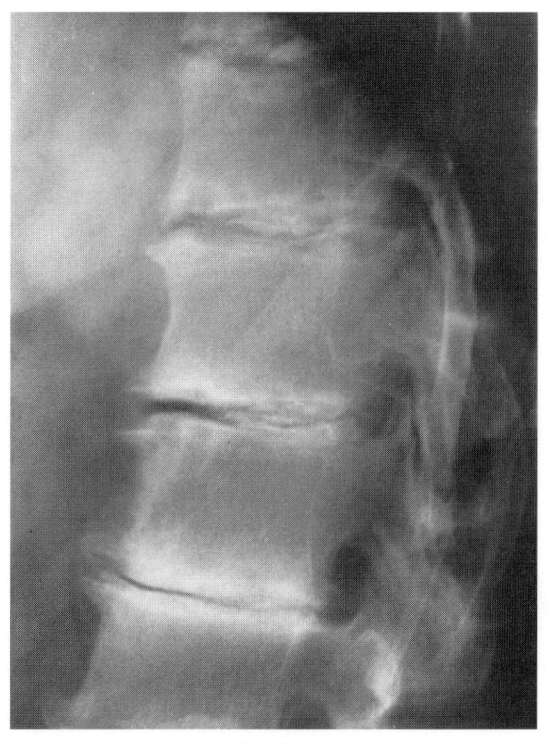

Fig. 82.1

Answer 82

a Alkaptonuria.
b Detection of homogentisic acid in urine.

Discussion

Alkaptonuria is an autosomal recessive disorder characterized by deficiency of the enzyme homogentisic acid oxidase. This results in an excess of homogentisic acid, which is excreted in the urine, confirming the diagnosis. The urine becomes black on standing – hence the term alkaptonuria. Ochronosis refers to the accumulation of homogentisic acid pigment in soft tissues and the subsequent arthropathy.

In mild cases, patients are usually asymptomatic. A brownish pigmentation occurs in the sclera and a bluish tinge in the cartilaginous structures of the nose and ears. Spondylosis is the main skeletal manifestation. Pigmented intervertebral discs and articular cartilage become brittle and calcify. The intervertebral discs narrow and show the vacuum phenomenon. There is marked subchondral sclerosis. The shoulders, hips and knees may also be affected.

QUESTION 83

This is a T1-weighted coronal magnetic resonance image of the brain in a 50-year-old woman with fluctuating conscious level.

a What is the diagnosis?

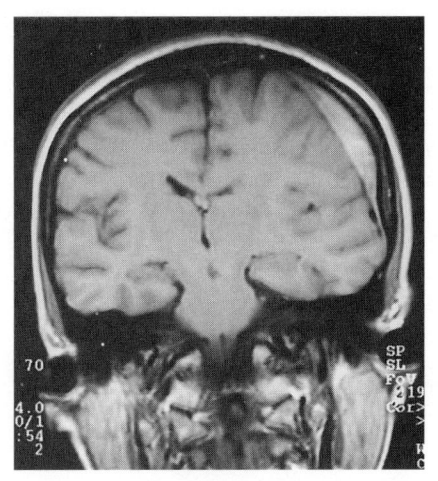

Fig. 83.1

ANSWER 83

a Acute left subdural haematoma with midline shift.

Discussion

Acute haematoma will appear as a high signal on T1-weighted imaging. There is midline shift of the third ventricle, a vertically orientated slit-like structure. There is also compression of the left lateral ventricle. (Note that CSF appears black on a T1-weighted image.)

QUESTION 84

A 43-year-old lady has right iliac fossa pain.

a What abnormality is present on her barium enema examination?
b What is the next investigation?

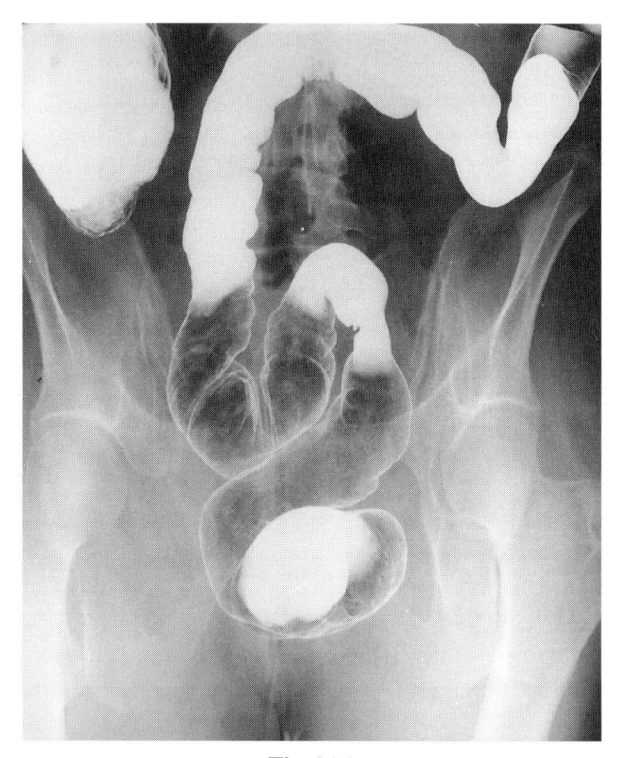

Fig. 84.1

Answer 84

a There is destruction of the right ischium.
b Isotope bone scan.
   Chest radiograph.

Discussion

It is very important to check the bones and soft tissues whenever a barium examination is studied. In this case, the cause of the patient's right iliac fossa pain was a destructive lesion in the ischium. An isotope bone scan is the single most important investigation. In metastatic bone disease, the bone scan will show multiple 'hot' areas throughout the bony skeleton. Common causes of metastases to bone are carcinoma of the bronchus, breast, kidney, prostate and thyroid. Do not forget myeloma as a cause of irregular bone destruction. A solitary lesion on the bone scan suggests either an infective process or a primary bone tumour. A chest radiograph is a useful investigation for ruling out a primary bronchial carcinoma.

Question 85

This 2-year-old boy has exophthalmos and polyuria.

a What radiological abnormalities are present?
b What is the cause of the polyuria?
c What is the diagnosis?

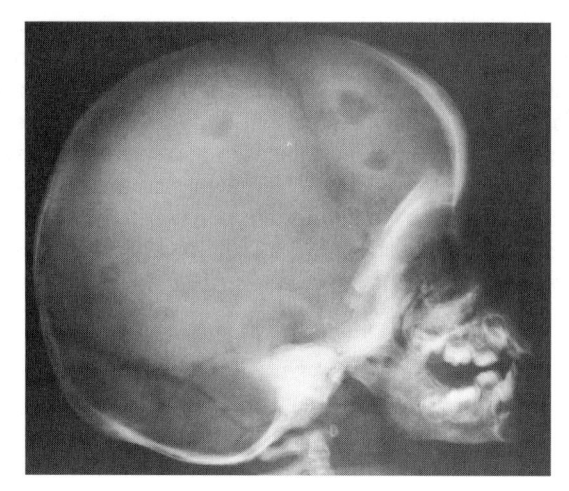

Fig. 85.1

ANSWER 85

a Multiple geographical lytic lesions in the skull vault.
b Cranial diabetes insipidus.
c Langerhans, cell histiocytosis (Hand–Schuller–Christian disease).

Discussion

Hand-Schuller-Christian disease, a granulomatous disorder characterized by histiocytic proliferation, is a variant of Langerhans cell histiocytosis (LCH) affecting infants below the age of 5 years. Up to 50% of patients develop diabetes insipidus because of granulomatous infiltration in the posterior pituitary. Twenty-five per cent of cases are associated with unilateral or bilateral exophthalmos, due to orbital infiltration. The skull vault contains destructive lytic lesions which have a 'geographical' appearance. Some lytic lesions have a button sequestrum which is an island of normal bone within a sea of lytic destruction. A good example is seen in the posterior calvarium in this case (Fig. 85.1). The calvarial lesions are associated with soft tissue swelling. Other bones affected are vertebrae, the mandible with 'floating' teeth and the medullary cavities of long bones.

There are two other variants of LCH. The first is Letterer-Siwe disease, which is often fatal and predominantly involves viscera in children under 2 years of age. The second is eosinophilic granuloma, in which bony lesions predominate. It is seen mainly before 10 years of age and in adolescents and young adults. The lungs may be affected in eosinophilic granuloma, causing a 'honeycomb' appearance. Lung involvement requires steroid therapy. Bone lesions in all three variants may heal spontaneously.

Question 86

This is a contrast-enhanced CT scan of the abdomen in a 50-year-old man.

a What is the radiological diagnosis?

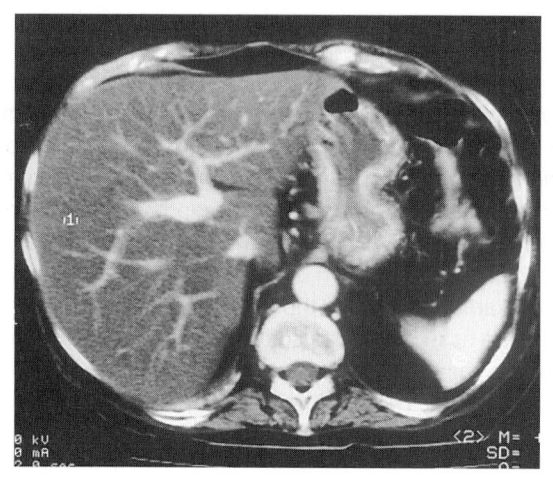

Fig. 86.1

ANSWER 86

a Fatty infiltration of the liver.

Discussion

Fatty liver is an accumulation of fat within hepatocytes greater than 5% of total weight. The commonest cause is alcohol excess.

On CT in normal subjects, the liver has approximately the same attenuation as spleen both before and after intravenous contrast medium. In fatty infiltration of the liver, the attenuation of the liver is reduced with respect to the spleen and therefore appears blacker. When intravenous contrast medium has been administered, the hepatic veins stand out as white, branching structures against a dark liver parenchyma. The architecture of the liver is preserved in fatty infiltration, further distinguishing it from neoplastic causes.

The other causes of fatty liver are:

- obesity;
- starvation;
- diabetes;
- steroids and chemotherapy;
- pregnancy.

QUESTION 87

This is a liver ultrasound scan in a 50-year-old woman with right upper quadrant pain and jaundice.

a What abnormality is shown in Fig. 87.1a?
b What complication has occurred in Fig. 87.1b?
c What investigation is indicated?

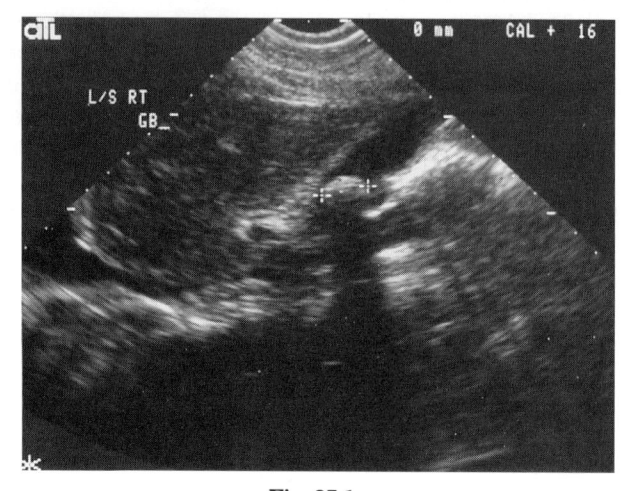

Fig. 87.1a

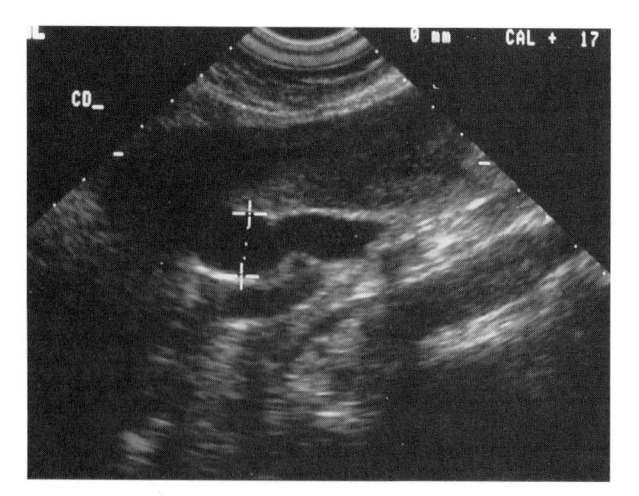

Fig. 87.1b

Answer 87

a A calculus within the gall bladder.
b Obstruction of the common duct by a calculus.
c Endoscopic retrograde cholangiopancreatography (ERCP).

Discussion

Gallstones are typically echogenic (white) and cause a posterior acoustic shadow (black). The gallbladder itself is echo poor and will appear black on ultrasound images. Ultrasound is the investigation of choice in patients with jaundice and/or upper quadrant pain, and is 98% accurate in the detection of gallstones. The common duct is usually easily recognized as it lies anterolateral and parallel to the portal vein. When the former is dilated (normal up to 7 mm) the typical 'shotgun' appearance occurs (Fig. 87.1b). Occasionally the calculus responsible for the duct dilatation can be shown. In any event, an ERCP should be undertaken to confirm the presence or absence of a calculus and relieve the obstruction.

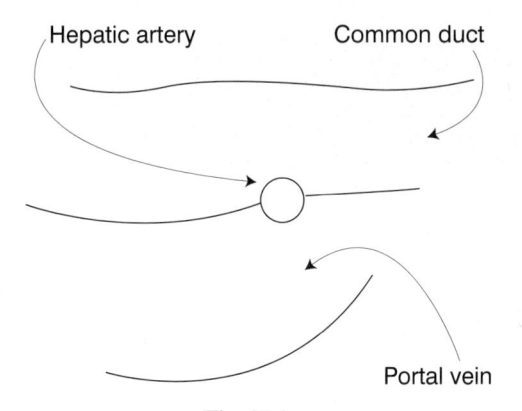

Fig. 87.2
Schematic demonstration of common duct on ultrasound.

QUESTION 88

This 65-year-old woman sustained a fracture of the femoral neck after minimal trauma. Four years earlier she underwent a partial gastrectomy for peptic ulcer disease.

a What other abnormalities are shown?
b What is the diagnosis?
c What is the underlying cause?

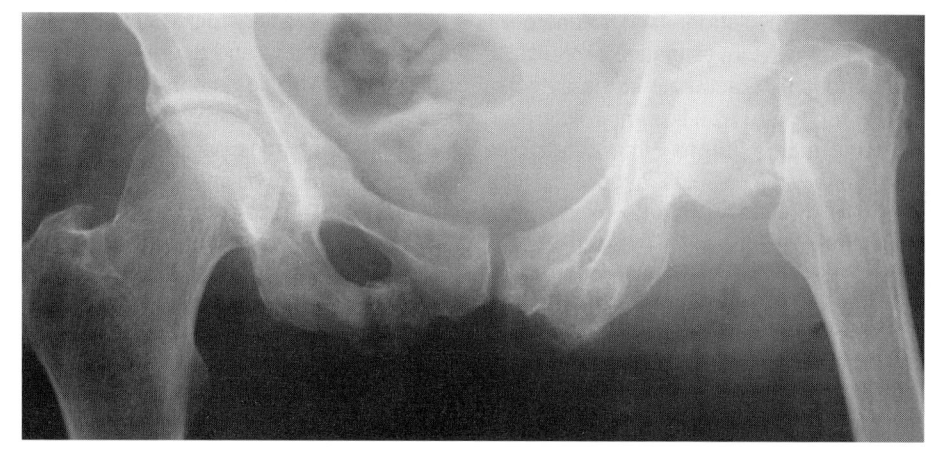

Fig. 88.1

Answer 88

a Looser's zones in both inferior pubic rami.
b Osteomalacia.
c Malabsorption of vitamin D due to partial gastrectomy.

Discussion

Osteomalacia has an identical pathological basis to rickets (see Fig. 41.1), except that the latter occurs in the growing skeleton. Osteomalacia is a bone-softening process due to an excess of demineralized osteoid. Bowing can occur in long bones in advanced cases. There is an increased incidence of pathological fractures, especially the femoral neck in all cases. Looser's zones are characteristic pseudofractures of osteomalacia and represent seams of unossified osteoid, typically appearing as an incomplete fracture line with sclerotic margins. They occur in the pubic rami, femoral necks, scapulae, ribs and long bones, and tend to be bilateral. Osteopenia and softening of the vertebral end plates causes compression fractures with central loss of vertebral body height (codfish vertebrae).

The main biochemical features in osteomalacia are:

- plasma calcium – normal or low;
- serum alkaline phosphatase – high;
- plasma phosphate – normal or low;
- plasma PTH – normal or low.

Note that in osteoporosis, biochemistry is normal although there is a reduction in total body calcium.

QUESTION 89

A 38-year-old air hostess presented with breathlessness and a dry cough.

a What is the most likely diagnosis?
b How could this be confirmed?
c What investigation would you consider next?

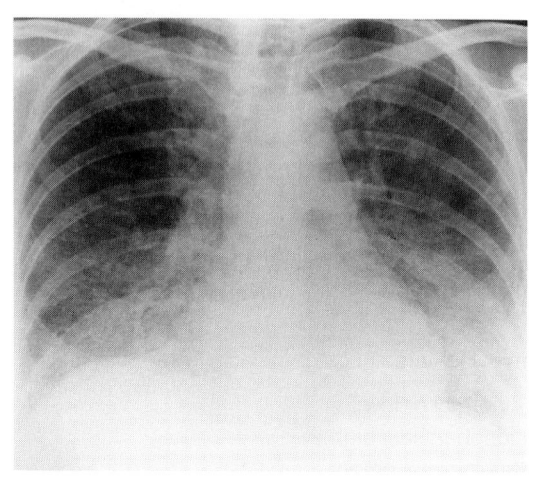

Fig. 89.1

ANSWER 89

a *Pneumocystis carinii* pneumonia (PCP).
b Induced sputum subjected to Grocott silver stain.
c HIV test.

Discussion

Pneumocystis carinii is a fungus and is the commonest cause of pneumonia in AIDS patients. Prior to routine use of prophylaxis, 80% of AIDS patients developed PCP. Clinically, patients experience a dry, irritating cough with dyspnoea. Fever and tachypnoea commonly occur, but there are usually no auscultatory signs.

Radiologically, there are bilateral symmetrical perihilar ground glass opacities. They have a predilection for the upper zones but spare the extreme apices and bases. Occasionally, in the early stages of PCP, the perihilar shadowing may be subtle and overlooked. In up to 40% of patients with PCP there are associated thin-walled cysts and coarse fibrosis may result from repeated infections. It is unusual to produce sputum in

PCP, but this can be obtained by sputum induction with a 3% saline nebulizer or bronchoalveolar lavage via bronchoscopy. If a patient is known to have AIDS, it is now customary in many centres to treat empirically for PCP based on the clinical and radiological findings.

The lung may be the site for other opportunistic infections and malignancies in AIDS cases. Table 89.1 summarizes their radiographic appearances.

Table 89.1 Radiographic appearances of various infections and malignancies in AIDS

Ground glass shadowing	*Consolidation*
PCP	Pyogenic pneumonia
Pyogenic pneumonia	Tuberculosis (TB)
Cytomegalovirus (CMV) pneumonitis	Atypical microbacterial infections (MAC)
Lymphocytic interstitial pneumonitis (LIP)	Cryptococcosis
	AIDS-related lymphoma

Nodules (bronchovascular distribution)
Kaposi's sarcoma

Nodules (random distribution)
TB
MAC
Toxoplasmosis
Fungal pneumonia
Septic embolic (peripheral)
PCP (rare)
CMV (rare)

Lymphadenopathy
TB (characteristically show rim enhancement on CT)
KS
AIDS-related lymphoma

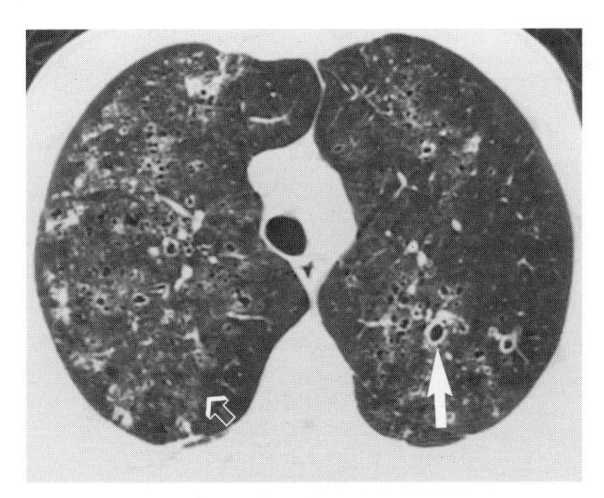

Fig. 89.2
Pneumocystis carinii pneumonia. HRCT. Note cysts (arrow) and ground glass shadowing (open arrow).

Question 90

A 40-year-old woman has bone pain after alcohol ingestion.

a What abnormality is shown on this contrast-enhanced thoracic CT?
b What is the most likely diagnosis?
c What additional radiological investigation would you advise?

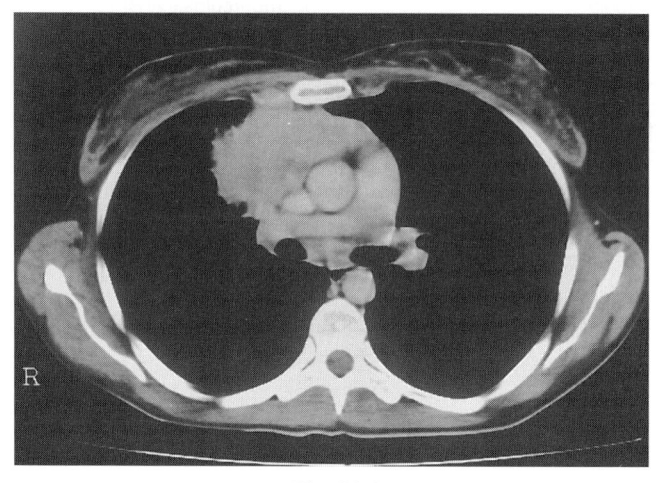

Fig. 90.1

Answer 90

a Large anterior mediastinal mass.
b Hodgkin's disease.
c Abdominal and pelvic CT scan.

Discussion

Bone pain following alcohol ingestion in a patient with an anterior mediastinal mass is virtually diagnostic of Hodgkin's disease (HD). Other systemic features include fever, weight loss, anorexia and night sweats. Lymph node enlargement is typically firm and painless. The liver and spleen may be enlarged. Unless there are specific symptoms, HD is radiologically indistinguishable from non-Hodgkin's lymphoma (NHL). A biopsy is therefore always required prior to treatment. This should be obtained, wherever possible, from an extrathoracic site, preferably by excising a cervical lymph node. In thoracic HD, involvement of anterior mediastinal nodes is usual and may be accompanied by hilar lymph node enlargement. Involvement of the lung occurs three times more frequently in HD than in NHL. In HD there is invariably associated lymph node enlargement, but isolated pulmonary involvement occurs in up to 50% of cases of NHL.

Further radiological investigation requires continuation of the CT scan below the diaphragm to stage this disease.

QUESTION 91

A 45-year-old mentally retarded man presented with rectal bleeding.

a What abnormalities are shown on the barium enema examination (Figs 91.1a and 91.1b)?
b What is the diagnosis?
c With which skin pathology is this associated?

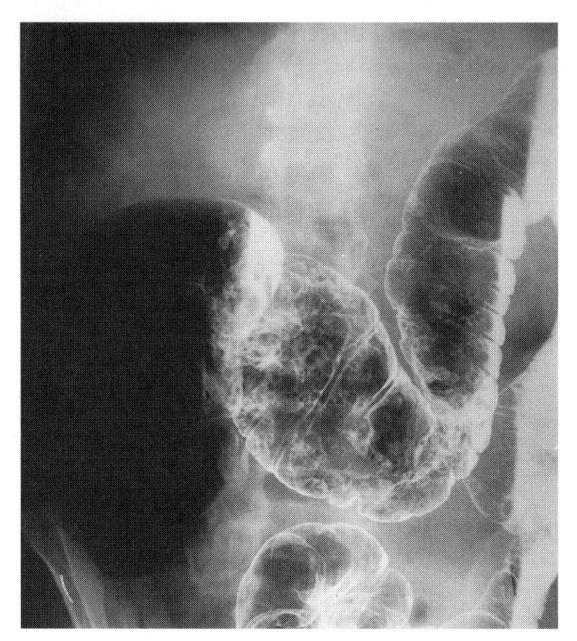

Fig. 91.1a

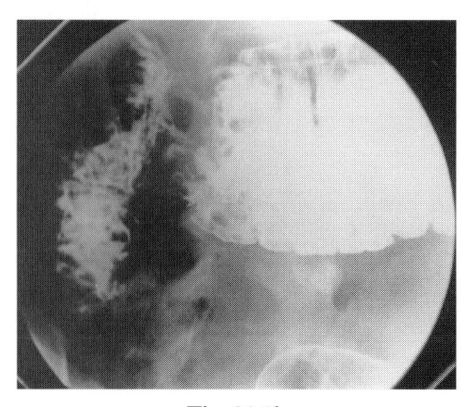

Fig. 91.1b

ANSWER 91

a Multiple polyps throughout the large bowel.
  Apple-core stricture in the proximal transverse colon (there is a stricture in the descending colon).
b Familial polyposis coli complicated by colonic carcinoma.
c Multiple sebaceous cysts.

Discussion

Familial polyposis coli is an autosomal dominant condition characterized by multiple adenomatous polyps throughout the colon. Unless treated, malignant transformation occurs before the age of 40 years. A subtotal colectomy with ileorectal anastomosis is the treatment of choice. Rectal polyps, if present, will regress following surgery, but endoscopic surveillance is mandatory. Polyposis coli is associated with osteomas of the mandible (Fig. 91.2) and skull in Gardner's syndrome. Additional features of this syndrome include desmoid tumours and sebaceous cysts.

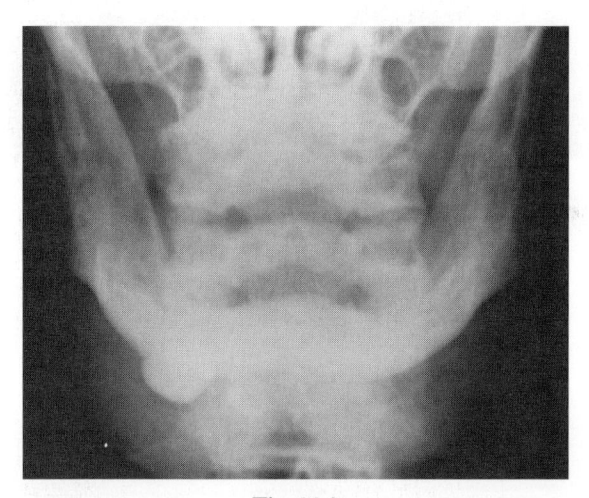

Fig. 91.2
Osteoma of the mandible in another patient.

Question 92

This is the HRCT scan of the lungs in a patient with a restrictive ventilatory defect.

a What abnormality is shown?
b Suggest two possible causes.
c What two pulmonary complications may occur?

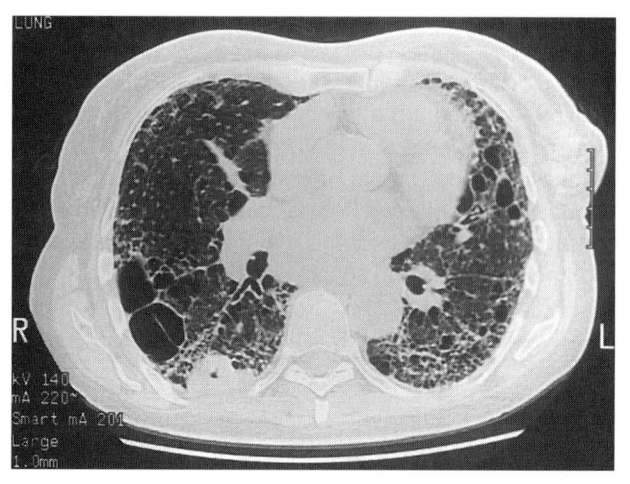

Fig. 92.1

Answer 92

a Honeycomb lung.
b Cryptogenic fibrosing alveolitis.
  Fibrosing alveolitis associated with connective tissue disorders.
  Drug-induced pulmonary fibrosis.
  Asbestosis.
c Bronchogenic carcinoma.
  Pneumothorax.

Discussion

Honeycomb lung signifies end-stage interstitial fibrosis with architectural distortion and cyst formation. A basal distribution suggests cryptogenic fibrosing alveolitis, rheumatoid or scleroderma lung, asbestosis or drug sensitivity. An upper zonal distribution is suggestive of silicosis or Langerhans' cell histiocytosis. Cystic bronchiectasis may mimic honeycomb lung, but is readily recognized by the absence of 'honeycombing' in the periphery of the lung.

Longstanding interstitial fibrosis increases the risk of developing bronchogenic carcinoma. Any cell type may be associated. Cystic lung disease, whatever its aetiology, may be associated with spontaneous pneumothorax. In this case there was an associated carcinoma in the apical segment of the right lower lobe seen posteriorly in the periphery.

Question 93

An 82-year-old woman was involved in a road traffic accident. This is her scanogram whilst waiting for a formal CT of the chest. She is intubated and has an intercostal drain in each hemithorax.

a What major life-threatening complication is shown?
b How would it be recognized clinically?
c How was it treated?

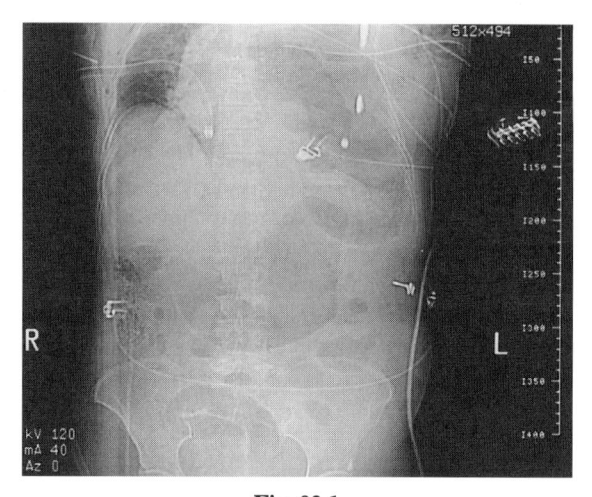

Fig. 93.1

Answer 93

a Left-sided tension pneumothorax.
b Tachypnoea, tachycardia, hypotension and cyanosis.
c Insertion of a cannula into the pleural space.

Discussion

Tension pneumothorax is a life-threatening situation in which the intrapleural pressure becomes positive, leading to compression of both lungs. Cardiovascular collapse occurs as a result of respiratory failure. A tension pneumothorax should probably be recognized clinically before the need for a chest radiograph. When a radiograph (or scanogram in this case) is done, the most reliable sign of tension is depression of the hemidiaphragm. The presence of mediastinal shift is not as sensitive, as it is also seen in pneumothorax without tension. It should also be noted that the lung may not collapse in patients with pneumothorax if there is underlying lung disease such as fibrosis or consolidation.

In this patient, a combination of lung laceration and positive pressure ventilation was thought to account for the development of the tension pneumothorax, despite the presence of a left intercostal tube. Immediate insertion of a cannula into the left second intercostal space resulted in an immediate decompression with a rush of air through the cannula.

Question 94

This 70-year-old woman has bone pain and impaired renal function. The serum alkaline phosphatase was normal.

- **a** What abnormalities are present?
- **b** What is the most likely diagnosis?
- **c** What other diagnosis would you consider?

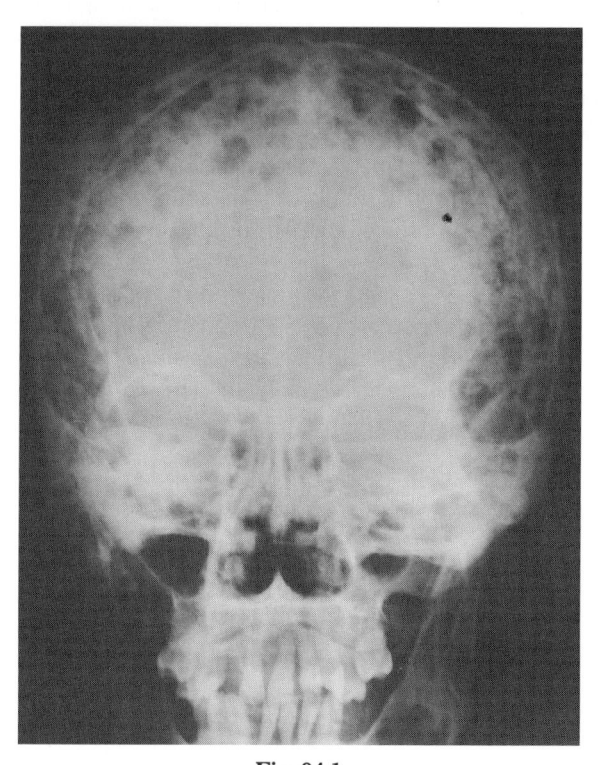

Fig. 94.1

ANSWER 94

a Multiple 'punched-out' lytic lesions in the skull vault and mandible.
b Multiple myeloma.
c Multiple bony metastases.

Discussion

Multiple myeloma is a neoplastic proliferation of plasma cells in the bone marrow with an excess production of monoclonal immunoglobulins, and is associated with osteopenia and multiple lytic defects in the axial skeleton, skull (Fig. 94.2), mandible, ribs, clavicle, spine and pelvis, humeri and femora. Osteolysis of the mandible is more suggestive of myeloma than bony metastases. The latter are often associated with elevated serum alkaline phosphatase. Renal impairment in myeloma results from hypercalcaemia, uric acid nephropathy, amyloid kidney and interstitial fibrosis (myeloma kidney), and only occasionally from renal tubular blockage by excreted paraproteins.

Classically, myeloma causes 'punched-out', expansile and focal lytic lesions in marrow-filled bone. In the skull, the occiput is spared as it contains no marrow (Fig. 94.2).

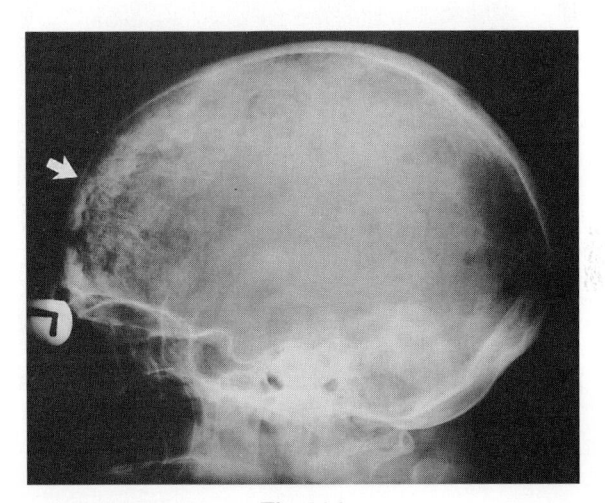

Fig. 94.2
Lateral skull radiograph. Multiple myeloma. 'Punched-out' lesions in the vault with sparing of the occiput, which contains no marrow. Note hyperostosis frontalis interna (arrow), a common incidental finding in elderly females.

QUESTION 95

This is an unenhanced CT scan of the brain in a 60-year-old man with dementia.

a Describe the abnormalities.
b What is the diagnosis?
c Suggest two possible aetiological factors that could be responsible.

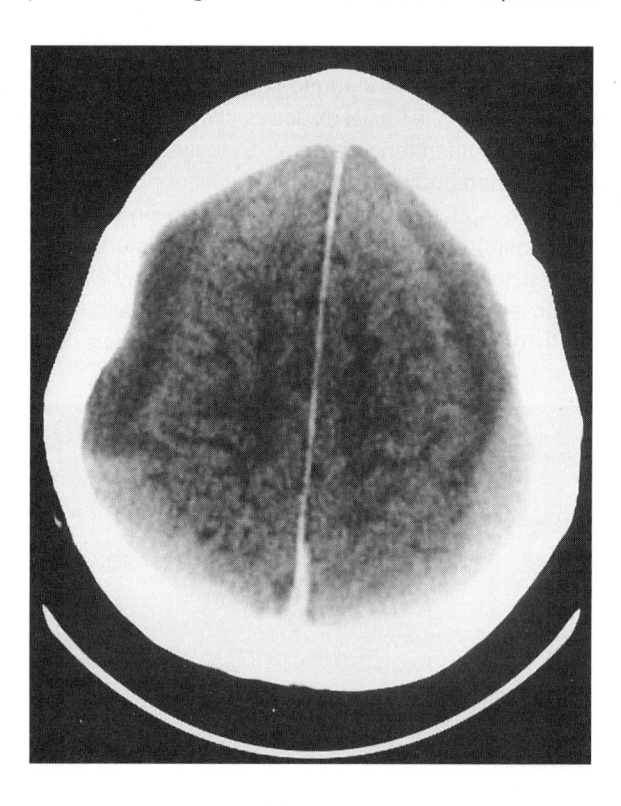

Fig. 95.1

Answer 95

a Bilateral crescenteric collections of high and low attenuation lateral to the brain.
b Acute on chronic bilateral subdural haematomas.
c Alcohol.
  Anticoagulants.

Discussion

Chronic subdural haematomas are hypodense relative to brain on CT. In this case, the dependent areas of the collections are hyperdense, indicating some recent haemorrhage (see also Answer 83).

QUESTION 96

This 45-year-old man was involved in a road traffic accident 10 years previously.

a What abnormality is shown?
b What is the most likely diagnosis?
c Suggest three other causes for this appearance.

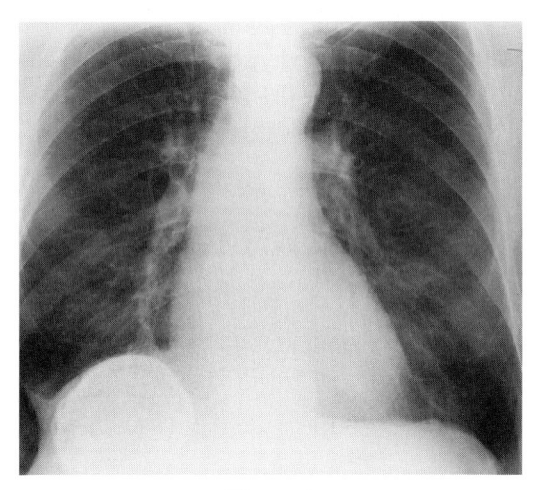

Fig. 96.1

Answer 96

a Calcified spherical lesion in the liver.
b Old calcified hepatic haematoma.
c Congenital liver cyst.
   Old pyogenic or amoebic abscess.
   Hydatid disease.
   Hepatic artery aneurysm (if considerably smaller in size).

Discussion

The history is vital for arriving at the correct diagnosis and avoiding unnecessary further investigations.

Other causes of hepatic calcification (not necessarily spherical) include:

- infection; TB (see Fig. 53.2); histoplasmosis; gumma; schistosomiasis (see Fig. 47.2b);
- vascular – portal vein thrombosis;
- biliary tract – intrahepatic duct calculi; porcelain gallbladder;
- primary neoplasms: haemangioma; haemangio-endothelioma; hepatoblastoma; cholangiocarcinoma;
- metastases: mucinous carcinoma of colon, stomach, breast, ovary; melanoma; osteosarcoma and carcinoid.

QUESTION 97

This is a radiograph of the foot in a 40-year-old man.

a What abnormalities are present?
b What is the diagnosis?

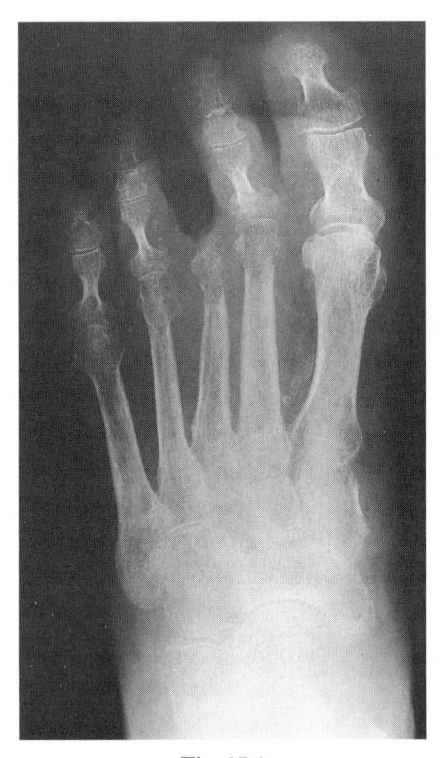

Fig. 97.1

ANSWER 97

a Calcified dorsalis pedis artery and digital artery to little toe.
   Amputation of third toe.
b Diabetic foot.

Discussion

Diabetic foot is the commonest reason for hospital admission when there are chronic complications. Ulceration develops after repeated trauma in the insensitive foot.

Proprioceptive and vascular impairment exacerbates this process. Soft tissue infection may occur, especially at pressure points, and may spread to involve bone. A combination of neuropathy, ischaemia and infection may produce the classical radiological features of a diabetic foot. Neuropathic changes result in bone fragmentation, loss of alignment at joints and eventually absorption of bone. Neuropathy in the tarso-metatarsal joints may produce a Lisfranc deformity – loss of alignment of the metatarsals with the tarsal bones (Fig. 97.2). Soft tissue infection in diabetes may result in gas bubbles being visible on radiographs. Calcification of small arteries is very common in diabetes.

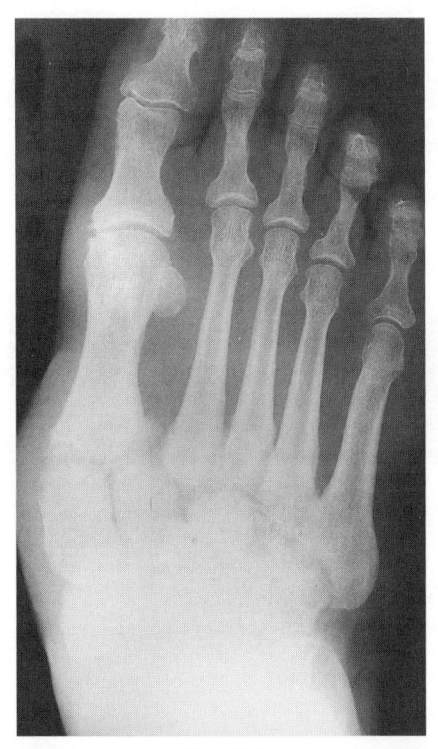

Fig. 97.2
Lisfranc deformity. Diabetic foot. There is lateral slip of the metatarsals away from the tarsal bones. Note the sclerosis and hypertrophic bone formation.

QUESTION 98

This 5-week-old male infant has abnormal serum electrolytes and failure to thrive.

a What investigation is shown?
b What is the diagnosis?
c What electrolyte imbalance would you expect to find?

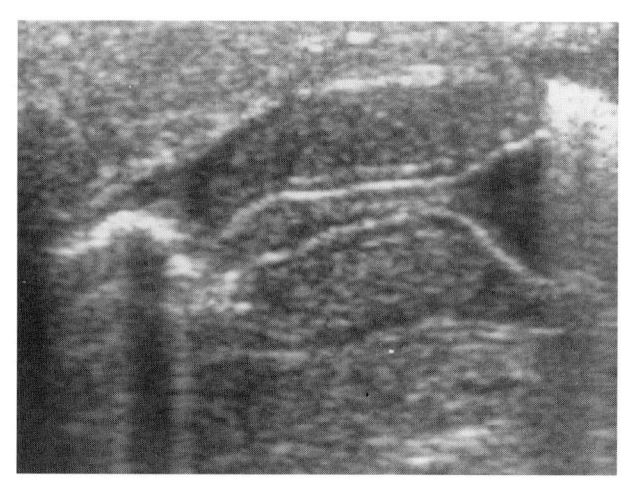

Fig. 98.1

Answer 98

a Pyloric ultrasound.
b Pyloric stenosis.
c Metabolic alkalosis.

Discussion

Hypertrophic pyloric stenosis is caused by thickening of antral and pyloric muscles, and results in gastric outlet obstruction in newborns. It presents at 4–6 weeks of age with projectile vomiting which, if severe, can be associated with a metabolic alkalosis and failure to thrive. Males are affected four times more frequently than females. The diagnosis is usually obvious from the history. Examination will reveal a pyloric 'tumour' which can be confirmed on ultrasound. Figure 98.1 shows the classical sonographic features of a hypertrophied muscle with a central track of echogenic mucosa. Ultrasound has virtually replaced barium studies (Fig. 98.2), which are now reserved for borderline cases.

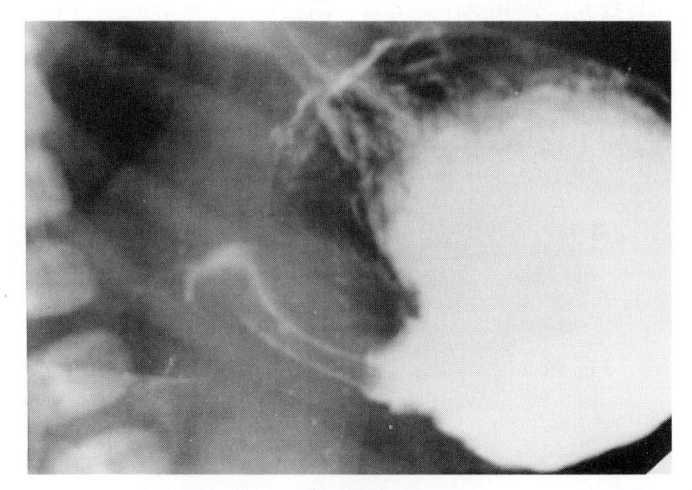

Fig. 98.2
Barium meal. Pyloric stenosis. The antrum is tapered and the narrowed pyloric canal produces a tram-track or parallel channel sign.

QUESTION 99

This child has delayed growth and hepatosplenomegaly.

a Describe two radiological features.
b What is the diagnosis?
c Suggest an alternative cause for the radiological features.

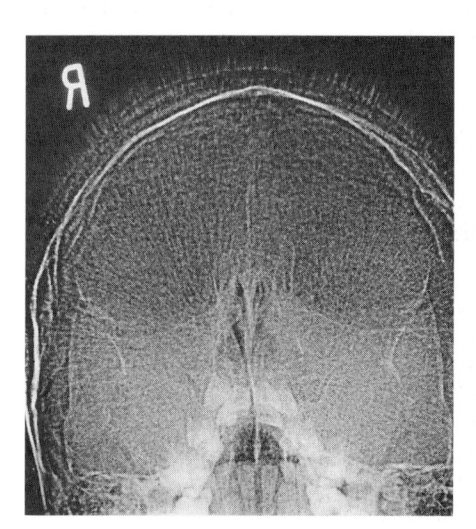

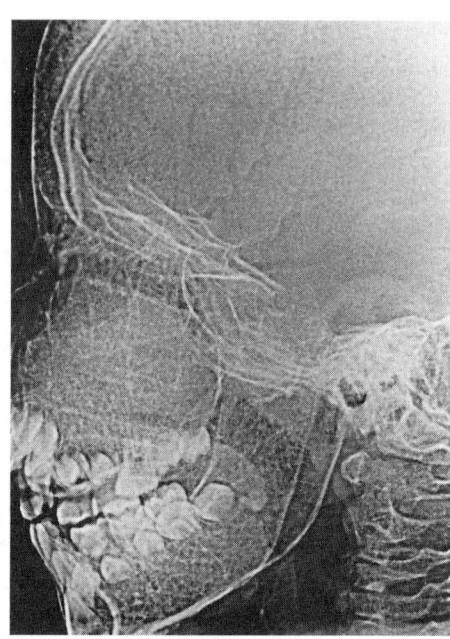

Fig. 99.1a   Fig. 99.1b

Answer 99

a 'Hair-on-end' appearance of skull vault opacification of maxillary sinuses.
b Thalassaemia major.
c Severe sickle cell anaemia.

Discussion

Thalassaemia major, also known as Mediterranean or Cooley's anaemia, is due to a deficiency in beta-chains and an excess of alpha-chains. The latter precipitate in immature and mature red cells, resulting in defective erythropoiesis and haemolysis. Severe anaemia occurs at 3 months. Hepatosplenomegaly occurs because of excess red cell destruction and extramedullary haematopoiesis. Gross marrow hyperplasia results in bone expansion, giving rise to the 'hair-on-end' appearance of the skull vault (Fig. 99.1). The occiput is spared as it contains no marrow (Fig. 99.2a). The maxillary sinuses become a source of extramedullary haematopoiesis. They opacify and expand, causing prominence of the maxilla and the so-called 'rodent' facies of thalassaemia. Expansion of the long bones of the hands gives a characteristic appearance with loss of minor trabeculae, giving a lace-like appearance, and medullary expansion (Fig. 99.2b).

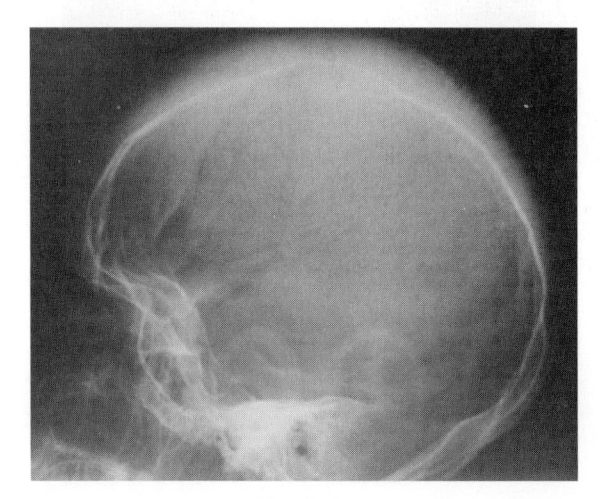

Fig. 99.2a
Thalassaemia major. Skull. Note the thinning of the outer table in the vault with sparing of the occiput.

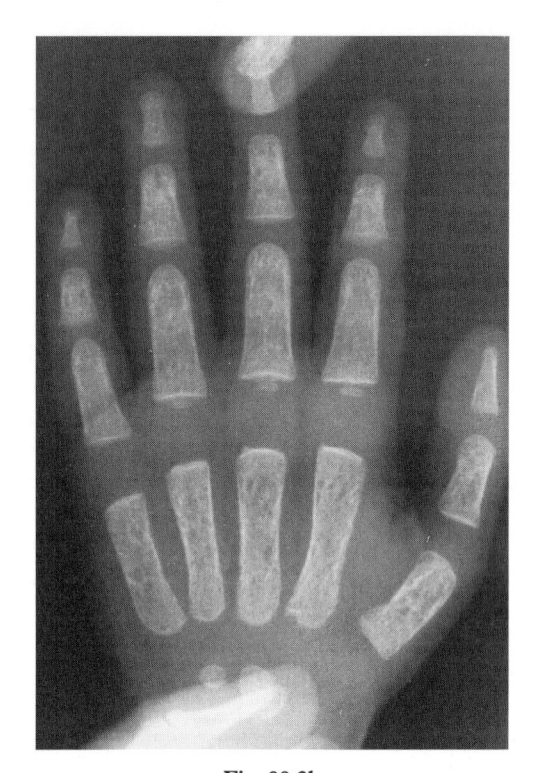

Fig. 99.2b
Thalassaemia major. Hands.

Question 100

A 51-year-old Mexican had recently noticed thinning of his eyebrows.

a What is the diagnosis?

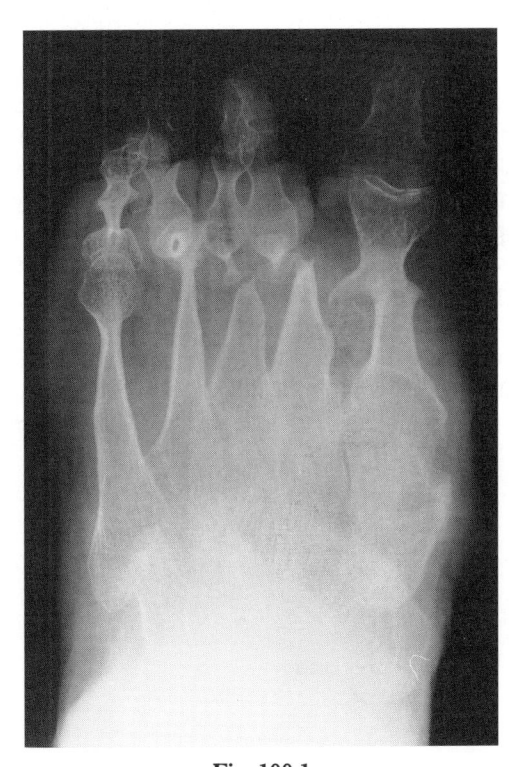

Fig. 100.1

Answer 100

a Lepromatous leprosy.

Discussion

Leprosy, caused by the acid-fast bacillus *Mycobacterium leprae,* is common in Africa, the Far East, and in Central and Southern America. The bone may be directly affected by infection or secondarily involved as a complication of neuropathy. Figure 100.1 shows resorption of the distal ends of the metatarsals (acro-osteolysis) with preserved bone density typical of leprosy. Rarely, peripheral nerves will calcify.

Leprosy represents a spectrum of disease: tuberculoid leprosy; borderline leprosy and lepromatous leprosy. In tuberculoid leprosy there is a strong cell-mediated immunity and the disease is localized to a few sites – hypopigmented anaesthetic skin patches and enlarged peripheral nerves. Lepromatous leprosy, on the other hand, causes symmetrical nodules laden with acid-fast bacilli, and is commonly associated with peripheral neuropathy in the extremities. There is no cell-mediated immunity in this form of leprosy. Facial skin becomes nodular and classically the eyebrows are lost. The borderline type has features common to both ends of the spectrum.

QUESTION 101

A 34-year-old female with abdominal cramps underwent a small bowel meal.
a What is the diagnosis?
b What intestinal complication may occur?
c What other organ is usually affected?

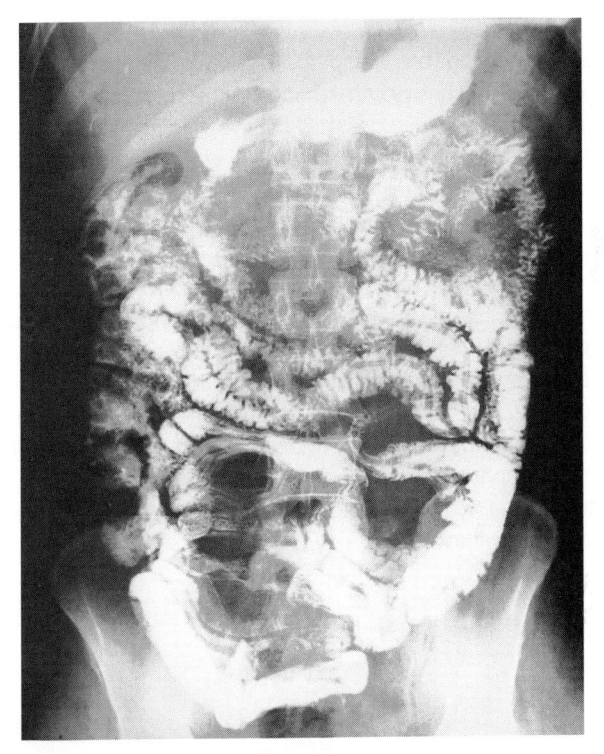

Fig. 101.1

Answer 101

a *Ascaris lumbricoides* infection of the small bowel (ascariasis).
b Intestinal obstruction.
  Malabsorption.
c Lungs.

Discussion

Ascariasis occurs worldwide, but is especially prevalent in warm areas of poor sanitation. It is endemic in Central and South America, Africa and South-East Asia. Eggs of the large roundworm *Ascaris lumbricoides* may survive in the soil for years. Ingestion of soil (pica) and poor sanitation provide the oral route of egg ingestion. Once the larvae hatch they migrate through the intestinal wall into the bloodstream, where they are carried to the lungs and liver. Once in the lungs, they pass into the alveoli and ascend the respiratory tract, only to be swallowed again. The larvae undergo maturation and the adult worm rests in the jejunum. The adult female worm can grow up to 50 cm in length.

The clinical features include fever, cough, wheezing, and eosinophilic and pulmonary infiltrates which are present during pulmonary transit of larvae. The intestinal phase produces anorexia, abdominal cramps and malabsorption. Life-threatening complications can occur, including acute intestinal obstruction, appendicitis, perforation, biliary tract involvement, pancreatic duct involvement and even tracheal obstruction as the larvae migrate through the upper respiratory tract.

On barium studies, the worms appear as negative filling defects in the intestine. Some worms contain barium within their own central canal (see jejunum in Fig. 101.1).

QUESTION 102

This is a CT scan of the chest in a 52-year-old woman with cough, haemoptysis and weight loss.

a What radiological abnormalities are present?
b What is the differential diagnosis?
c What investigation would you do next?

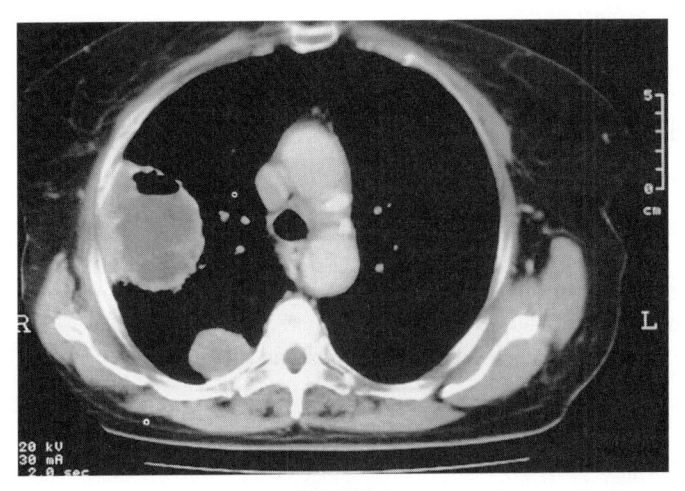

Fig. 102.1

Answer 102

a Two large pulmonary mass lesions, the larger of which is cavitating.
b Squamous carcinoma primary neoplasm with metastatic deposit.
   Metastases.
   Multiple abscesses.
   Wegener's granulomatosis.
   Rheumatoid arthritis.
c Sputum cytology.
   Serum c-ANCA.
   Percutaneous needle biopsy.

Discussion

There are many causes of multiple pulmonary masses:

- neoplasia – metastatic carcinoma or sarcoma; lymphoma; lymphomatoid granulomatosis; Kaposi's sarcoma and alveolar cell carcinoma;
- inflammation – progressive or tuberculous abscesses; Wegener's granulomatosis and rheumatoid arthritis;
- others – pulmonary infarction; haematomas and hamartomas.

All of these conditions may be associated with cavitation, with the exception of hamartomas.

In this example, the diagnosis was a cavitating primary bronchial neoplasm (squamous carcinoma) with a pulmonary metastasis. Cavitating metastases may be seen in squamous cell carcinoma, colon carcinoma and in sarcomas.

QUESTION 103

A 53-year-old man has night sweats, backache and impaired renal function.

a What abnormalities are present on this unenhanced abdominal CT scan?
b What is the differential diagnosis?
c What further investigation is indicated?

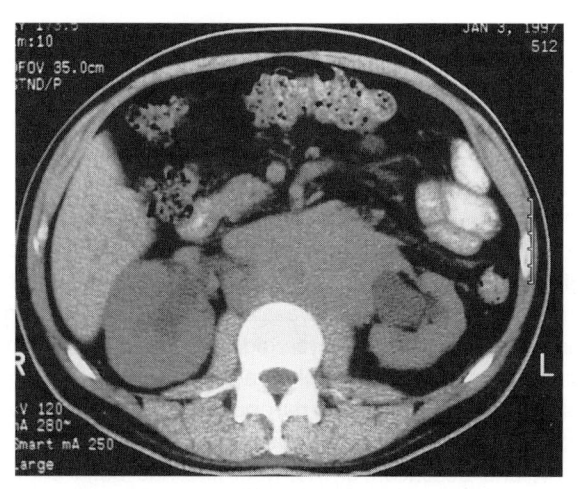

Fig. 103.1

Answer 103

a Bilateral hydronephrosis.
 Para-aortic soft tissue mass.
b Lymphoma.
 Retroperitoneal fibrosis (RPF).
c CT-guided percutaneous needle biopsy.

Discussion

Extrinsic obstruction of the ureters may occur anywhere along their length. Causes include pelvic malignancy or prostatic enlargement. In retroperitoneal fibrosis the ureters become enveloped in a 'mass' of tissue, usually at the L4/5 level. The ureters are pulled medially at this level with focal narrowing. While a number of conditions may be responsible for retroperitoneal fibrosis (RPF), approximately 50% of cases are of the idiopathic variety, which is associated with fibrosing mediastinitis and sclerosing cholangitis.

Causes of RPF include aortic surgery and aortitis, retroperitoneal inflammation (e.g. from inflammatory bowel disease or extravasated urine), trauma causing retroperitoneal haemorrhage, and drugs such as methysergide and practolol. An important cause of retroperitoneal mass is malignancy. Lymphoma is suggested by the history. Carcinoma of the colon or bladder may give rise to a retroperitoneal mass. It is mandatory to obtain histology for exclusion of a malignant cause. Steroid therapy may improve ureteric obstruction in RPF, and cessation of methysergide has been shown to reverse the changes.

QUESTION 104

This 55-year-old woman has an abnormal peripheral blood film.

a What radiological abnormalities are present in
   i Fig. 104.1a?
   ii Fig. 104.1b?
b What is the diagnosis?
c How do you explain the findings in Fig. 104.1b?
d What abnormalities are in the peripheral blood film?

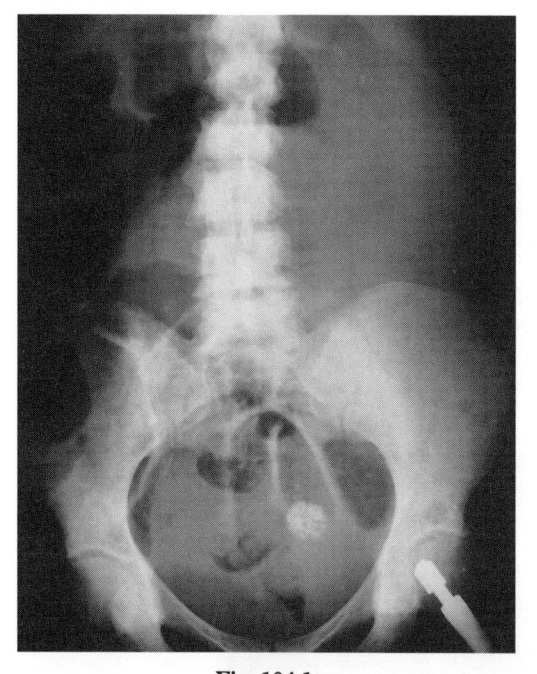

Fig. 104.1a

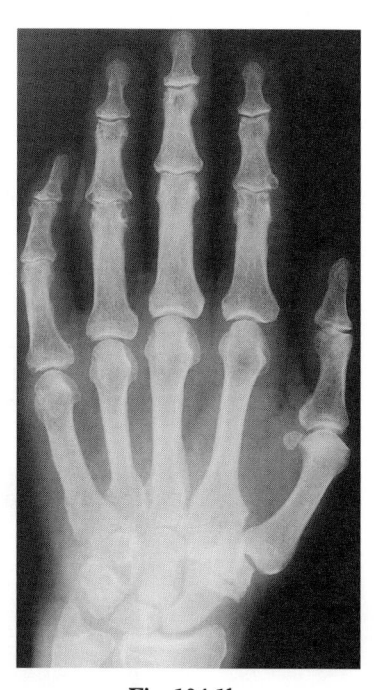

Fig. 104.1b

ANSWER 104

a i Generalized osteosclerosis.
      Splenomegaly.
      Dynamic hip screw, left hip.
      Calcified fibroid.

ii Soft tissue swelling and juxta-articular erosions of the PIP joints of index and ring fingers.
b Myelofibrosis. Gout secondary to hyperuricaemia.
c Hyperuricaemia secondary to increased cell turnover.
d Nucleated RBCs, poikilocytosis (tear drop), immature granulocytes. Leukoerythroblastic anaemia.

Discussion

Myelofibrosis is characterized by bone marrow fibrosis, splenomegaly and a leukoerythroblastic anaemia with tear-drop poikilocytes. The primary pathology is proliferation of haemopoietic stem cells in the bone marrow, liver and spleen. Over a third of patients will give a previous history of polycythaemia rubra vera. Myelofibrosis has an insidious onset in middle age, usually with anaemia or massive splenomegaly. In a few patients gout, bone pain and bleeding may be the presenting feature.

Radiological patterns of osteosclerosis include generalized or patchy areas of increased bone density. On abdominal radiographs it is important to inspect the left flank for splenic enlargement, which is usually moderate to massive. The bone density may be normal in some patients with myelofibrosis. Gout occurs as a result of unchecked hyperuricaemia and has similar appearances to classical gout.

Other causes of generalized osteosclerosis include:

- metastases from prostate, breast, gastrointestinal tract, carcinoid;
- sickle cell disease, mastocytosis, polycythaemia rubra vera;
- metabolic causes – fluorosis, renal osteodystrophy, primary hyperparathyroidism;
- others – osteopetrosis, Paget's disease.

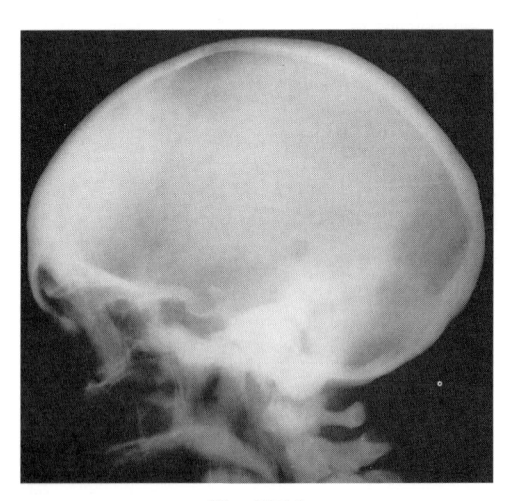

Fig. 104.2
Myelofibrosis. Skull. Note the generalized sclerosis with loss of trabecular markings in the vertebrae.

QUESTION 105

This is a barium swallow in a 46-year-old man with dysphagia for 3 months.

a What abnormality is shown?
b What investigations would you consider?
c What is the most likely diagnosis?

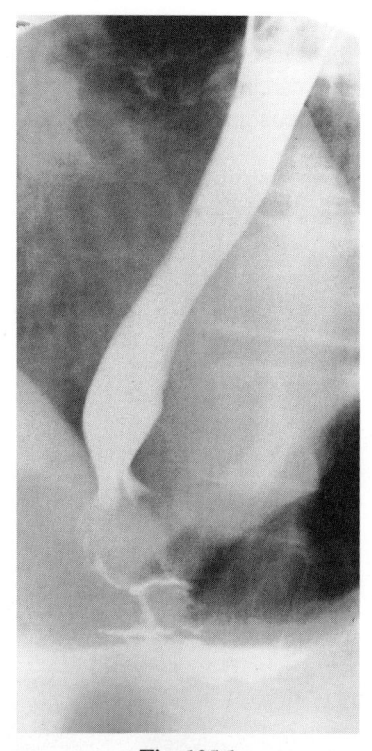

Fig. 105.1

ANSWER 105

a There is a well-defined spherical filling defect in the lower oesophagus.
b Endoscopy.
 CT thorax.
c Leiomyoma of the oesophagus.

Discussion

Leiomyomas are the commonest benign tumours in the oesophagus, and are frequently discovered as incidental findings during endoscopy, barium studies and autopsy. They only rarely give symptoms of dysphagia or pain. Radiologically they appear smooth and have a sharp border with the oesophageal mucosa, which is clearly delineated. Leiomyomas are intramural extraluminal lesions and arise in the submucosa. If large, they may mimic an extrinsic lesion. Endoscopy and CT are useful investigations. It is not often possible to biopsy these lesions if they cannot be seen deep to normal mucosa. Unlike leiomyomas of the stomach, they rarely bleed.

Carcinoma of the oesophagus causes narrowing and an irregular 'shaggy' mucosa. Fifty per cent are located at the level of the carina (Fig. 105.2) and 25% in the lower third. Eighty per cent are squamous carcinomas and the remainder are adenocarcinomas, which tend to occur in the lower oesophagus and cardia.

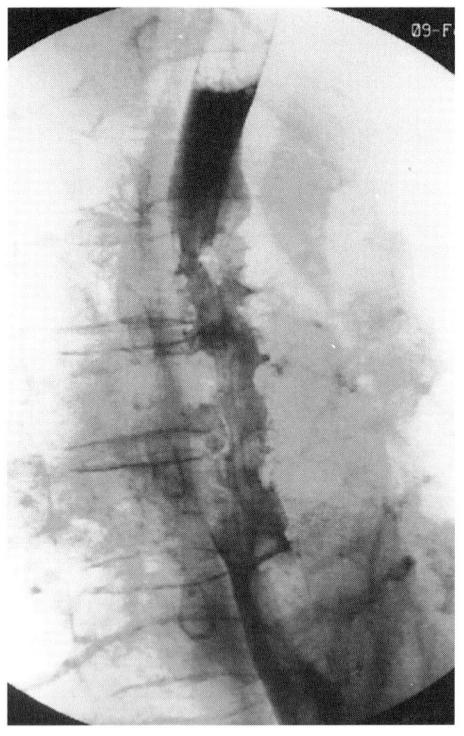

Fig. 105.2
Carcinoma of oesophagus. Barium swallow. Irregular stricture mid-oesophagus.

QUESTION 106

This 8-year-old boy has iron deficiency anaemia.

a What investigation is shown?
b What is the diagnosis?
c List two possible complications.

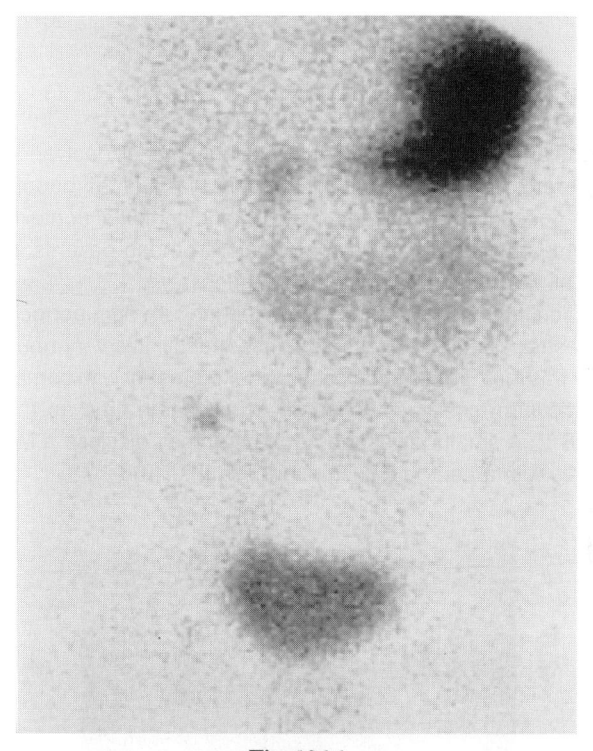

Fig. 106.1

Answer 106

a Meckel's scan.
b Meckel's diverticulum.
c Bleeding.
   Intussusception.
   Perforation.
   Infection (diverticulitis).
   Ulceration.

Discussion

Meckel's diverticulum is a remnant of the vitello-intestinal duct and arises from the antimesenteric side of the distal ileum. It is present in 2% of the population and occurs 2 feet from the caecum. Approximately 20% of diverticula contain ectopic gastric mucosa, and these are likely to be symptomatic. In those patients who present with bleeding almost all will contain ectopic gastric mucosa.

Meckel's diverticulum may be diagnosed on technetium-99m pertechnetate scanning only if ectopic gastric mucosa is present. Consequently, it is very unusual for adults to be diagnosed by this method, as such cases tend to present with complications in childhood. The diverticulum takes up the tracer at the same time as the normal gastric mucosa (Fig. 106.1). A small bowel enema or meal may disclose a Meckel's diverticulum in those cases without ectopic gastric mucosa (Fig. 106.2).

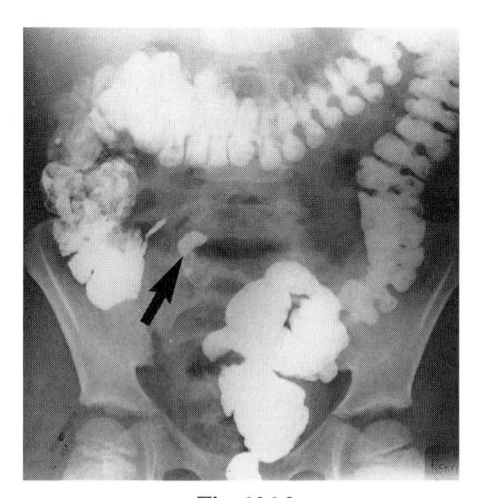

Fig. 106.2
Barium follow through from small bowel meal. Meckel's diverticulum retaining barium (arrow).

QUESTION 107

This 12-year-old girl has a chronic medical condition.

a What is the skeletal abnormality?
b What is the chronic medical condition and how is it being treated?

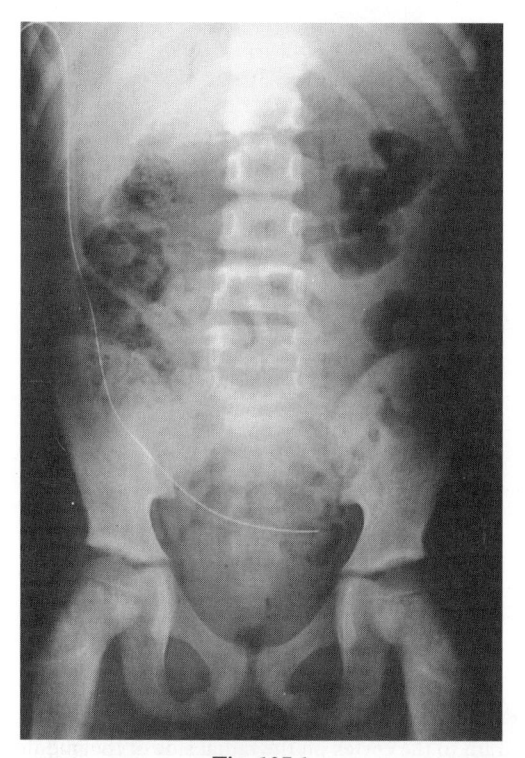

Fig. 107.1

ANSWER 107

a Renal osteodystrophy (renal rickets).
b Chronic renal failure.
Peritoneal dialysis.

Discussion

Renal osteodystrophy in children gives classical appearances. In Fig. 107.1 the proximal femoral growth plates are widened with an irregular metaphyseal margin – the so-called 'rotting fence' appearance. The pubic syndesmoses are unossified and the trabeculae are ill-defined. There is a peritoneal dialysis catheter with its tip in the pelvis.

Advanced renal osteodystrophy in an adult gives classical changes of hyperparathyroidism (Figs 107.2a and 107.2b).

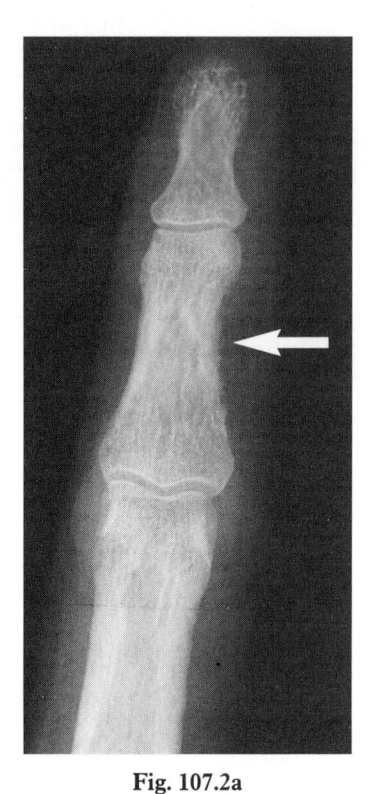

Fig. 107.2a
Left index finger. Renal osteodystrophy. Note the subperiosteal resorption (arrow) giving an ill-defined margin to the cortex on the radial side of the middle phalanx, a classic appearance and distribution.

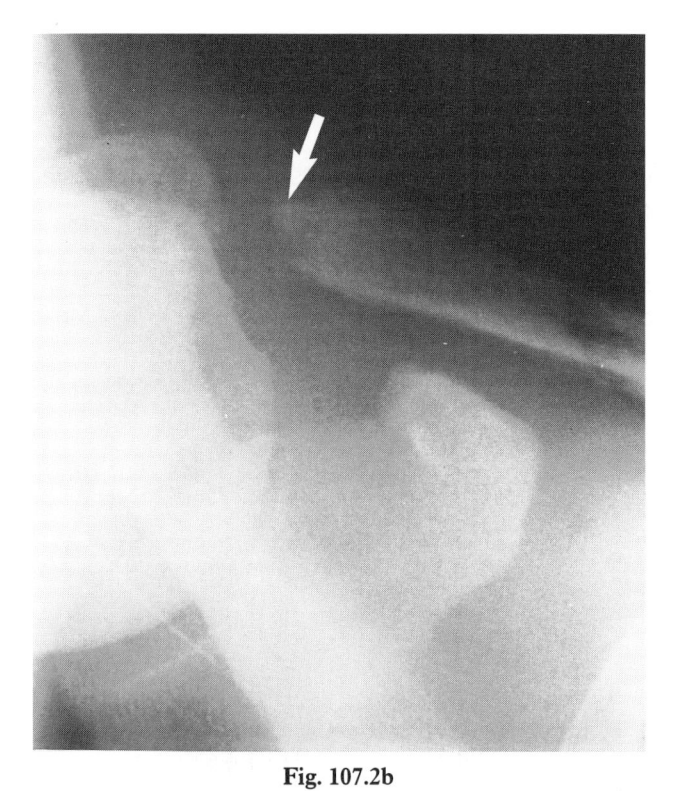

Fig. 107.2b
Right shoulder coned view. Renal osteodystrophy. There is erosion of the outer end of the clavicle (arrow). Other causes of absorption of the outer end of clavicle include trauma, rheumatoid arthritis and scleroderma.

QUESTION 108

This is a high-resolution CT of the lungs in a 29-year-old man with asthma and peripheral blood eosinophilia.

a What major abnormality is shown?
b What is the most likely diagnosis?
c How would you confirm it?

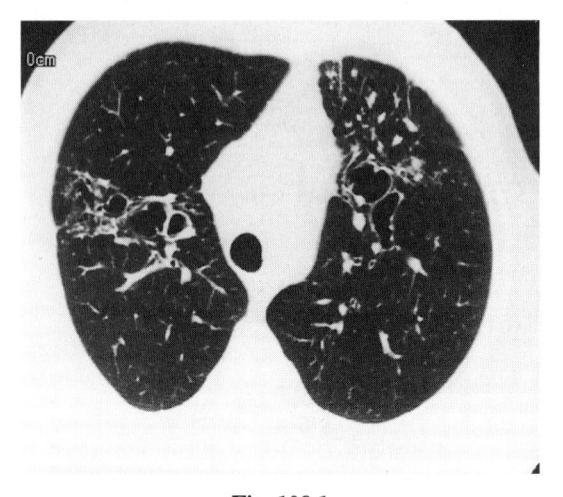

Fig. 108.1

Answer 108

a Central bronchiectasis.
b Allergic bronchopulmonary aspergillosis (ABPA).
c Instant reaction to *Aspergillus* skin prick test.

Discussion

Allergic bronchopulmonary aspergillosis (ABPA) is characterized by asthma, peripheral eosinophilia and shadowing in the lung parenchyma. It is a hypersensitivity reaction to *Aspergillus* species which plug proximal airways. Recurrent episodes damage the surrounding lung tissue and lead to bronchiectasis. Steroids halt the progress of disease and reduce the associated bronchospasm.

The various radiographic changes in ABPA are numerous. In the acute phase, *Aspergillus* species plug proximal airways. This results in bronchial wall thickening which appears as 'tramline' shadows. Consolidation and mucoceles result from airway obstruction. In the latter stages of the disease the mucous plugs resolve only to leave bronchiectatic airways and localized fibrosis. In chronic ABPA the lungs are hyperinflated in association with segmental volume loss in areas of bronchiectasis.

QUESTION 109

A 35-year-old woman presents with orthopnoea, paroxysmal nocturnal dyspnoea and fever. Examination revealed a loud first heart sound and bilateral basal crackles. She was in sinus rhythm.

a What is the diagnosis?
b What complications can occur?
c What treatment is indicated?

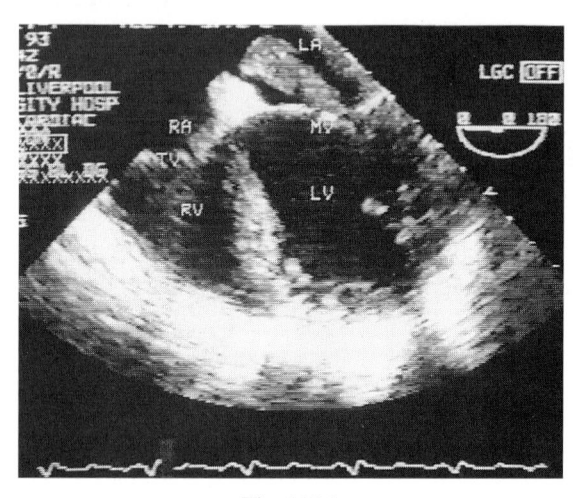

Fig. 109.1

ANSWER 109

a Left atrial myxoma.
b Pulmonary oedema.
  Systemic emboli (in 40% of patients).
  Anaemia (haemolysis).
  Polycythaemia.
c Urgent surgical excision.

Discussion

Atrial myxomata are rare benign tumours. Seventy-five per cent occur in the left atrium. Females outnumber males by a ratio of 2:1, and most patients are aged between 30 and 60 years. Atrial myxomata are polypoid masses of amorphous, gelatinous material. The base of the pedicle arises near the fossa ovalis. During diastole the tumour descends through the mitral valve orifice into the left ventricle and causes a 'tumour plop' and loud first heart sound. Poor left ventricular infilling results in pulmonary oedema. Adherent thrombus on the surface of the tumour is at high risk of detaching and embolizing. Large thrombi of clot and tumour may dislodge and occlude the aortic bifurcation (Fig. 109.2).

Clinical features of left atrial myxoma include symptoms of left atrial hypertension – orthopnoea, PND and pulmonary oedema. Systemic emboli occur in 40% of cases and may be the presenting feature. Emboli in young patients in sinus rhythm should always prompt a search for atrial myxomata. Twenty-five per cent of patients are febrile. Weight loss, Raynaud's phenomenon, finger clubbing and raised ESR may be present. Treatment is by surgical excision.

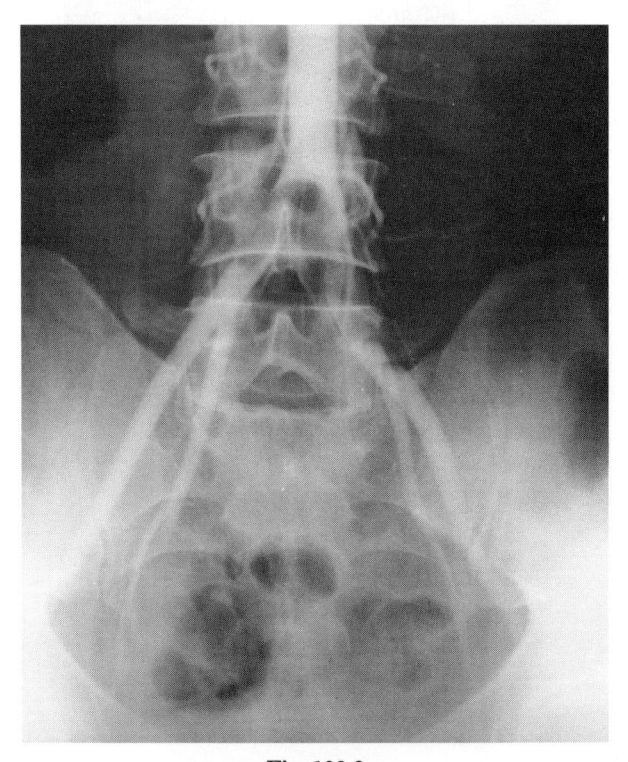

Fig. 109.2
Saddle embolus at aortic bifurcation. Inverted V-shaped filling defect at the aortic bifurcation in another patient.

QUESTION 110

This is a T2-weighted sagittal image of the cervical spine in a 38-year-old female heroin addict with loss of bowel control and urinary retention.

a What abnormality is shown?
b What is the diagnosis?

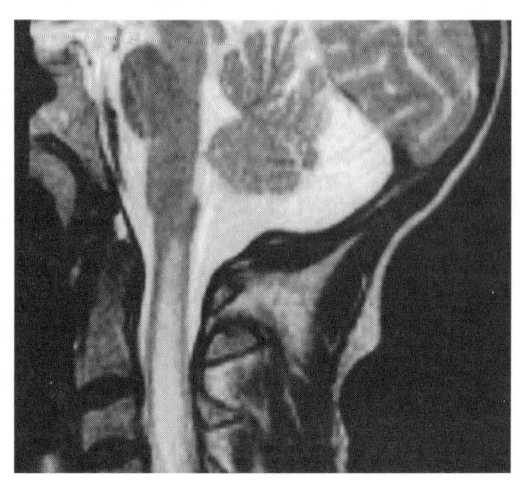

Fig 110.1

Answer 110

a Swelling of the cervical cord with a uniform high-signal intensity.
b Transverse myelitis.

Discussion

Transverse myelitis is a demyelinating disorder of the spinal cord without an intramedullary space-occupying effect. It affects the young and middle-aged, and usually involves two to three adjacent vertebral segments. The cause may remain unknown. Symptoms develop over a few hours, leading to loss of sensation below the lesion with flaccid paralysis and areflexia. Complete respiratory paralysis will result if the myelitis involves C3. Complete or partial recovery may occur.

Recognized causes of transverse myelitis include multiple sclerosis, epidural abscess, post-viral causes, mycoplasma infection, intravenous heroin abuse, radiation and vascular impairment.

Figure 110.1 demonstrates cord oedema and swelling extending from C2.

QUESTION 111

This 70-year-old man has intermittent dysphagia and substernal chest pain.

a What is the descriptive term for the radiological appearance on this barium swallow examination?
b List two causes.
c What investigation is indicated next?

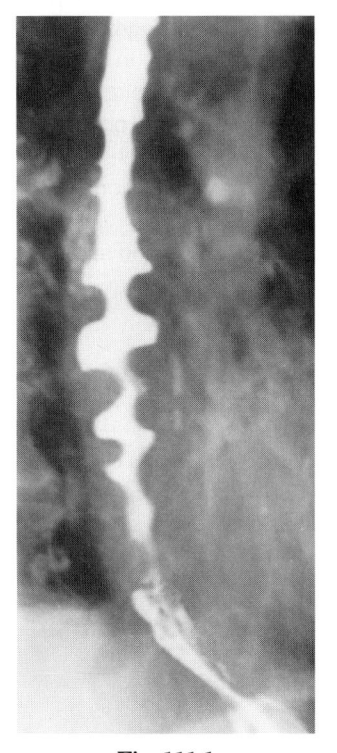

Fig. 111.1

Answer 111

a Corkscrew oesophagus (rosary bead oesophagus or spastic pseudodiverticulosis).
b Gastro-oesophageal reflux.
Achalasia.
Autonomic neuropathy (diabetes).
Distal oesophageal obstruction.
c Endoscopy.
Oesophageal manometry.

Discussion

Corkscrew oesophagus is a descriptive term applied to the radiological appearances encountered in diffuse oesophageal spasm. A cause may occasionally be found on barium swallow, e.g. distal obstruction by carcinoma or gastro-oesophageal reflux, but in the majority of patients no cause is found. Endoscopy is important in order to exclude a neoplasm. Manometry will define the spasm with a high degree of specificity and sensitivity. Diffuse oesophageal spasm is difficult to treat, but symptomatic relief may be gained with calcium-channel blockers, dilatations and, in severe cases, myotomy.

226

QUESTION 112

This is the abdominal CT scan in a 70-year-old lady with haematemesis.

a What are the two radiological abnormalities?
b What is the diagnosis?
c List three possible causes.

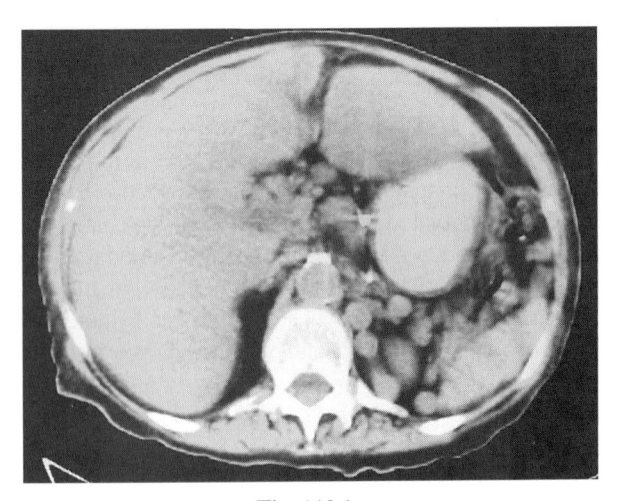

Fig. 112.1a
Pre-contrast

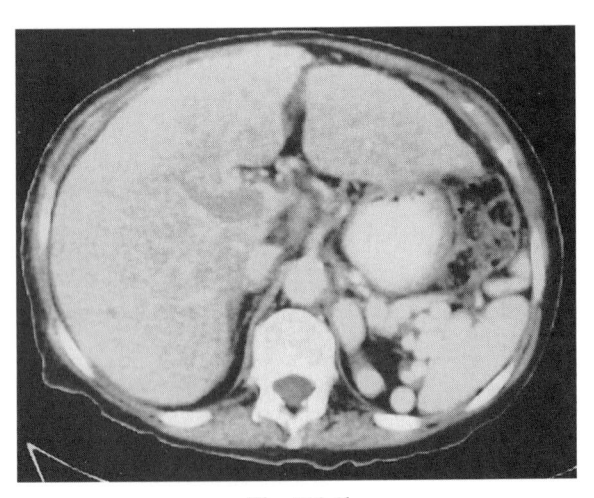

Fig. 112.1b
Post-contrast

Answer 112

a Filling defect in portal vein.
Extensive splenic varices.
b Portal hypertension secondary to portal vein thrombosis.
c Neonatal umbilical sepsis.
Intra-abdominal sepsis.
Pancreatic cancer invading portal vein.
Polycythaemia rubra vera.
Contraceptive pill.
Inflammatory bowel disease.

Discussion

Extrahepatic portal hypertension due to portal vein obstruction has a number of causes, listed above. There is usually a history of umbilical catheterization or infection when presenting in infancy. In adults, there may be a history of intra-abdominal sepsis or symptoms specific to other causes. In some patients no prior history is obtained and they present with haematemesis or rectal bleeding. Splenomegaly can be a feature, although ascites and liver failure are unusual.

Oesophageal varices can be demonstrated on barium swallow (Fig. 112.2). They are shown as serpiginous filling defects in the lower third of the oesophagus. In severe cases they may extend up to involve the upper third.

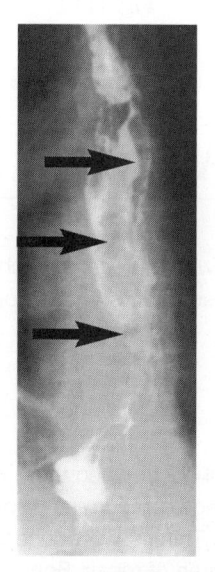

Fig. 112.2
Barium swallow. Severe oesophageal varices. Serpiginous filling defects (arrows) extending up into the upper third of the oesophagus.

QUESTION 113

This 63-year-old woman has a broad-based gait.

a What two abnormalities are shown?
b What is the diagnosis?
c What is the most likely cause?

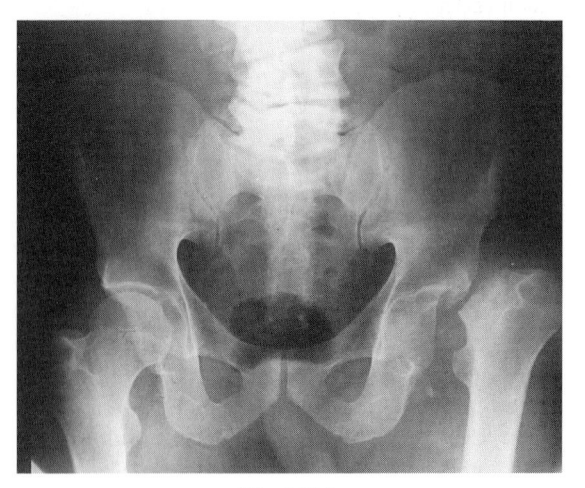

Fig. 113.1

ANSWER 113

a Sclerosis of lumbar vertebrae with degenerative change.
  Dislocated left hip joint with resorption of the femoral head and intra-articular debris.
b Neuropathic spine and hip.
c Tabes dorsalis (syphilis).

Discussion

A Charcot or neuropathic joint will occur when there is loss of pain and position sense. Ligamentous laxity results, leading to recurrent painless trauma, culminating in bone destruction with or without repair. This may produce either a hypertrophic joint or bone resorption, depending on the degree of repair. Bone resorption is thought to result from hyperaemia and is illustrated in the left hip in Fig. 113.1. A hypertrophic neuro-arthropathy will result when there is marked osteoblastic activity. Classically the joint will show disorganization, debris, dislocation, sclerosis and effusion (Fig. 113.2). In tabes dorsalis there is a 5% incidence of neuro-arthropathy. The knee (Fig. 113.2) is the most commonly affected joint (70%), followed by the ankle, hip and feet (30%). The lumbar or lower thoracic vertebrae are affected in approximately 15% of cases.

Neuropathic shoulder is typically due to syringomyelia.

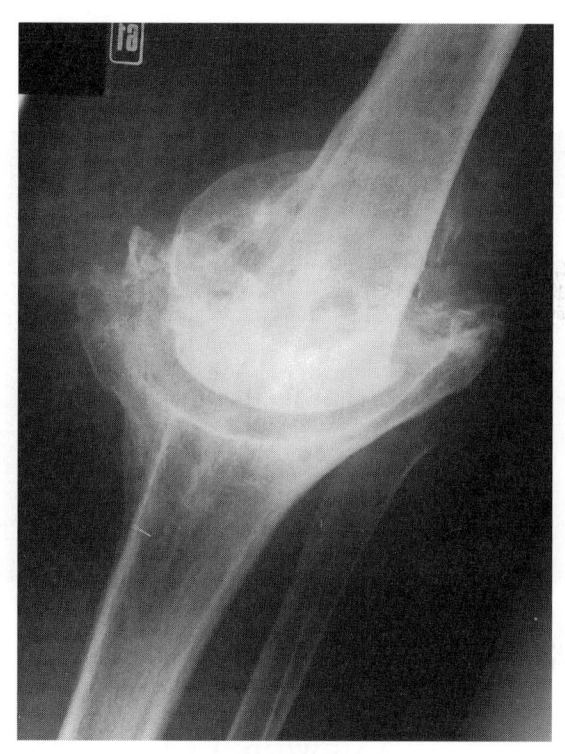

Fig. 113.2
Tabes dorsalis knee joint.

QUESTION 114

a What abnormalities are present in this skull radiograph of a 54-year-old man?
b What is the likely cause?
c What complication has occurred?
d Name an additional complication of this disease.

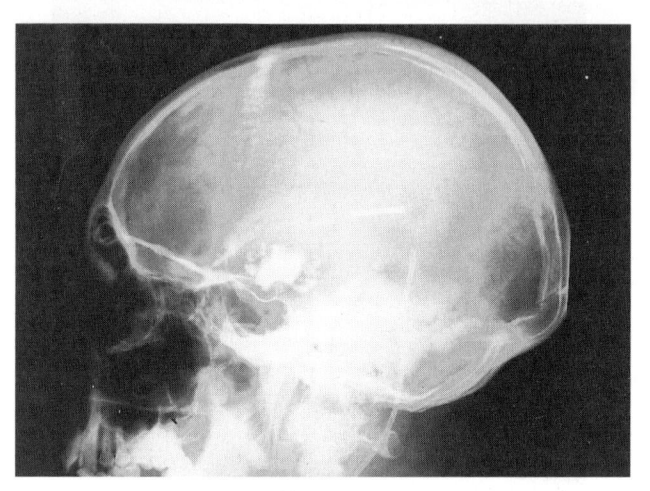

Fig. 114.1

ANSWER 114

a Ventricular shunt.
   Basal cistern calcification.
b Tuberculous meningitis.
c Obstructive hydrocephalus.
d Cranial nerve palsies.
   Cerebral and brainstem infarction secondary to arteritis.

Discussion

Tuberculous meningitis is invariably associated with a focus of infection outside the central nervous system. In children, infection is acquired from dissemination of primary pulmonary TB. In adults, miliary TB or reactivation TB is usually the cause. Tubercles seed to the pia-arachnoid by haematogenous spread (Rich foci). Only when the tubercle bursts into the subarachnoid space does meningism result.

The onset of illness is insidious. Patients complain of anorexia and symptoms of a viral illness. Headache and vomiting herald the meningitic phase which, if left untreated, leads to cranial nerve destruction, and brainstem and cerebral infarction as a result of endarteritis. Tuberculous meningitis can be overlooked because of vague symptoms and its indolent course. Following successful treatment of tuberculous meningitis, meningeal calcification often results, especially around the basal cisterns. Obstruction to CSF flow here and at the cerebral aqueduct leads to hydrocephalus, causing stupor and coma. Chest radiograph will show evidence of recent or old TB in 70% of cases.

In the acute illness CT may be used to exclude cerebral abscess, hydrocephalus and infarction, especially of the brainstem. Figures 114.2a and 114.2b demonstrate marked meningeal enhancement and thickening in a case of acute tuberculous meningitis. Other causes of meningeal enhancement are pyogenic meningitis, sarcoid meningitis and fungal meningitis.

The CSF has the following characteristics in tuberculous meningitis: clear appearance; lymphocytic pleocytosis with a cell count of 400 cells/mm^3; glucose concentration less than 3 mmol/L and protein concentration 1–5 g/L; tubercle isolation in 80% of cases.

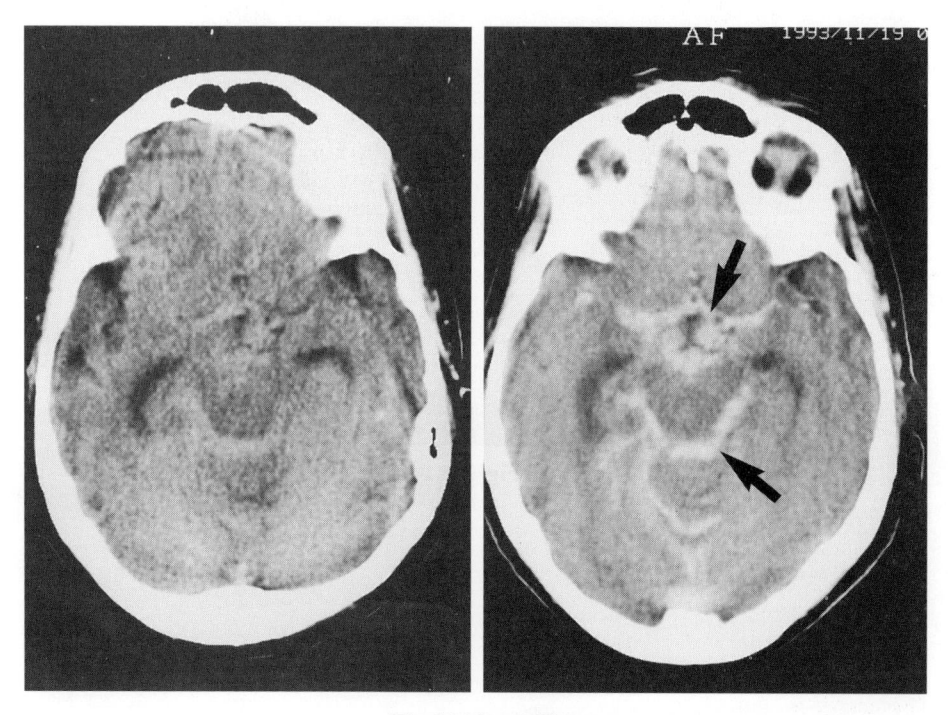

Fig. 114.2a and b
Tuberculous meningitis. Pre and post i.v. contrast medium. Note the marked enhancement of thickened basal meninges.

QUESTION 115

A 53-year-old woman has abdominal cramps and diarrhoea.

a What is the diagnosis?
b With what diseases is it associated?

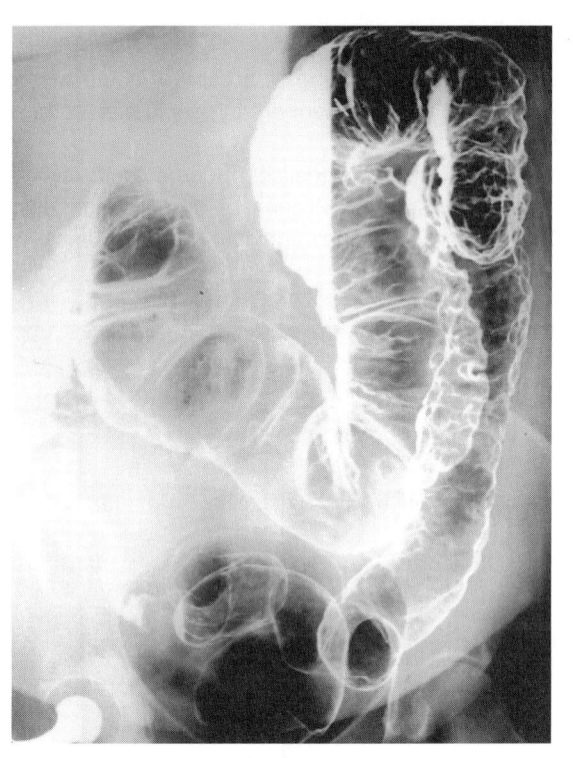

Fig. 115.1

Answer 115

a Pneumatosis cystoides intestinalis (pneumatosis coli).
b Chronic obstructive pulmonary disease.
Scleroderma.
Peptic ulceration.

Discussion

Pneumatosis cystoides intestinalis (PCI) can affect small and large bowel. It is most commonly seen in the distal colon (pneumatosis coli). Symptoms include abdominal pain, altered bowel habit, mucus discharge and occasionally rectal bleeding. Air-containing cysts are found in the submucosa and serosa of the intestine. There is a strong association with chronic obstructive pulmonary disease (COPD). There is also an association with scleroderma and peptic ulceration. No specific treatment is required, although oxygen therapy for COPD causes the cysts to deflate. PCI is associated with pneumoperitoneum without peritonitis if there is cyst rupture.

QUESTION 116

This 59-year-old man complains of headaches. On examination he is icteric and has an enlarged liver.

a What abnormality is shown in Fig. 116.1a?
b What abnormalities are shown in Fig. 116.1b?
c What is the most likely diagnosis?

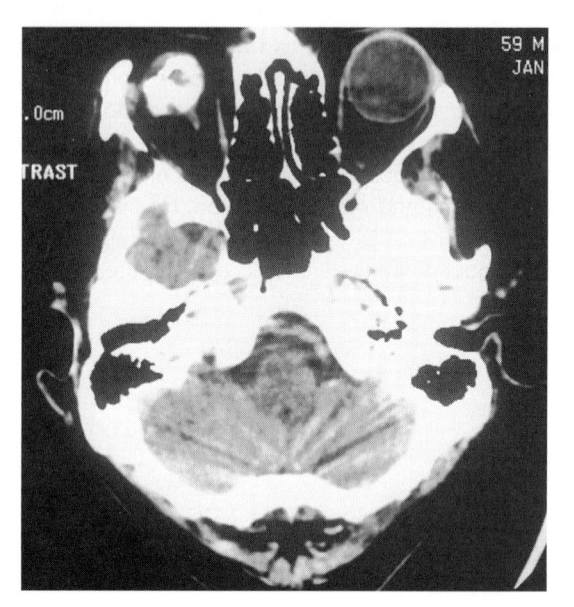

Fig. 116.1a

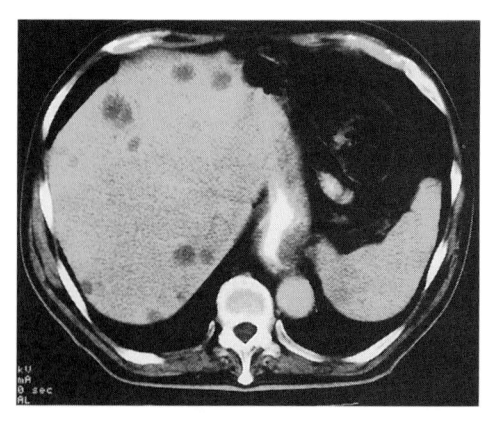

Fig. 116.1b

Answer 116

a Prosthesis in right orbit.
b Multiple liver metastases.
c Ocular melanoma with liver metastases.

Discussion

Choroidal melanoma is the commonest primary ocular neoplasm. If diagnosed early, it may be treated with enucleation, although there is often microscopic spread at the time of presentation. This may be local, involving tissues of the orbit, or it may be distant with spread via the lymphatics to the bloodstream and then to the lungs, liver and brain.

Remember the aphorism 'Beware the man with the glass eye and large liver'!

QUESTION 117

This is a T1- weighted sagittal image through the chest in a 6-year-old girl.

a What abnormalities are shown?
b What is the diagnosis?
c How may this condition present?
d List four associated conditions.

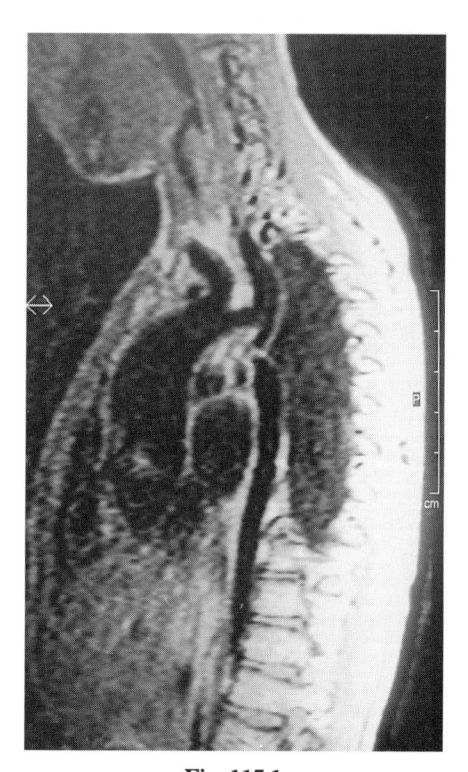

Fig. 117.1

Answer 117

a Dilated ascending aorta and great vessels. Narrowed segment of aorta distal to left subclavian artery.
b Coarctation of the aorta.
c Asymptomatic.
Stroke.
Endocarditis.
Hypertension.
Claudication.
d Bicuspid aortic valve.
Endocarditis.
Berry aneurysms.
Patent ductus arteriosus, ventricular septal defect.

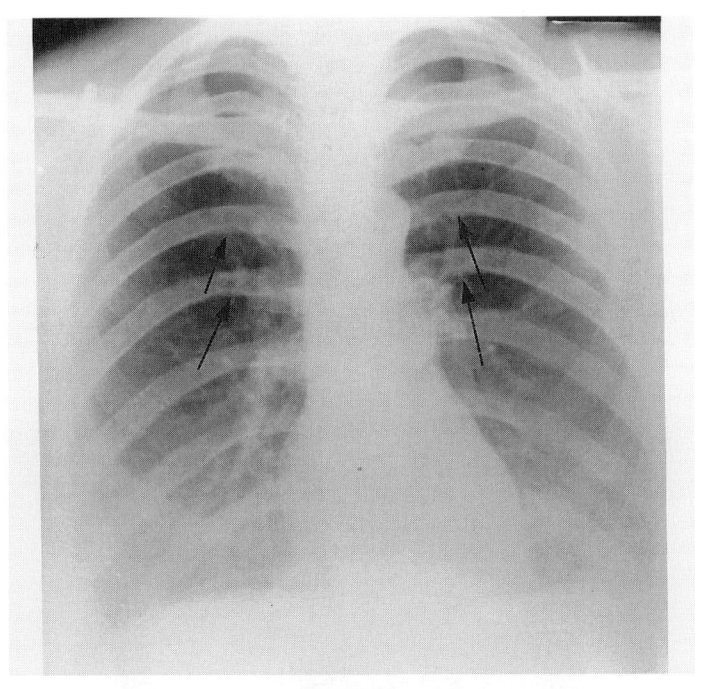

Fig. 117.2a
Coarctation of the aorta. Note rib notching (arrows). Note also air under the right hemidiaphragm indicating pneumoperitoneum.

Marfan's syndrome.
Turner's syndrome.

Discussion

Coarctation is a localized stenosis of the aorta leading to obstruction; 98% occur distal to the left subclavian artery. Coarctation may present in infancy with heart failure, and then requires urgent repair. In older children and adults presentation is insidious. Up to 60% of the total cases are asymptomatic. The remainder may present with hypertension, endocarditis, stroke and lower limb claudication. Males are affected twice as frequently as females. The most classical physical signs are delay and reduction in volume of the femoral pulses with upper limb hypertension. Thrills may be elicited over collateral vessels posteriorly. Notching will develop by the age of 10 years and affects the posterior inferior aspects of the third to eighth ribs due to dilatation of intercostal arteries (see Fig. 117.2a). Rib notching is only right-sided if the coarctation is proximal to the left subclavian artery, and only left-sided if associated with a Blalock shunt (subclavian – pulmonary artery anastomosis).

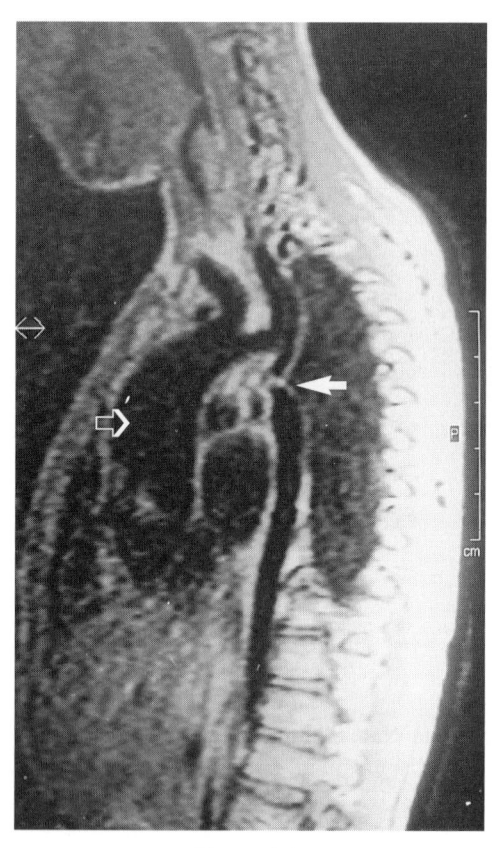

Fig. 117.2b
Coarctation of the aorta (arrow). Note dilated ascending aorta (open arrow).

Other important causes of rib notching include neurofibromatosis (multiple neurofibromas involving the intercostal nerves), superior vena caval obstruction and rheumatoid arthritis.

Coarctation is associated with bicuspid aortic valves in 25% of cases (which provides the site of infection in endocarditis), berry aneurysms and cerebral haemorrhage, ventricular septal defect, Turner's syndrome and Marfan's syndrome.

QUESTION 118

A 30-year-old woman presents with a left hemiplegia and fever.

a What abnormality is shown in Fig. 118.1a?
b What abnormality is shown on a contrast-enhanced CT brain scan (Fig. 118.1b)?
c What is the underlying diagnosis?
d What treatment is indicated?

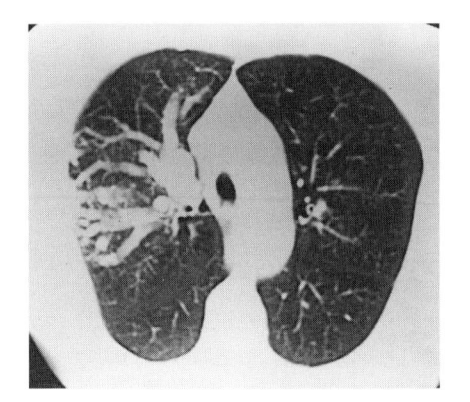

Fig. 118.1a

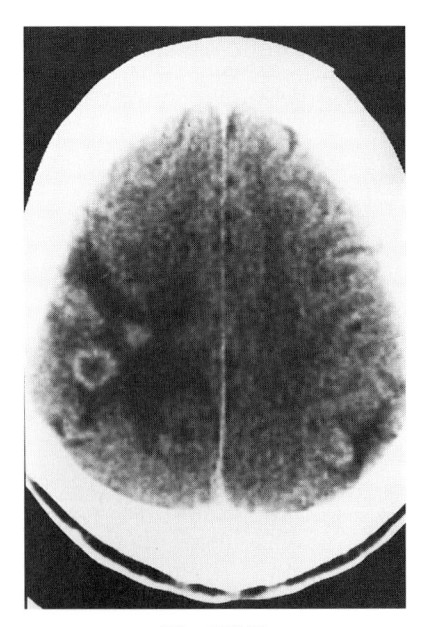

Fig. 118.1b

Answer 118

a A large pulmonary arteriovenous malformation (AVM).
b Enhanced abscess in right parietal lobe with marked surrounding oedema.
c Osler–Weber–Rendu syndrome.
d Intravenous antibiotics and/or surgical drainage.
  Embolization of the pulmonary AVM.

Discussion

Pulmonary AVMs may be simple or multiple. Nearly all cases are due to Osler-Weber-Rendu (OWR) syndrome (also known as hereditary haemorrhagic telangiectasia), whereas about 15% of patients with OWR have pulmonary AVMs. Pulmonary AVMs are sometimes large enough to cause cyanosis in children and hypoxia in adults due to right-to-left shunting. A major complication of this shunt is bypassing of the lungs as a filter – abscesses and paradoxical emboli may occur in the systemic circulation, notably to the brain. On CT, a cerebral abscess typically enhances with marked surrounding oedema (Fig. 118.1b).

OWR syndrome is inherited as an autosomal dominant condition and tends to present at puberty. Telangiectasia are found on the skin and mucous membranes and may occur anywhere in the gastrointestinal tract, where they may be associated with intussusception. Patients may present with iron deficiency anaemia and haemoptysis in those with pulmonary AVMs. The pulmonary lesions may be successfully treated by coil embolization.

QUESTION 119

a What abnormality is shown?
b What can be inferred from this observation?
c Would you expect a functional deficit if this was the only abnormality?

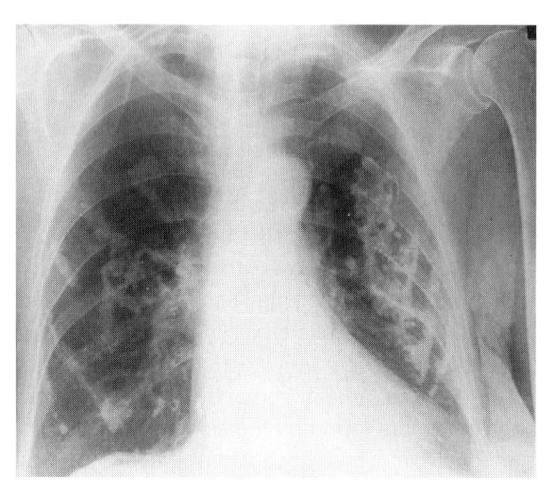

Fig. 119.1

ANSWER 119

a Bilateral pleural calcification.
b Asbestos exposure.
c No.

Discussion

Asbestos-related pleural plaques may be calcified or non-calcified. They tend to be bilateral, and the finding of unilateral calcified pleural plaques suggests an alternative diagnosis such as a previous tuberculous empyema or haemothorax. The dose of exposure and time interval from exposure are important factors determining the incidence of plaque formation. They tend to occur in the parietal pleura over the diaphragm and lateral chest wall. They calcify in a linear fashion along the periphery of the plaque, giving rise to the so-called 'holly-leaf' calcification (Fig. 119.2). Pleural plaques are not usually clinically significant enough to cause a restrictive defect, and are not known to transform into mesothelioma.

Other findings due to asbestos inhalation include:

- pleural effusions, which may be intermittent;
- pulmonary fibrosis, often coarse and extensive within the lower zones, causing a 'shaggy' heart;
- pleural mesothelioma – showing as a tumour encasing the lung, associated with lobulated pleural thickening and loculated pleural fluid.

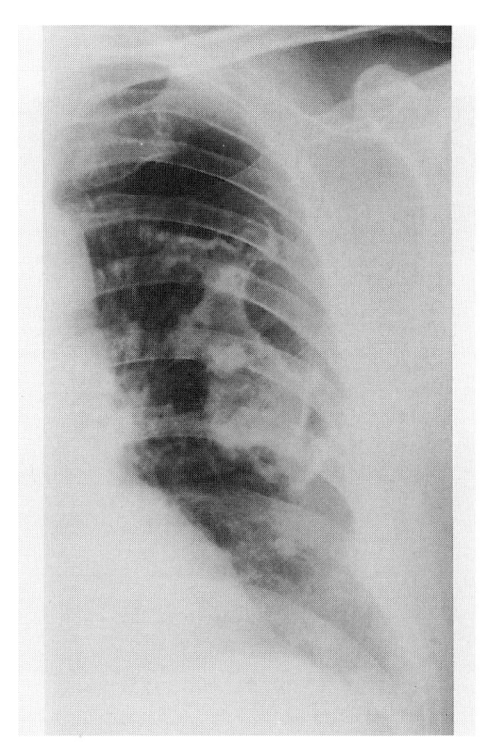

Fig. 119.2
Asbestos exposure. 'Holly-leaf' calcification of an asbestos-related pleural plaque.

QUESTION 120

This 63-year-old woman has recurrent chest infections.

a What abnormality is shown?
b What is the diagnosis?
c Name two complications of this disorder.

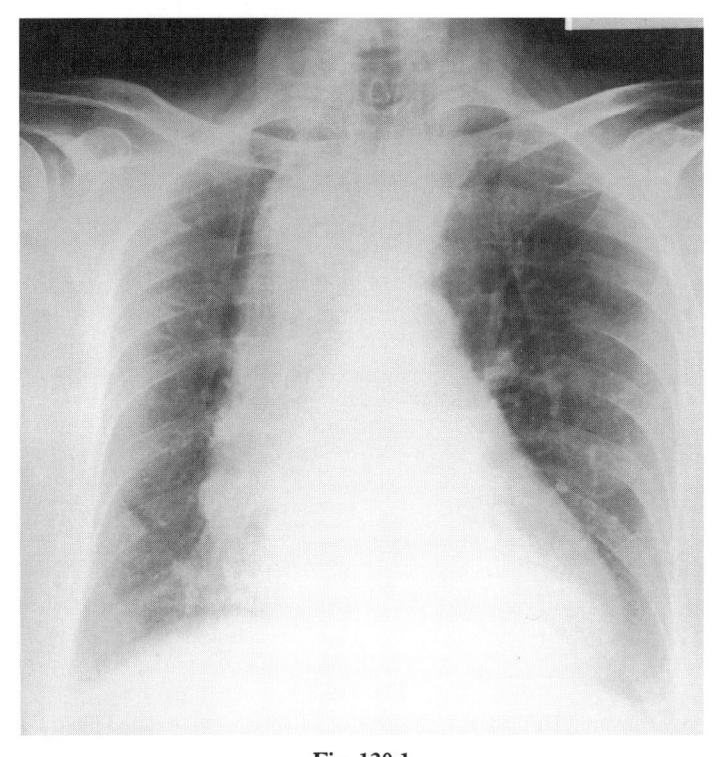

Fig. 120.1

Answer 120

a Dilated food-filled oesophagus. Absent gastric bubble.
b Achalasia.
c Overspill pneumonitis. Carcinoma of the oesophagus.

Discussion

Achalasia is due to a depletion of ganglion cells in the lower oesophagus. This results in failure of the lower oesophageal sphincter to relax. Classically the primary and secondary peristaltic waves are lost in the distal oesophagus. Most cases are idiopathic, but in South America achalasia may result from Chaga's disease due to *Trypanosoma cruzi*. Achalasia may also be caused by carcinoma involving the ganglion cells.

Radiologically there is dilatation of the oesophagus, which may be filled with food debris or fluid. Characteristically the gastric bubble is absent. On barium studies the lower oesophagus has a bird's-beak appearance – barium empties intermittently through the sphincter. Patients are at risk of overspill pneumonitis, and there is an increased risk of developing oesophageal carcinoma.

QUESTION 121

This is a barium enema in a 43-year-old lady with bloody diarrhoea.

- **a** What is the exact diagnosis?
- **b** What treatment is she receiving?
- **c** Name two colonic complications.

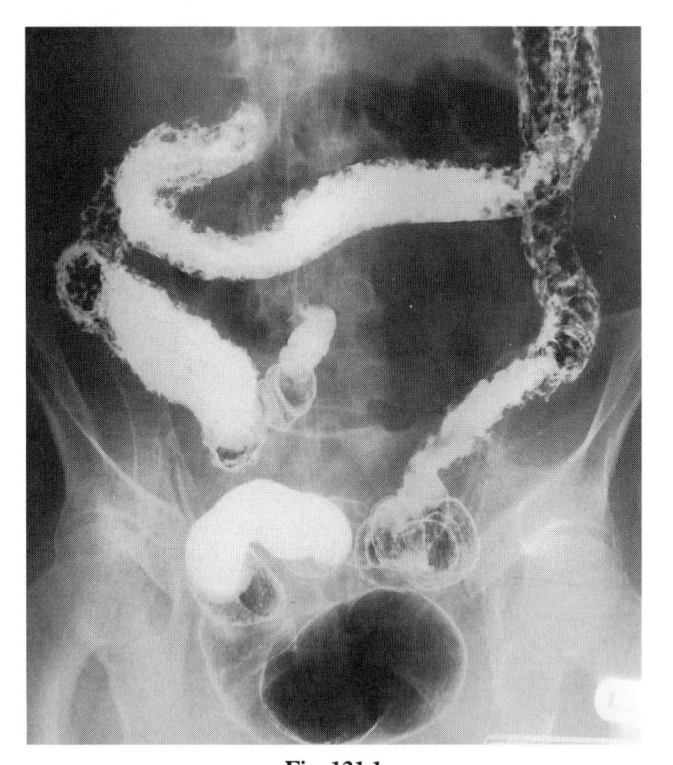

Fig. 121.1

ANSWER 121

- **a** Ulcerative colitis.
- **b** Rectal steroids.
- **c** Perforation.
  Toxic megacolon.
  Carcinoma.
  Stricture (benign).

Discussion

Ulcerative colitis (UC) has an annual incidence of 6 per 100 000 members of the population. It is due to chronic inflammation confined to the mucosa, unlike Crohn's disease (CD), which extends to involve the submucosa and bowel wall. UC typically presents with diarrhoea and increased stool frequency.

The radiological features strongly suggestive of UC are loss of haustra, colitis in continuity, granular mucosa, rectal involvement, generalized narrowing and symmetrical involvement. In this case there is relative sparing of the recto-sigmoid due to topical steroids. The narrowed proximal colon contains multiple pseudopolyps and 'collar-stud abscesses'. Closer inspection of the rectum on this examination shows granularity of the mucosa. CD, in contrast, tends to be asymmetrical, discontinuous, and associated with fistulae. Aphthoid ulceration with fissuring is characteristic of CD.

Radiolabelled white-cell scanning (Fig. 121.2) may be used to evaluate disease activity in inflammatory bowel disease and complicating intra-abdominal sepsis such as abscess formation.

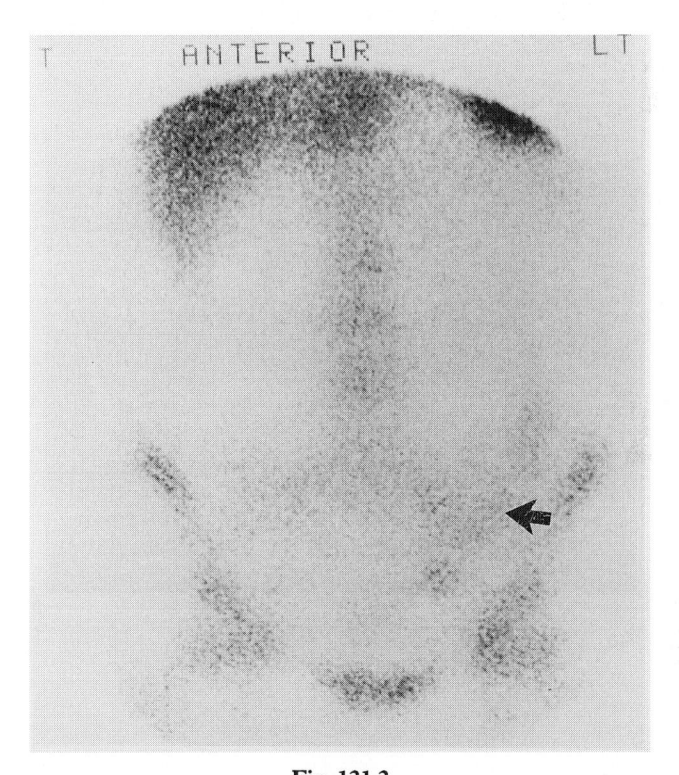

Fig. 121.2
Tc99m – HMPAO scan. Ulcerative colitis. There is increased activity in the sigmoid colon (arrow) indicating active colitis.

QUESTION 122

A 28-year-old HIV-positive man has a 7-day history of headache, fever and confusion, followed by right-sided weakness.

- **a** What pulse sequence is shown on this axial MR image through the brain?
- **b** What abnormality is shown?
- **c** List the differential diagnoses.
- **d** How would you manage this patient?

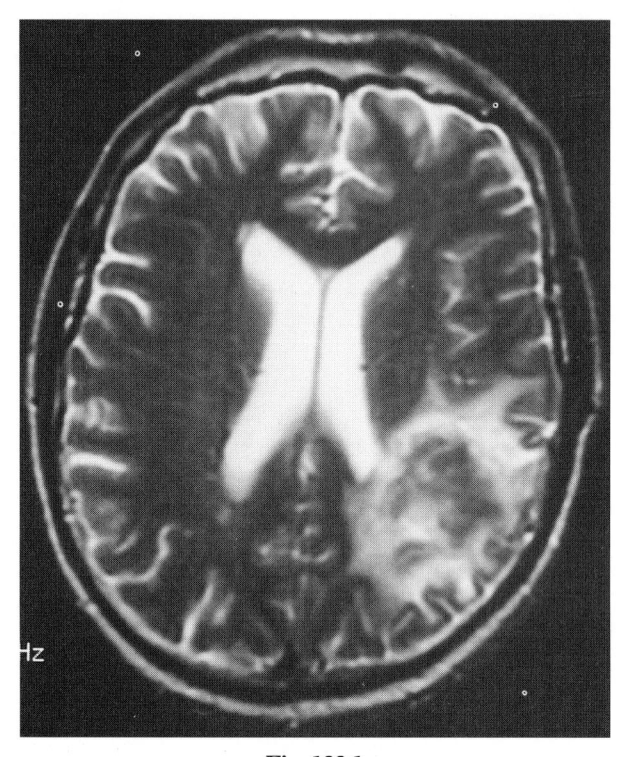

Fig. 122.1

ANSWER 122

a T2-weighted sequence.
b Space-occupying lesion with surrounding oedema in the left parietal lobe.
c Toxoplasma abscess.
Lymphoma.
Pyogenic, tuberculous or fungal abscess.
Kaposi's sarcoma (KS).
d Treatment with pyrimethamine (with or without dexamethasone).
Repeat MRI scan in 2 weeks.

Discussion

Cerebral toxoplasmosis is the commonest focal encephalopathy, occurring in up to 15% of AIDS patients. The causative agent is the protozoan *Toxoplasma gondii,* which may give a diffuse or focal encephalitis.

In AIDS patients, encephalitis may be due to dissemination or reactivation of latent infection. Diffuse involvement causes headache, confusion and fever. A more focal encephalitis or a toxoplasma abscess will give symptoms of a space-occupying lesion. Classically there is a short clinical history. Elevated serum IgG may be negative in immunocompromised individuals and is of little use. Radiologically, it is often impossible to differentiate a toxoplasma abscess from other lesions (see above). Classically there is one single mass or multiple ring-enhancing masses with surrounding oedema. Empirical treatment with pyrimethamine, an antiprotozoal agent, should be commenced and response to treatment assessed by MRI.

AIDS may be associated with neurological complications in up to 50% of patients throughout the course of illness. The most important intracranial complications are:

- meningitis   – cryptococcal
human immunodeficiency virus (HIV)
viral
tuberculosis (TB);
- encephalopathy – diffuse (metabolic, chronic HIV, cytomegalovirus)
focal (toxoplasmosis, lymphoma, progressive multifocal leucoencephalopathy, KS).

QUESTION 123

This is a coronary arteriogram taken in the right anterior oblique position in a 60-year-old man with angina.

a Which coronary artery has been examined?
b What are the two branches of this artery?
c What abnormalities would you expect to observe on an ECG?

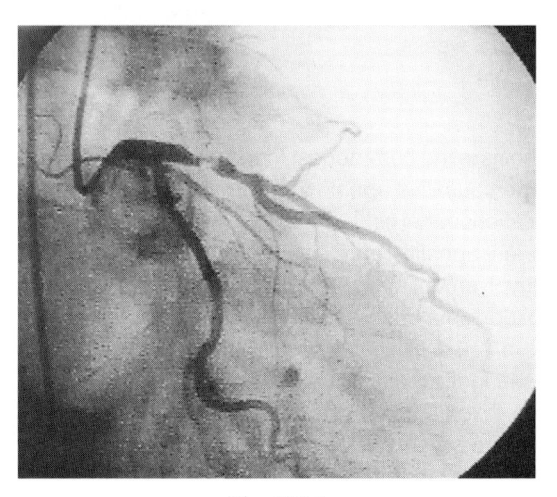

Fig. 123.1

Answer 123

a Left coronary artery.
b The left mainstem artery gives rise to the left anterior descending and circumflex arteries.
c ST-segment depression and/or T-wave inversion in the anterior chest leads. Q-waves may be present in old infarction.

Discussion

Figure 123.1 demonstrates a tight stenosis in the left anterior descending artery. This vessel supplies the interventricular septum and apex. It gives rise to diagonal branches which supply the lateral wall of the left ventricle.

Coronary angiography is employed to identify patients with angina who may benefit from coronary artery bypass grafting or angioplasty. These patients may be resistant to anti-anginal treatment. Coronary angiography may sometimes be used to establish the diagnosis in patients with atypical chest pain.

QUESTION 124

This 40-year-old man has adult respiratory distress syndrome (ARDS). His oxygen saturation has suddenly dropped.

a What two complications have occurred?
b What treatment must be given?
c List four causes of ARDS.

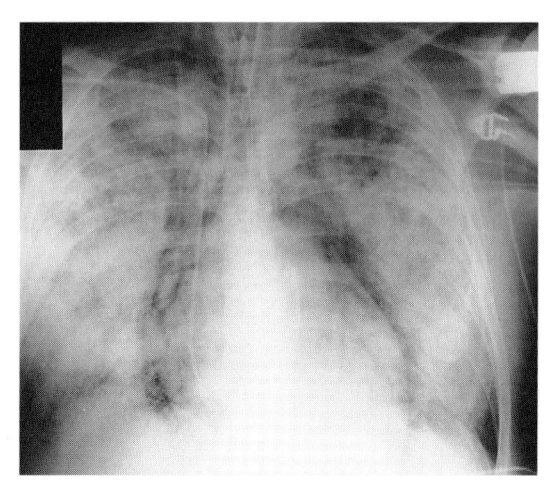

Fig. 124.1

ANSWER 124

a Pneumomediastinum.
   Left-sided pneumothorax.
b Left intercostal tube.
c Sepsis.
   Shock.
   Major surgery, e.g. aortic aneurysm repair.
   Burns.
   Trauma.
   Fat embolism.
   Aspiration.
   Toxic inhalation.
   Drug overdose (heroin, aspirin).

Pancreatitis.
Diabetic ketoacidosis.

Discussion

ARDS, or non-cardiogenic pulmonary oedema, is respiratory failure associated with a variety of injuries to the lung parenchyma. The characteristic triad of oedema, respiratory distress and hypoxia is present in all cases. ARDS develops within 48 hours of the insult to the lungs. The capillary membranes of the alveolus are damaged, causing increased permeability to protein and tissue fluid which results in oedema. There is also a reduction in surfactant.

On the chest radiograph, widespread nodular or alveolar shadows resemble pulmonary oedema. The heart is not usually enlarged, which helps to distinguish ARDS from cardiogenic oedema. ARDS has a high mortality and is refractory to diuretic treatment. Pneumonia is often a complication and may be difficult to establish radiologically. Positive pressure ventilation may cause barotrauma which manifests as pneumomediastinum, pneumothorax or interstitial emphysema.

It is important to recognize pneumothoraces in these patients. The lungs are stiff and do not collapse to the same degree as more compliant lungs. In Fig. 124.1, the pneumomediastinum is shown as a band of lucency which parallels the contours of the heart and superior mediastinum. The evidence for a left-sided pneumothorax is surgical emphysema in the left pectoralis major muscle and deepening of a lucent costophrenic sulcus. The latter sign is important because it denotes a pneumothorax in a supine patient.

It is important to note the position of the endotracheal tube in all patients on intensive care who desaturate. A careful inspection will allow prompt recognition that an endotracheal tube has been misplaced (Fig. 124.2).

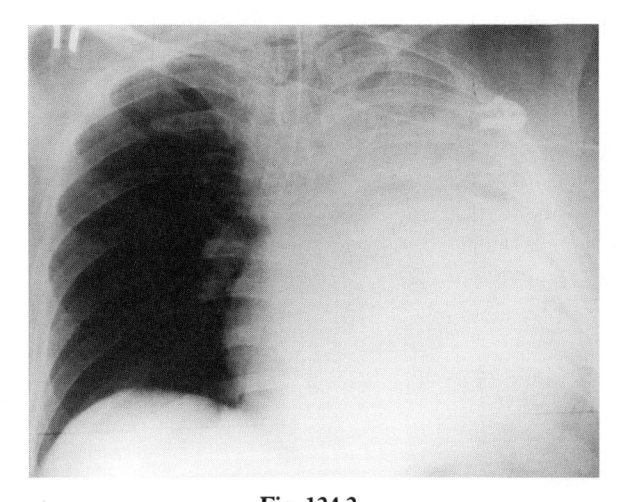

Fig. 124.2
Misplaced ET tube in the right main bronchus, causing acute collapse of the left lung.

QUESTION 125

a What procedure has been performed?
b List two indications for this procedure.
c What abnormality is shown?

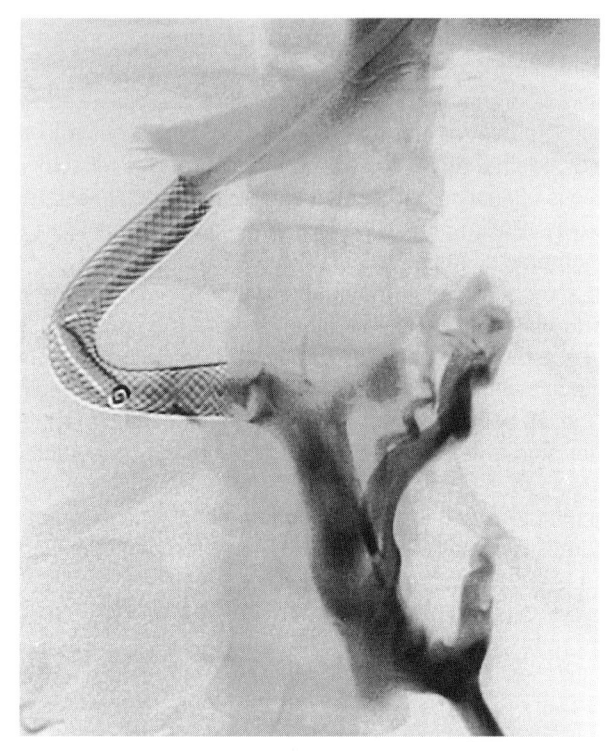

Fig. 125.1

Answer 125

a Transjugular intrahepatic portosystemic stent shunt (TIPSS).
b Variceal bleeding.
   Intractable ascites.
c Gastric varices.

Discussion

TIPSS was first performed in 1989. It is a procedure in which a communication is formed between the hepatic vein (systemic circulation) and the portal vein. It involves puncturing the right internal jugular vein. A catheter is manipulated into the right hepatic vein from the inferior vena cava. A cutting wire 'drills' through the liver substance from the hepatic vein down to the portal vein. The resulting track is dilated with a balloon catheter (similar to balloon angioplasty) and a metallic stent is positioned. TIPSS has now replaced the old surgical treatment of porto-caval shunts.

The indications for TIPSS are:

- uncontrolled variceal haemorrhage;
- intractable ascites;
- trial of shunt therapy in patients awaiting liver transplantation;
- Budd–Chiari syndrome (only if hepatic vein is patent).

The advantages of TIPSS over surgery are:

- it is less invasive;
- it is cheaper than surgery;
- TIPSS does not preclude liver transplantation, unlike surgical treatment.

The complications of TIPSS are:

- fatal haemoperitoneum (5% of procedures);
- hepatic encephalopathy (5–30% of procedures);
- intimal hyperplasia of the endothelialized stent.

Coils may be deployed within varices to induce thrombosis.

Question 126

a What investigation is shown?
b What abnormality is present?
c Suggest two possible causes.

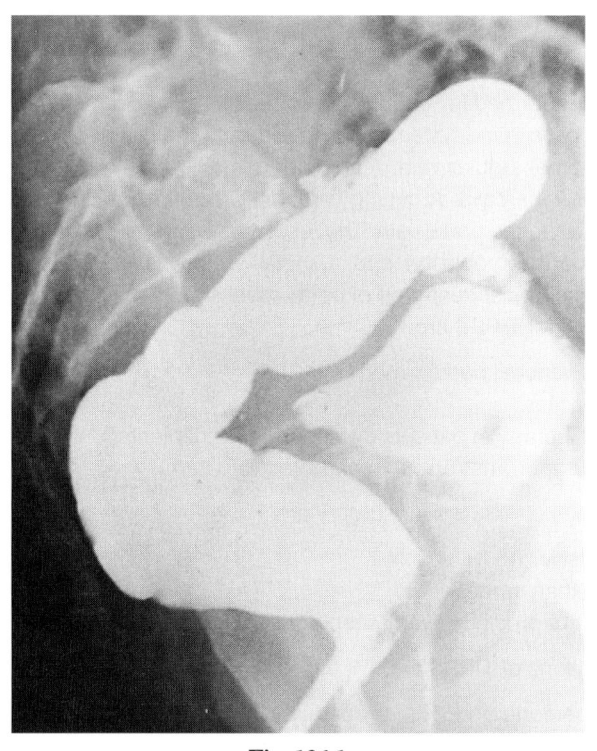

Fig. 126.1

Answer 126

a Barium enema.
b Colo-vesical fistula.
c Diverticular disease of sigmoid colon.
   Carcinoma of colon.
   Crohn's disease.

Discussion

The commonest cause of a colo-vesical fistula is diverticular disease of the sigmoid colon. Men are five times more frequently affected than women, as the uterus is often interposed between the bladder and sigmoid. Carcinoma of the sigmoid colon is the next commonest cause. Primary bladder cancer rarely causes fistulae. Other causes include Crohn's disease, tuberculosis of the ileocaecal region or bladder, bilharzia (schistosomiasis) and calculous disease. Symptoms of a colo-vesical fistula include dysuria, frequency, haematuria, pneumaturia and faecuria. A colo-vesical fistula is one of the causes of gas in the bladder on a plain radiograph.

QUESTION 127

This 54-year-old woman has back pain, loin pain and haematuria.

a What abnormality is shown?
b What is the most likely diagnosis?
c What three investigations would you consider?

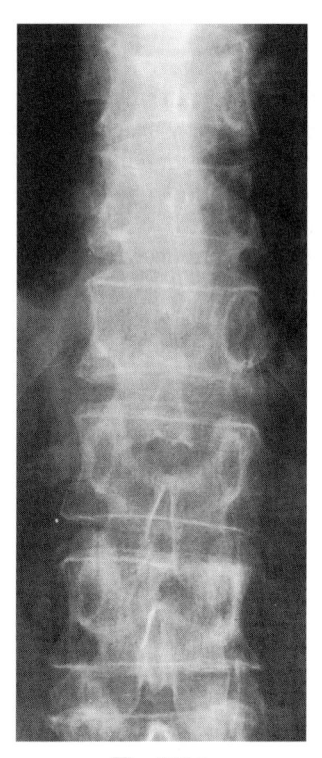

Fig. 127.1

ANSWER 127

a Absent right pedicle of T12 vertebra.
b Metastasis from hypernephroma.
c Isotope bone scan.
   Chest radiograph.
   Ultrasound or CT of the kidneys.

Discussion

Primary tumours which classically metastasize to bone are from the breast, bronchus, kidney, thyroid and prostate. Up to 80% of metastases are located in the axial skeleton and skull, and about 40% are located in the ribs. Only 20% of metastases are located in the extremities. Bone metastases from a hypernephroma are often solitary, showing rapid lytic bone expansion with a soft tissue mass. Metastases from the prostate are invariably sclerotic, from the breast they are mixed lytic and sclerotic, and from the remainder they are lytic. The loin pain and haematuria point towards a renal neoplasm as the primary. In these circumstances CT or ultrasound of the kidneys may confirm the diagnosis. CT has the added advantage of assessing the destroyed pedicle and demonstrating any associated soft tissue mass.

QUESTION 128

a What is the radiological diagnosis?
b What is the most likely cause?

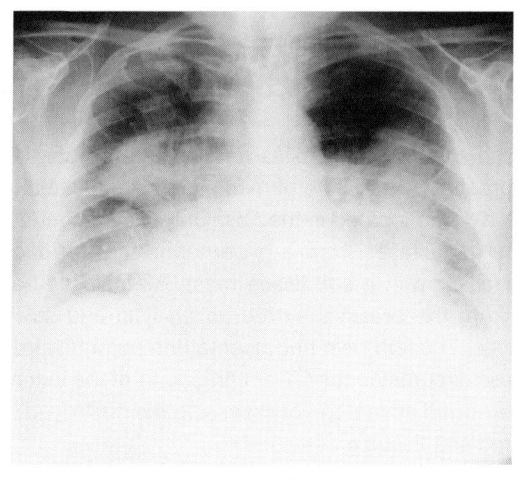

Fig. 128.1

ANSWER 128

a Alveolar (bat's-wing) pulmonary oedema.
b Left ventricular failure.

Discussion

Left ventricular failure results in pulmonary oedema because of pulmonary venous hypertension. This produces typical signs on the chest radiograph, namely upper lobe blood diversion, septal lines (Kerley B lines), pleural effusion, often with fluid in the fissures, bat's-wing air-space shadowing and cardiomegaly. Kerley B lines are not well seen in this case of severe perihilar alveolar oedema. Figure 128.2 demonstrates Kerley A and B lines. Kerley A lines radiate towards the hilar regions and B lines align perpendicular to the lateral chest wall. Kerley lines represent engorged lymphatics.

Cardiomegaly, the predominantly perihilar nature of the oedema and pleural effusions are the major features that are absent in non-cardiogenic pulmonary oedema (ARDS).

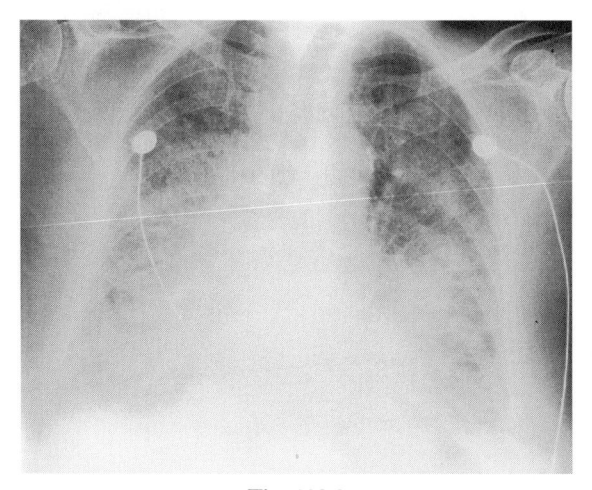

Fig. 128.2
Chest radiograph. Interstitial and alveolar pulmonary oedema. Prominent Kerley A and B lines, cardiomegaly and perihilar alveolar oedema.

QUESTION 129

A 24-year-old woman complains of chest pain after gastroscopy.
a What complication has occurred?
b How would you manage the patient?

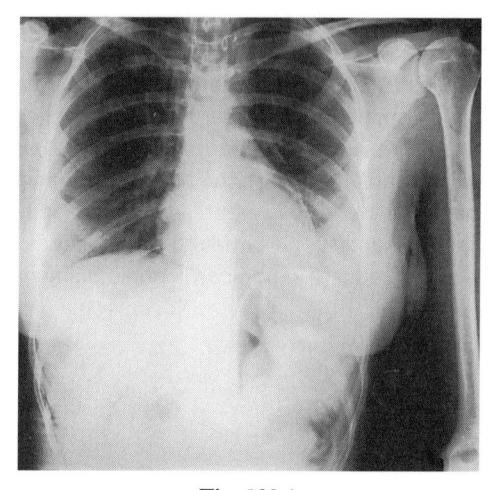

Fig. 129.1

Answer 129

a Oesophageal rupture.
b Nil by mouth.
   Intravenous antibiotics.
   Primary surgical repair if conservative measures fail.

Discussion

Figure 129.1 shows pneumomediastinum as a linear lucency of air paralleling the cardiac contour. This is demarcated laterally by a thin pleural line. Air has tracked through the diaphragm into the retroperitoneal spaces. The medial end of the left hemidiaphragm meets the descending thoracic aorta, forming a triangular lucency projected over the heart shadow.

Other causes of pneumomediastinum are as follows.

Spontaneous causes include:

- oesophageal neoplasm;
- tracheal neoplasm;
- asthma;
- aspiration pneumonia;
- vomiting/coughing;
- diabetic ketoacidosis (DKA).

Traumatic causes include:

- bronchial rupture;
- oesophageal rupture (DKA, alcoholics, violent vomiting, Boerhaave's syndrome);
- endoscopy (gastroscopy, bronchoscopy);
- positive pressure ventilation;
- mediastinoscopy;
- central venous cannulation.

QUESTION 130

A 53-year-old man, previously well, develops sudden cardiac failure 5 days after an extensive myocardial infarct.

a What does the echocardiogram show?
b What is the diagnosis?
c How would you treat this condition?

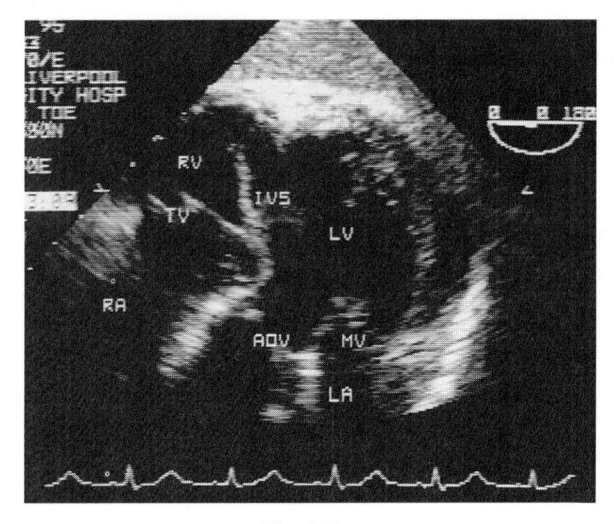

Fig. 130.1

Answer 130

a There is separation of the interventricular septum (IVS) from the myocardial wall.
b Acute septal rupture following myocardial infarction.
c Surgical repair.

Discussion

Rupture of the interventricular septum complicates up to 2% of all myocardial infarcts. It occurs between 4 and 21 days following infarction and presents with heart failure. There is right-sided enlargement of the heart and plethoric lungs due to a left-to-right shunt. Unlike rupture of a papillary muscle, pulmonary oedema is not a prominent feature. Rupture of the interventricular septum carries a high mortality unless it is treated surgically.

QUESTION 131

A 54-year-old woman presents with pyramidal signs in the right leg.

a What investigation has been performed?
b What abnormality is shown?
c Give the most likely diagnosis.

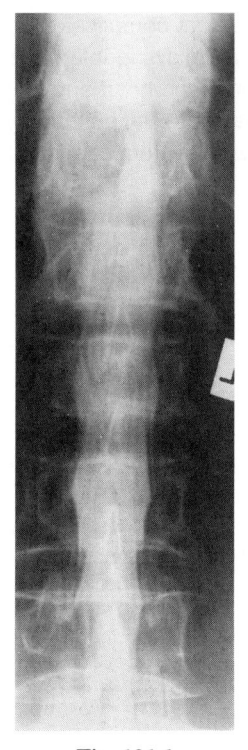

Fig. 131.1

Answer 131

a Lumbar myelogram.
b Extradural mass on the right side at T11 level.
c Spinal meningioma.

Discussion

Spinal meningiomas classically occur in middle-aged females; 80% occur in the thoracic spine and arise on the lateral aspect of the spinal canal. They may be intradural extramedullary or extradural, or a combination of both. They may present with myelopathy or radiculopathy, depending on their size and position. Meningiomas may calcify (Fig. 131.2) or may have the same attenuation as muscle, with marked contrast enhancement.

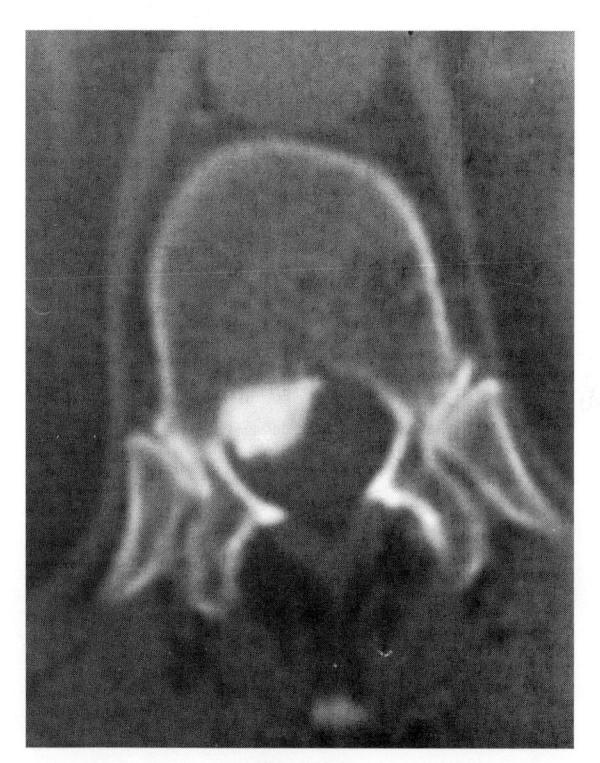

Fig. 131.2
Axial CT T11 on bone window. There is calcified meningioma arising from the right anterolateral aspect of the spinal canal. Note the compression on the cord.

Question 132

A 12-month-old boy develops vomiting and a palpable mass in the abdomen.

a   What procedure is this?
b   What is the diagnosis?
c   List three causes of this condition.

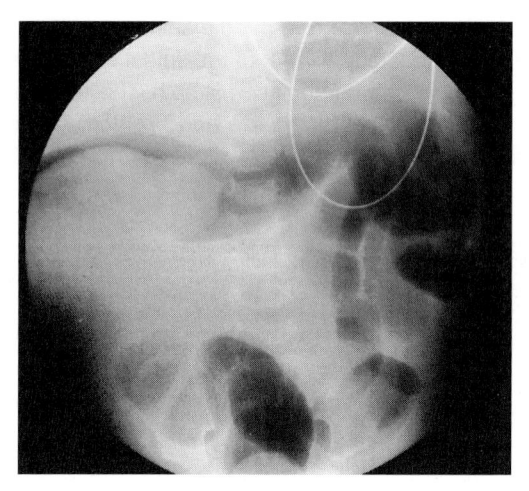

Fig. 132.1

Answer 132

a Pneumatic reduction of ileo-colic intussusception.
b Ileo-colic intussusception.
c Idiopathic (95%).
   Meckel's diverticulum.
   Polyp.
   Enterogenous cyst.
   Henoch–Schönlein purpura.

Discussion

Intussusception is the invagination of a segment of bowel within the lumen of contiguous bowel. It tends to occur in children aged between 6 months and 2 years, and is commonly idiopathic (thought to be lymphoid hyperplasia associated with viral infection). If an intussusception occurs before 6 months or after 2 years of age, a specific cause should be ruled out. Local small bowel pathology such as Meckel's diverticulum may act as a lead point and precipitate ileo-colic intussusception. Ileo-ileal and colo-colic intussusceptions are very rare. Patients present with abdominal pain, vomiting, abdominal mass and, classically, 'redcurrant jelly' stools. Hydrostatic or pneumatic reduction can be attempted by instilling air, oxygen or barium via the rectum under pressure. Figure 132.1 shows the column of oxygen (in this case) outlining the intussusception, which appears as a soft tissue mass in the right flank. Reduction should never be attempted if there is free peritoneal air, peritonism or hypovolaemia.

QUESTION 133

a What type of arthropathy is present?
b What alternative might you consider?

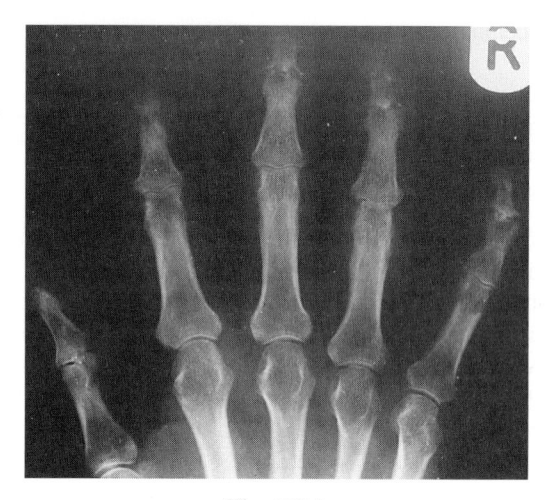

Fig. 133.1

Answer 133

a Psoriatic arthropathy.
b Erosive osteoarthritis.

Discussion

Psoriatic arthropathy is relatively uncommon, affecting less than 5% of patients with psoriasis. Joint changes may pre-date skin changes in a minority of patients. Psoriatic arthropathy is a disease of synovium and ligamentous attachments and is characterized by asymmetrical erosion in the distal interphalangeal (DIP) joints of the hands and feet. Characteristically, severe erosive change in the DIP joints results in 'pencil-in-cup' deformities (Fig. 133.2). New bone proliferation occurs at sites of ligamentous insertions.

Psoriatic arthropathy is usually distinguishable radiologically from rheumatoid arthritis in the hands and feet because the latter is usually bilaterally symmetrical, typically affects proximal interphalangeal and metacarpophalangeal joints, and is characterized by marginal erosions. Absorption of the terminal phalangeal tufts sometimes occurs in psoriatic arthropathy, and is associated with nail dystrophy.

Ankylosing spondylitis and sacro-iliitis may complicate psoriatic arthropathy. Like rheumatoid disease, arthritis mutilans may be a feature of psoriatic arthropathy.

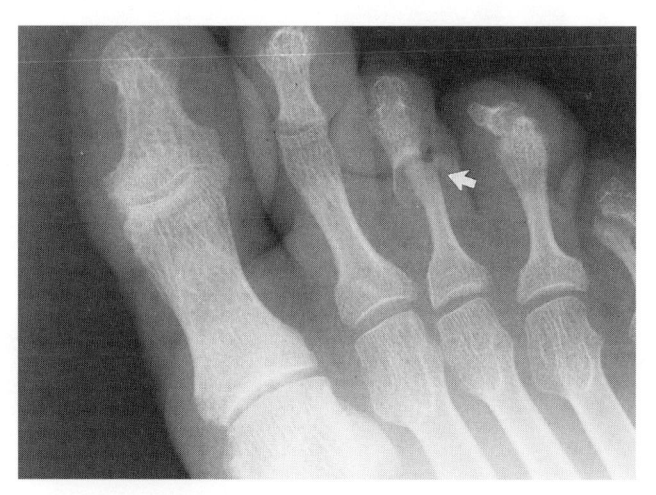

Fig. 133.2
Psoriatic arthropathy. 'Pencil-in-cup' deformity (arrow).

Question 134

This 56-year-old woman with bladder cancer and impaired renal function develops acute left loin pain and fever.

a What is shown on ultrasound examination of the left kidney?
b What treatment is necessary?

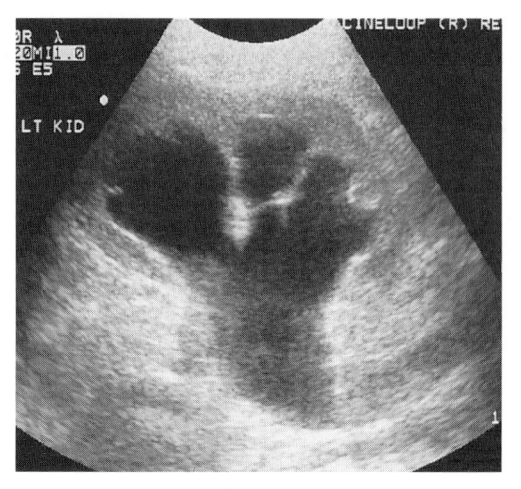

Fig. 134.1

Answer 134

a Gross hydronephrosis.
b Urgent nephrostomy left kidney.
  Elective nephrostomy right kidney.

Discussion

Hydronephrosis is dilatation of the collecting system, and it may be acute or chronic. Bladder cancer results in chronic hydronephrosis which is most likely to be bilateral, given the known renal impairment. The triad of hydronephrosis, loin pain and fever always requires an urgent nephrostomy to relieve a pyonephrosis (infected hydronephrosis). The right kidney needs to be decompressed in order to improve renal function whilst the contralateral kidney is recovering from sepsis.

On ultrasound, the dilated collecting system appears echo poor because it contains urine. Pyonephrosis is a clinical diagnosis, and may be indistinguishable from non-infected hydronephrosis on ultrasound.

Acute causes of hydronephrosis are:

- ureteric calculus;
- ureteric blood clot;
- inadvertent ligation at surgery;
- normal pregnancy;
- ureteral oedema following surgery.

Chronic causes may be congenital or acquired. Acquired causes are:

- ureteric neoplasms;
- ureteric strictures;
- benign prostatic cancer;
- retroperitoneal fibrosis;
- neurogenic bladder;
- bladder cancer;
- prostatic cancer;
- cervical cancer;
- pelvic mass (ovarian cancer, lymphoma);
- urethral strictures.

QUESTION 135

This is a frontal tomogram of the cervical spine in a 35-year-old woman.

a What abnormality is shown?
b What is the diagnosis?
c List four associated features in this condition.

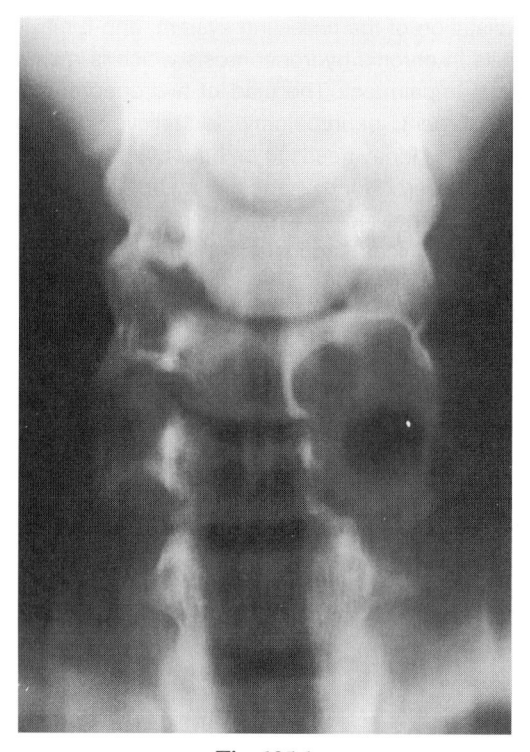

Fig. 135.1

Answer 135

a Enlargement of several bilateral intervertebral foramina due to 'dumb-bell' paraspinal neurofibromas.
b Neurofibromatosis.
c Optic and cerebral gliomas.
  Cranial nerve schwannomas (especially Vth, VIIIth).
  Plexiform neurofibromas.
  Meningiomas.
  Café-au-lait spots (more than five).
  Axillary freckling.
  Lateral thoracic meningoceles.
  Scoliosis.
  Ribbon-ribs and other bone dysplasia.
  Pulmonary fibrosis.
  Phaeochromocytomas.
  Parathyroid adenomas.
  Mucosal neurofibromas in the gastrointestinal tract.
  Lisch nodules (hamartomas) of the iris.

Discussion

'Dumb-bell' neurofibromas of spinal nerves are slow-growing neoplasms which can become large enough to cause cord compression. They slowly expand intervertebral foramina, producing characteristic appearances (Fig. 135.1). They may occur at any level, giving rise to muscle wasting and sensory loss. They may undergo malignant change (up to 16%). There are characteristic MRI features of intradural neurofibromas (Fig. 135.2a).

Neurofibromatosis is peripheral (type 1) in 90% of cases and in the remainder it is central (type 2). Peripheral neurofibromatosis or von Recklinghausen's disease (Fig.135.2b) is an autosomal dominant mesodermal dysplasia with systemic involvement. In contrast, central neurofibromatosis is characterized by a tendency to develop multiple Schwannomas, meningiomas and ependymomas. There is a predisposition to develop bilateral acoustic neuromas. Unlike peripheral neurofibromatosis, there is an absence (or reduced number) of many of the systemic features. Like the peripheral form, central neurofibromatosis is also an autosomal dominant disorder.

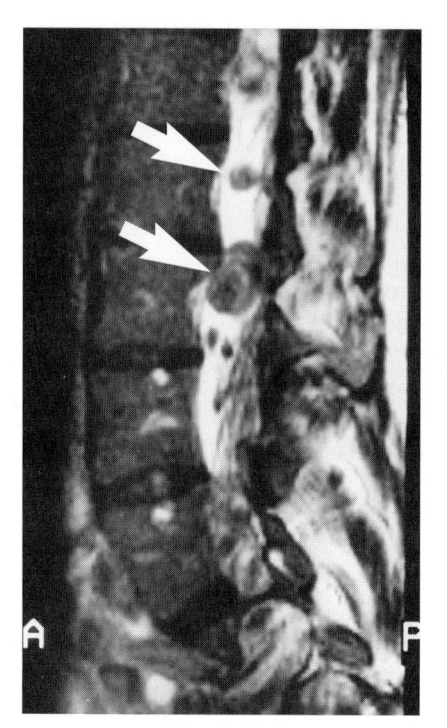

Fig. 135.2a
T2-weighted sagittal image of lumbar spine. Multiple 'dumb-bell' neurofibromas. Note the white CSF. The neurofibromas (arrows) have classical intermediate signal peripheries and low-signal cores.

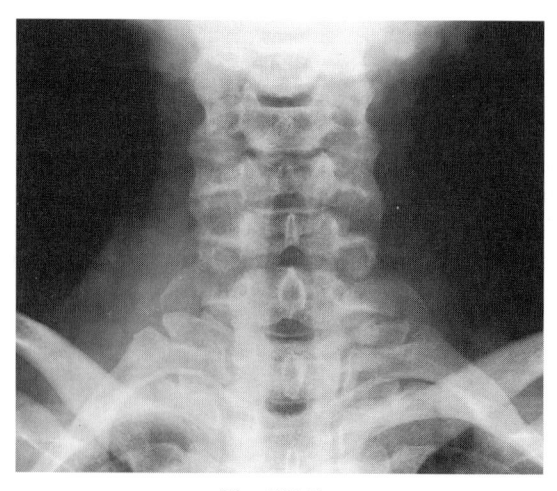

Fig. 135.2b
Cervical spine. Peripheral neurofibromatosis. Note multiple subcutaneous nodules.

QUESTION 136

A 30-year-old woman has epilepsy.

a What two abnormalities are shown on this unenhanced abdominal CT?
b What is the diagnosis?
c List four associated features in this condition.

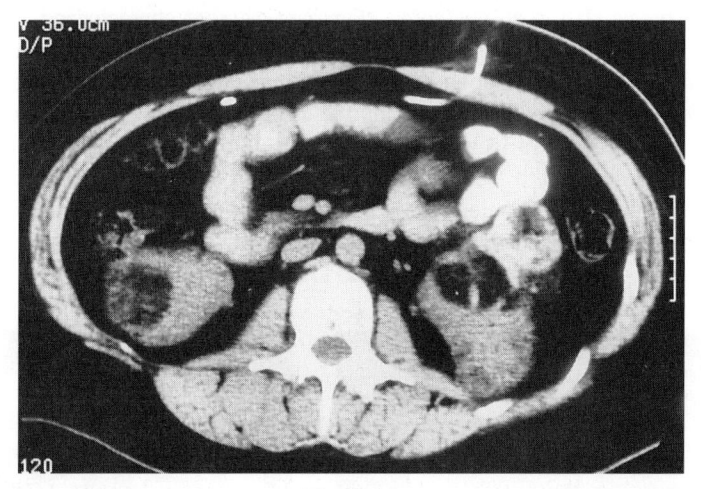

Fig. 136.1

ANSWER 136

a Fatty (low-attenuation) tumours in both kidneys (angiomyolipomas).
Intra-abdominal tubing (ventriculo-peritoneal shunt).
b Tuberous sclerosis complicated by hydrocephalus.
c Adenoma sebaceum.
Low IQ.
Fits (myoclonic).
Subependymal hamartomas.
Cortical hamartomas (tubers).
Giant cell astrocytoma.
Demyelination.
Ash-leaf patches.
Shagreen patches.
Subungual fibromas.

Café-au-lait spots.
Retinal hamartomas.
Renal angiomyolipomas.
Renal cysts.
Honeycomb lung (lymphangioleiomyomatosis).
Subendocardial rhabdomyoma.
Bone sclerosis.

Discussion

Tuberous sclerosis (TS) is an autosomal dominant disorder characterized by adenoma sebaceum, mental retardation and seizures. The central nervous system and almost every other system are involved. Subependymal hamartomas (Fig. 136.2a), found along the ventricular surface of both lateral ventricles, tend to calcify with time. Giant cell astrocytomas are serious complications of TS and occur in up to 15% of cases. They obstruct CSF flow from the lateral ventricles to the third ventricle, causing obstructive hydrocephalus (Fig. 136.2b). This patient has been treated with a ventriculoperitoneal shunt. Angiomyolipomas are renal tumours composed of three elements – fat, blood vessels and muscle. They occur in approximately 40% of cases of TS, and tend to be bilateral and multiple.

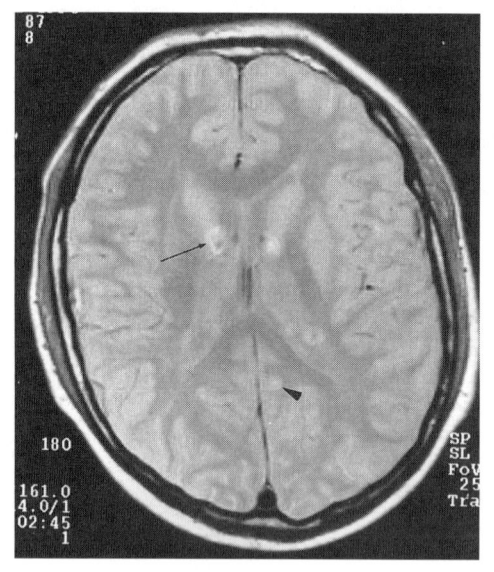

Fig. 136.2a
MR brain. Proton density sequence. Tuberous sclerosis. Multiple subependymal hamartomas (arrow) and cortical hamartoma (arrowhead).

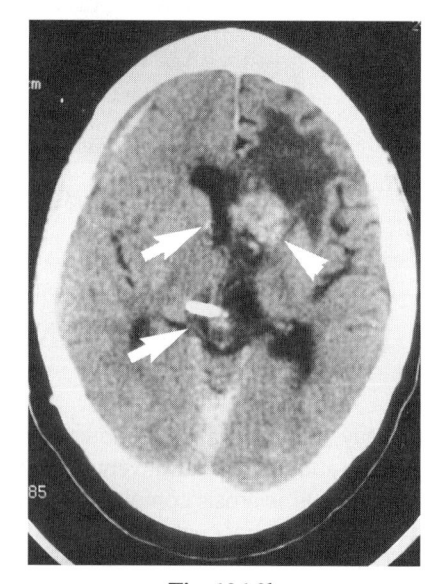

Fig. 136.2b
CT brain. Tuberous sclerosis. There is a ventricular shunt *in situ* (lower arrow) and a large subependymal nodule (arrowhead) near the foramen of Munro. Note also the small, calcified subependymal nodule on the ventricular surface of the right caudate nucleus (upper arrow).

QUESTION 137

An 80-year-old woman complains of intermittent rectal bleeding.
a What investigation is shown?
b What is the abnormality?
c What alternative investigation may identify a source of bleeding?

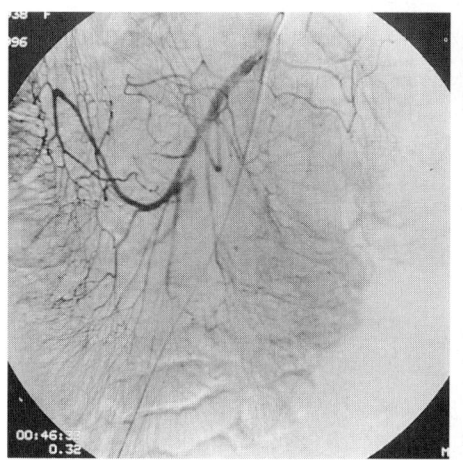

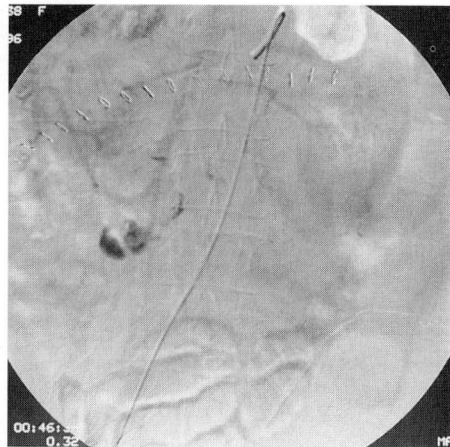

Fig. 137.1a

Fig. 137.1b

ANSWER 137

a Superior mesenteric arteriogram.
b Bleeding from a branch of the superior mesenteric artery.
c Red-cell-labelled isotope scan.
   Colonoscopy.
   Barium enema.

Discussion

Gastrointestinal bleeding has an overall mortality of approximately 10%, and is especially high in the elderly.

Upper gastrointestinal bleeding is usually investigated by endoscopy.

Lower gastrointestinal bleeding, defined as bleeding distal to the duodeno-jejunal junction, can be investigated in a number of ways.

Sustained bleeding is best demonstrated by mesenteric angiography. This technique requires blood loss of 1 mL/minute in order to give a positive result. Frequently blood loss is intermittent, and a negative result will be obtained if angiography is performed when bleeding has stopped. Isotope red cell scanning is useful for intermittent bleeding and may even detect blood loss at a rate of 0.5 mL/minute. It is more sensitive than mesenteric angiography, but less specific. The patient's own red blood cells are labelled with Tc-99m *in vitro* and reinjected intravenously. When bleeding is active, tracer accumulates over time (Fig. 137.2a) at the site of abnormality. Images may be obtained for up to 36 hours, giving a further advantage over mesenteric angiography.

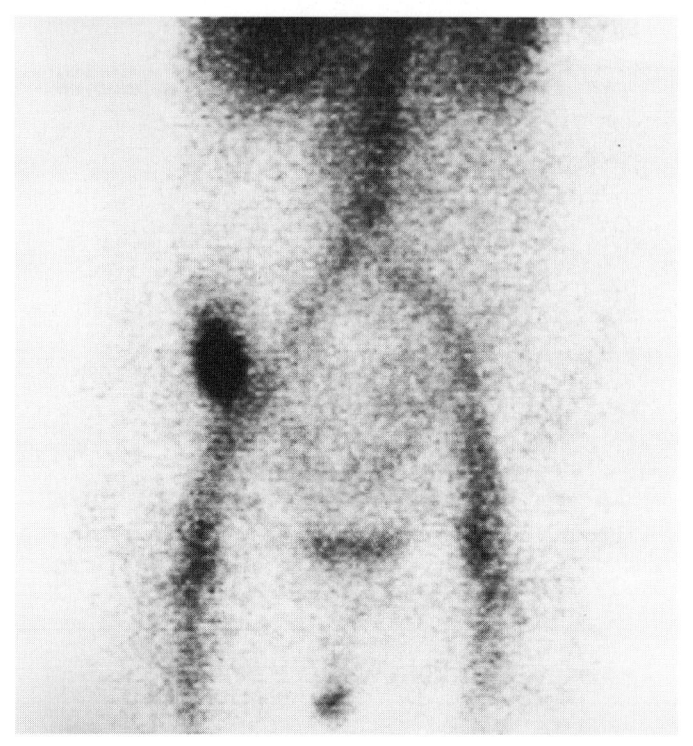

Fig. 137.2a
Tc-99m red blood cell scan. There is accumulation of tracer in the right flank conforming to the caecum/ascending colon region. Note the tracer activity in the liver, spleen, bladder and aorto-iliac vessels.

Table 137.1 Causes of gastrointestinal bleeding

Small bowel	Large bowel
Tumour	Diverticula
Ulceration	Angiodysplasia
Diverticulum	Colitis
Vascular malformation	Tumours
Visceral aneurysm	

Colonoscopy may occasionally be necessary, especially if bleeding is chronic and structural pathology is suspected. As a general rule, barium studies are reserved for those cases where angiography or isotope studies are deemed unnecessary. Barium will interfere with the interpretation of both of these tests. Figure 137.2b shows caecal angiodysplasia diagnosed on a mesenteric arteriogram.

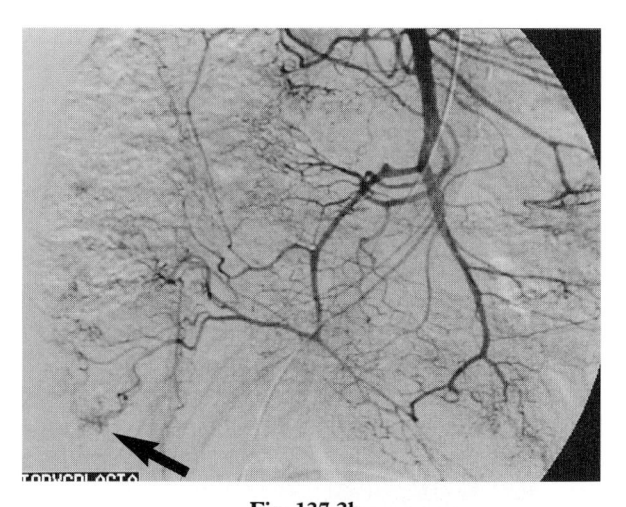

Fig. 137.2b
Superior mesenteric arteriogram in another patient showing angiodysplasia of the caecal pole (arrow).

QUESTION 138

This is a longitudinal ultrasound scan through the right lobe of the liver in a 63-year-old woman.

a What abnormality is shown?
b List the three most likely causes in a woman of this age.

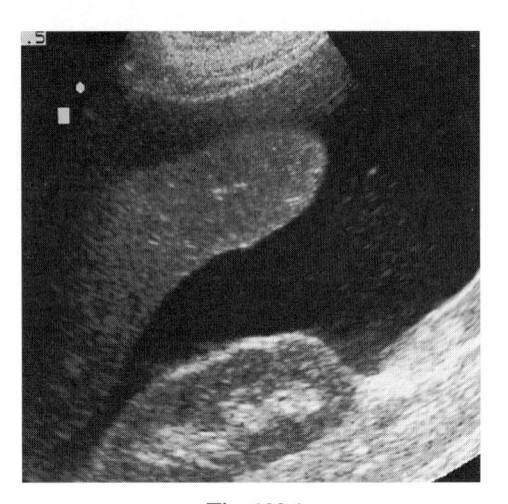

Fig. 138.1

ANSWER 138

a Ascites.
b Malignancy.
   Hypoalbuminaemia.
   Congestive cardiac failure.
   Cirrhosis and portal hypertension.

Discussion

Ascites causes an echo-poor or black image on ultrasound. Early ascites accumulates in the pelvis, but moderate to severe ascites causes bulging flanks and will be easily seen on ultrasound. Figure 138.1 demonstrates ascitic fluid around the liver and in the right subhepatic space (Morison's pouch) anterior to the right kidney. Note that the echoes beyond the ascites are 'bright'. This occurs because sound waves are relatively unimpeded as they travel through water, causing 'acoustic enhancement', which is also nicely demonstrated when examining the gallbladder (Fig. 87.1a).

QUESTION 139

a What investigation is this?
b What abnormality is shown?
c What is the most likely diagnosis?

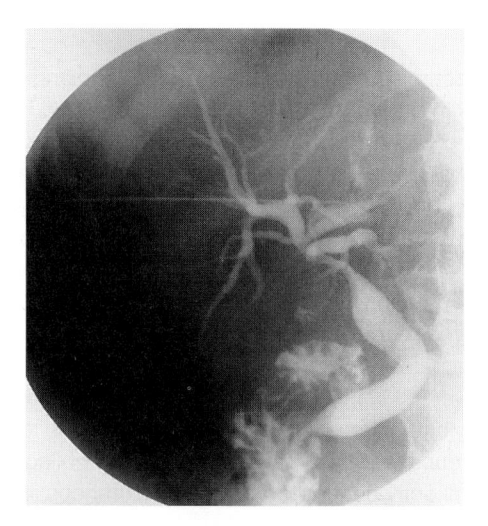

Fig. 139.1

Answer 139

a Percutaneous transhepatic cholangiogram (PTC).
b Stricture involving the junction of the common hepatic and common bile ducts.
c Extrahepatic cholangiocarcinoma (bile duct carcinoma).

Discussion

Extrahepatic cholangiocarcinoma represents 90% of all cholangiocarcinomas. It is common in the Far East, with a slight male predisposition and occurring mainly in the sixth decade of life. Typical presentations include intermittent painless jaundice, cholangitis, weight loss, tender hepatomegaly and elevated bilirubin and alkaline phosphatase. The tumour is commonly exophytic and occurs frequently in the distal common bile duct and common hepatic duct. Tumours may spread to periductal, coeliac and peripancreatic lymph nodes, liver and peritoneum. The prognosis is very poor unless it involves the ampulla of Vater, when presentation is earlier with jaundice.

There are a number of conditions that predispose to extrahepatic cholangiocarcinoma, including inflammatory bowel disease, sclerosing cholangitis, Crohn's disease, *Clonorchis sinensis* (liver fluke) infection, choledochal cysts and gallstones.

Intrahepatic cholangiocarcinoma is a term used to describe lesions which arise from small intrahepatic bile ducts. Lesions may be diffuse, resembling sclerosing cholangitis, or nodular. It carries a slightly better prognosis than extrahepatic cholangiocarcinoma.

Question 140

This man had his right arm amputated 12 months earlier.

a What abnormalities are shown on his chest radiograph?
b What is the most likely diagnosis?
c What might an isotope bone scan demonstrate?

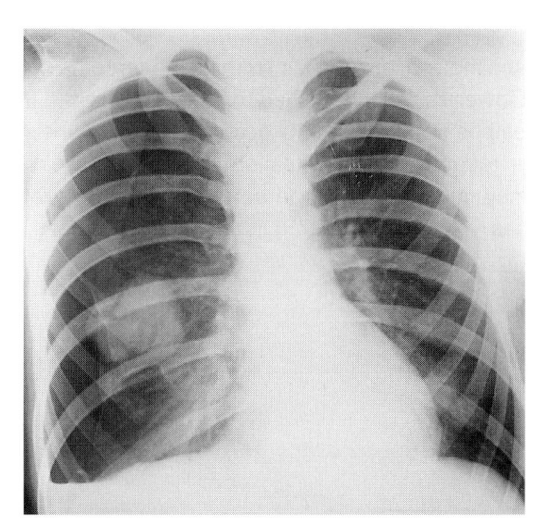

Fig. 140.1

ANSWER 140

a Large mass in right mid-zone. Cavitating mass in right lower zone. Right-sided hydropneumothorax.
b Osteosarcoma of right arm with pulmonary metastases.
c Absent tracer activity in right arm region. Tracer uptake within pulmonary masses.

Discussion

Cavitation may complicate a metastasis from osteosarcoma. This is shown in the deposit in the right lower zone, and has led to pneumothorax in this case. Pulmonary metastases from osteosarcoma tend to occur at the periphery of the lungs, and pneumothorax is a recognized complication. Metastases from osteosarcoma and chondrosarcoma may calcify. An isotope bone scan demonstrates increased tracer activity in metastases from osteosarcoma in up to 40% of cases, due to osteoblastic activity.

QUESTION 141

A 56-year-old woman with general malaise has prominent carotid pulses.

a What abnormality is shown on this echocardiogram?
b What is the diagnosis?
c What is the treatment?

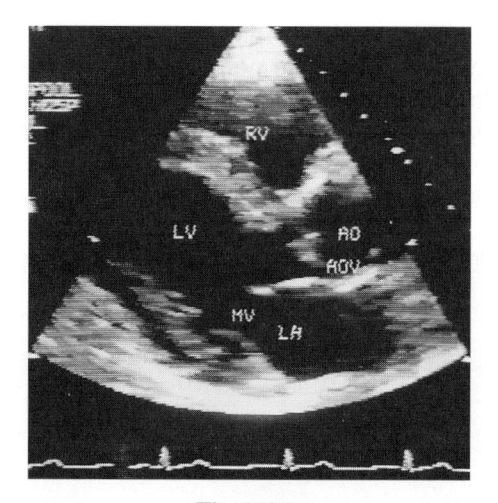

Fig. 141.1

Answer 141

a Vegetations on the aortic valve.
b Infective endocarditis.
c Benzypenicillin (intravenous).

Discussion

This parasternal echocardiogram demonstrates vegetations on the aortic valve, signifying endocarditis. Vegetations appear as mobile masses with a shaggy outline, and are often associated with valvular regurgitation. This explains the prominent carotid pulsations (Corrigan's sign) in this patient. Transthoracic echocardiography will demonstrate vegetations in 70% of cases, increasing to 80% when a transoesophageal study is performed. A negative echocardiogram does not exclude the diagnosis.

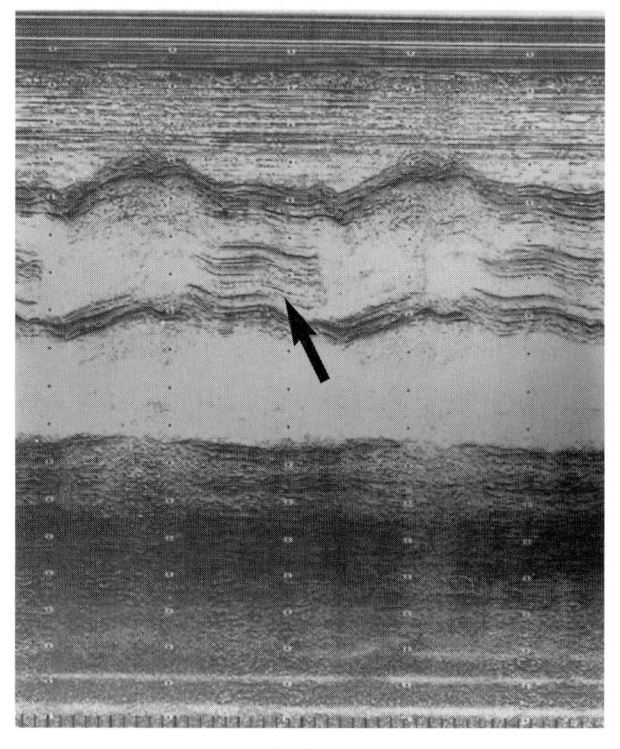

Fig. 141.2
Infective endocarditis. M-mode echocardiogram demonstrating vegetations on the aortic valve (arrow).

QUESTION 142

This is an isotope bone scan in a 60-year-old man.

a What is the most likely diagnosis?
b How do you explain photopenia in the renal areas?

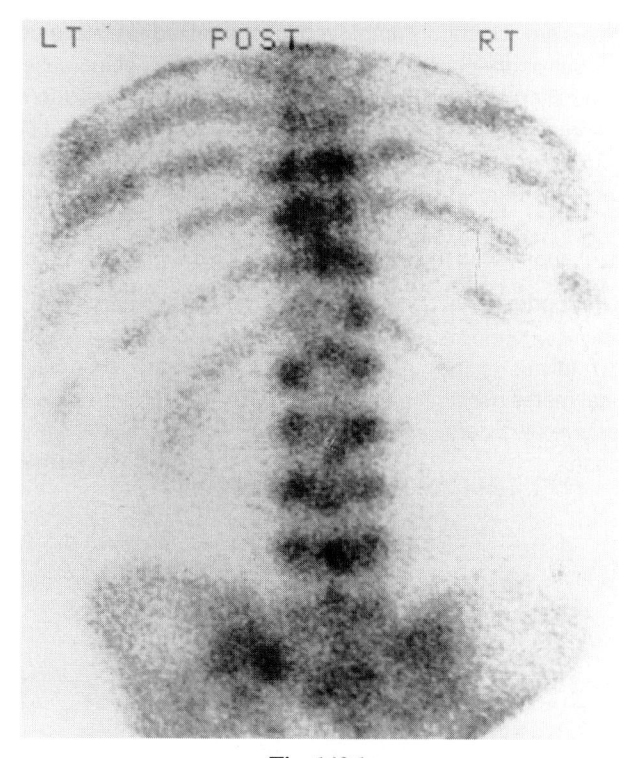

Fig. 142.1

Answer 142

a Multiple bone metastases.
b 'Super scan' effect.

Discussion

Isotope bone scans are commonly employed for suspected skeletal metastases, having a 95% sensitivity but poor specificity. Multiple scattered foci of increased tracer activity in the ribs are virtually diagnostic of metastases. Rib fractures tend to be symmetrical, very focal and aligned in a linear fashion. In a normal individual, about 50% of the radiotracer (Tc-99m-MDP) is excreted via the kidneys. When there is markedly increased bone turnover there is relative photopenia in the renal areas, producing the so-called 'super scan'.

Other causes of super scan include:

- renal osteodystrophy;
- osteomalacia;
- hyperparathyroidism;
- diffuse skeletal metastases;
- myeloproliferative disorders;
- Paget's disease.

QUESTION 143

A 35-year-old woman is clinically and biochemically hyperthyroid. This is her thyroid scan.

a What abnormality is shown?
b What is the most inferior hot spot?
c How should she be treated?

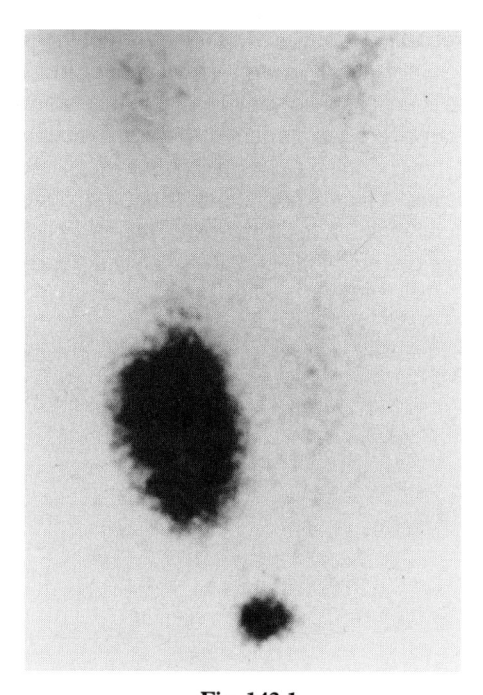

Fig. 143.1

Answer 143

a Large functioning nodule (adenoma) in the right thyroid lobe with suppression of extranodular tissue.
b The inferior 'hot spot' represents a radioactive marker at the suprasternal notch.
c Surgery.

Discussion

A solitary toxic nodule represents only 20% of the cases of thyrotoxicosis. It may present with a palpable neck lump, usually in females over the age of 40 years. Medical treatment for toxic adenomas is unsatisfactory in the long term. Radio-iodine is the treatment of choice, although in young females surgery may be desirable.

Approximately 3% of 'hot' nodules seen on technetium pertechnetate scanning are 'cold' on radio-iodine scans. A single hot nodule seen on technetium scanning should not be diagnosed as a functioning adenoma until confirmed with a radio-iodine scan or at surgery. A 'cold' nodule on radio-iodine scans is likely to represent a carcinoma.

QUESTION 144

This is a lumbar spine radiograph in a 65-year-old man.

a What two abnormalities are shown?
b What is the diagnosis?
c What is the commonest mode of presentation in this disorder?

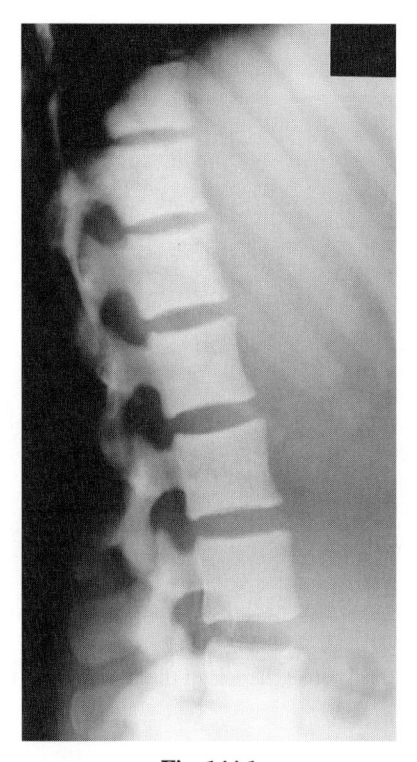

Fig. 144.1

ANSWER 144

a Diffuse osteosclerosis.
  Splenomegaly.
b Myelofibrosis.
c Anaemia.

Discussion

There are multiple 'ivory vertebrae' on the lateral lumbar spine film. See Answer 104 for further details on myelofibrosis.

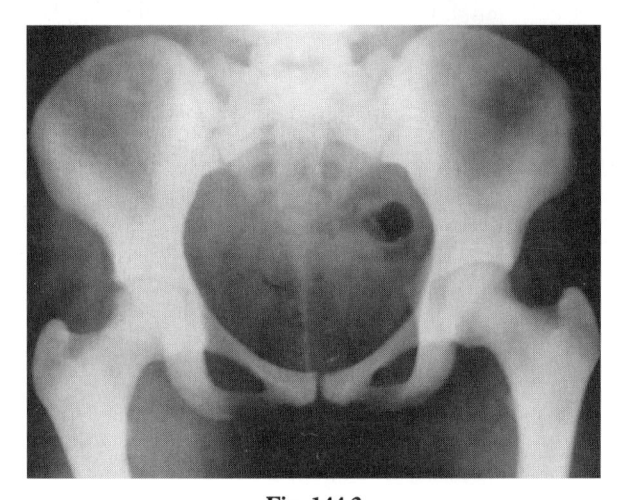

Fig. 144.2
Myelofibrosis. Generalized osteosclerosis of the pelvis. Note the loss of trabeculae.

QUESTION 145

This 42-year-old diabetic has a sterile pyuria.

a What is the diagnosis?
b List four other causes of this condition.
c Name two complications.

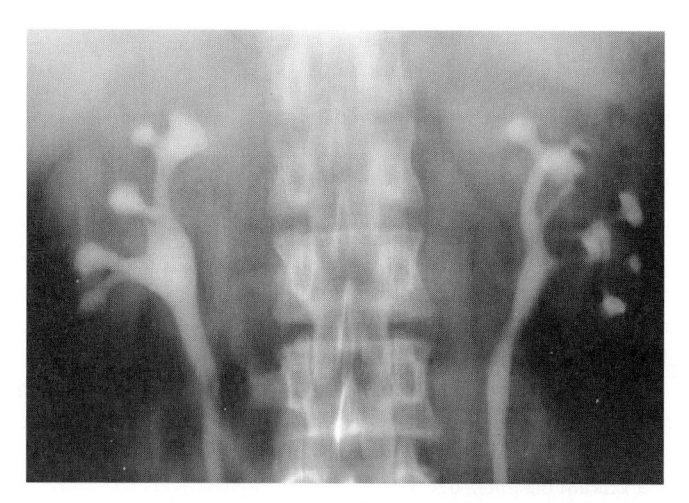

Fig. 145.1

Answer 145

a Renal papillary necrosis.
b Analgesic nephropathy.
  Pyelonephritis.
  Obstruction.
  Sickle cell disease/trait.
  Alcohol.
  Infants in shock.
c Ureteric colic from sloughed papilla.
  Hypertension.

Discussion

Renal papillary necrosis (RPN) is due to ischaemic necrosis of the papilla secondary to vascular obstruction or interstitial nephritis. It has many causes, listed above. Figure 145.1 demonstrates clubbing of the calyces on the right side. Pools of contrast medium adjacent to mid and lower pole calyces in the left kidney signify necrosed papillae.

RPN is an important diagnosis to make. It is essential to look closely at the bones for clues to the underlying cause. For example, central end-plate depression in sclerotic vertebrae suggests sickle cell disease. A calcified pancreas in association with RPN may have three causes – alcohol related, diabetes related or analgesic related (chronic pancreatitis is a painful condition).

There is a mnemonic to remind you of the causes of RPN: **ADIPOSE** (after Chapman, S. and Nakielny, R. 1995: *Aids to Radiological Differential Diagnosis*. 3rd edn. London: Saunders).

    A-   Analgesics
    D-   Diabetes
    I-   Infantile shock
    P-   Pyelonephritis
    O-   Obstruction
    S-   Sickle cell disease
    E-   Ethanol

QUESTION 146

This plain abdominal radiograph is from a 30-year-old woman being investigated for haematuria. She is normocalcaemic and her kidneys are slightly enlarged.

a What descriptive term is used for this appearance?
b What is the diagnosis?
c What are the other causes of this appearance?

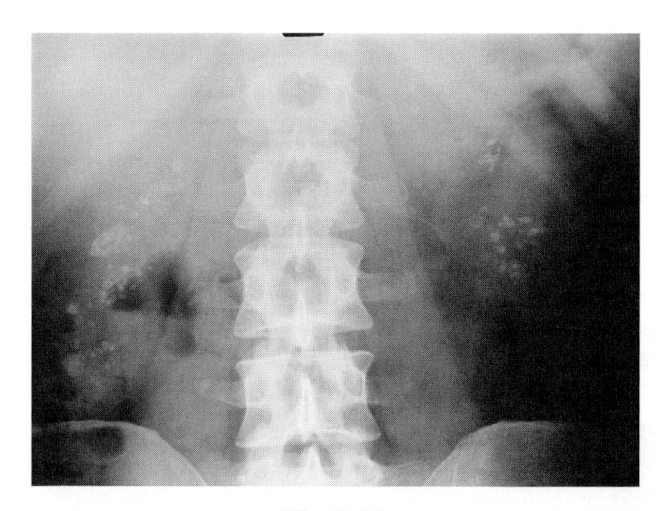

Fig. 146.1

Answer 146

a Nephrocalcinosis.
b Medullary sponge kidney (MSK).
c Hyperparathyroidism.
  Renal tubular acidosis.
  Idiopathic hypercalcuria.
  Renal papillary necrosis.
  Hypercalcaemia: milk alkali syndrome; sarcoidosis; idiopathic hypercalcaemia,
  Primary hyperoxaluria.

Discussion

Medullary sponge kidney (MSK) is a congenital anomaly characterized by cystic dilatation of the collecting tubules of the medullary pyramids. It presents in adults of any age and may be focal or diffuse, unilateral (25%) or bilateral (75%). It is frequently asymptomatic or may be associated with urinary colic, haematuria or infection. Cigar-shaped calculi develop within the dilated tubules (Fig. 146.1). The kidneys are often enlarged. There is a medullary 'blush' following intravenous contrast medium, well demonstrated in Fig. 146.2. MSK may be associated with hypercalciuria. The plasma calcium is normal.

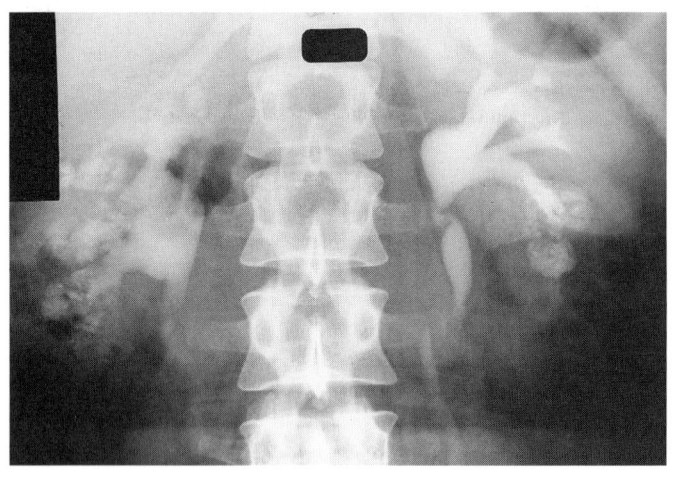

Fig. 146.2
Medullary sponge kidney. Pyelogram. Note the medullary 'blush' in the right kidney.

QUESTION 147

This is a contrast-enhanced abdominal CT in a 58-year-old man with an epigastric mass following an episode of severe abdominal pain. Water-soluble contrast medium (Gastrografin) fills the gastric antrum (arrow).

a What abnormality is labelled with curved arrows?
b Name one additional abnormality.
c What is the most likely underlying cause?

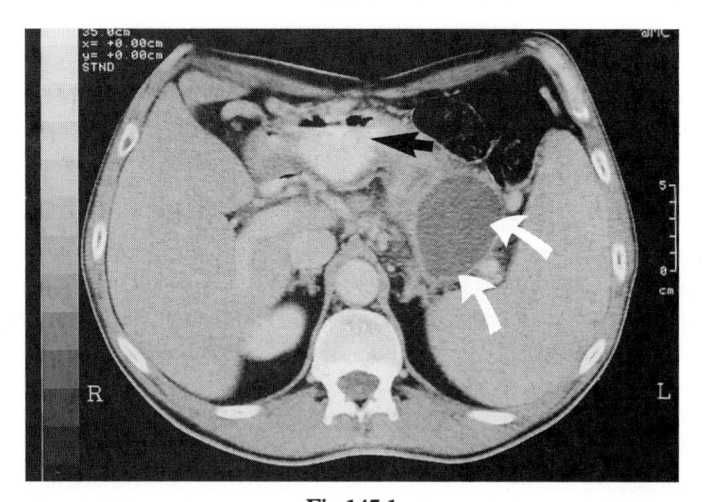

Fig 147.1

Answer 147

a Pancreatic pseudocyst.
b Splenomegaly. Varices.
c Alcohol excess.

Discussion

A pseudocyst is a collection of pancreatic fluid arising within or adjacent to pancreatic tissue. A third of pseudocysts are extrapancreatic in location – peritoneal, retroperitoneal, intraparenchymal (hepatic, renal, splenic) and mediastinal. Pseudocysts are associated with pancreatitis, trauma and pancreatic malignancy. In acute pancreatitis, pseudocysts reach their maximum size by about 6 weeks. The majority resolve in a further 6 weeks. Pseudocysts may persist in recurrent acute or chronic pancreatitis. They are lined by a fibrous capsule and may be complicated by infection, perforation or erosion into viscera.

In this case, the finding of a pseudocyst, splenomegaly and varices makes alcohol excess with portal hypertension the most likely explanation.

Pseudocysts can be drained via a percutaneous or transgastric approach under CT or ultrasound guidance. Indications for drainage include infection, recurrent pancreatitis and pressure symptoms.

QUESTION 148

A 33-year-old man presents with acute backache. A chest radiograph demonstrates an anterior mediastinal mass.

a What abnormalities are shown on MRI of the lumbar spine?
b What is the most likely diagnosis?
c Give an alternative diagnosis.

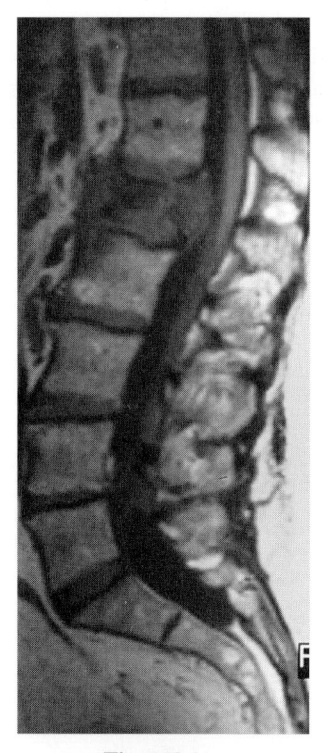

Fig. 148.1a
T1-weighted

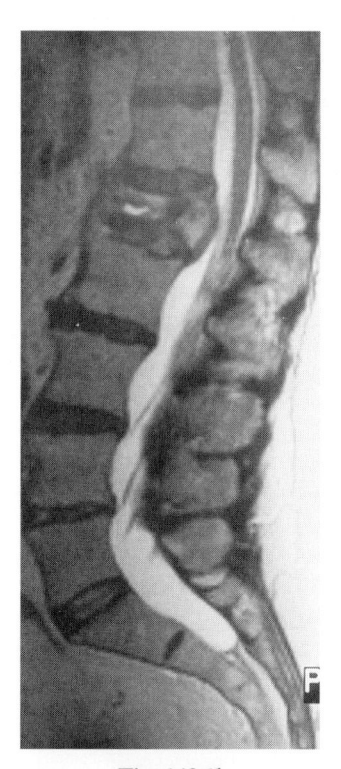

Fig. 148.1b
T2-weighted

Answer 148

a Wedge compression collapse of L1 with preservation of intervertebral discs. The vertebral body has been replaced by low signal on T1 and high signal on T2 weighting.
b Hodgkin's disease.
c Metastatic carcinoma.

Discussion

Hodgkin's disease (HD) is a very rare cause of primary bone neoplasm, being more commonly associated with primary lymph node involvement. About 20% of patients with HD have bony involvement and 75% of these occur in the axial skeleton. A solitary 'ivory' vertebral body is a typical radiographic manifestation of HD. An example of multiple ivory vertebral bodies is shown in Fig. 144.1. Typically, neoplasms of vertebral bodies cause sclerosis ('ivory vertebral body') or lysis with preservation of the disc spaces and end plates. This is unlike tuberculous or infective spondylitis, when destruction of the discs and end plates is usual.

Other causes of 'ivory' vertebral body are Paget's disease, prostatic carcinoma, lymphoma, myelofibrosis and osteoblastic metastases.

QUESTION 149

This is a supine abdominal radiograph of a 45-year-old psychiatric patient with an acute abdomen.

a What is the diagnosis?
b How is it treated?
c What other group of patients may be affected?

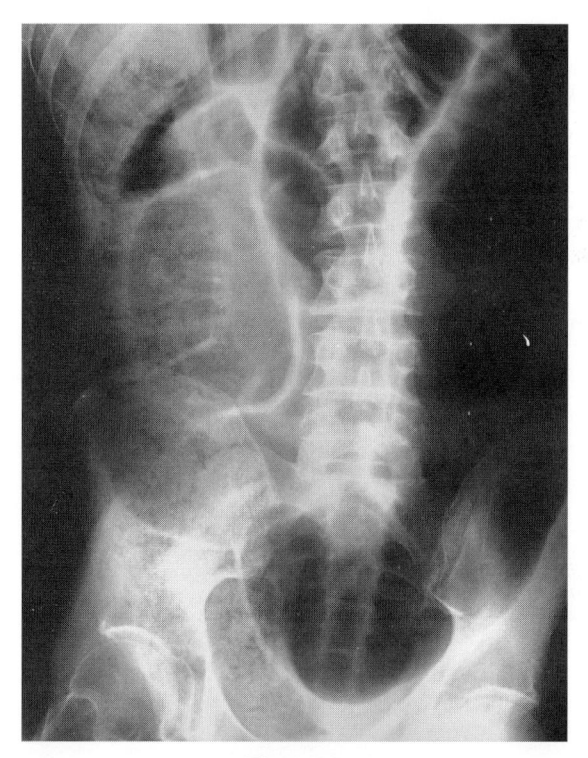

Fig. 149.1

Answer 149

a Sigmoid volvulus.
b Rectal tube insertion.
c Elderly; mentally handicapped.

Discussion

Volvulus is rotation of the large bowel in an anticlockwise direction around its mesenteric axis. The sigmoid colon is the commonest site, although the caecum may occasionally be involved. A sigmoid volvulus occurs in the elderly (in males more often than in females), mentally handicapped individuals and psychiatric patients on psychotropic drugs. Redundancy of the sigmoid colon allows it to twist on its mesentery. This process is usually chronic with acute intermittent attacks.

The dilated sigmoid loop resembles an inverted 'U' on a plain radiograph. The limbs of the loop converge in the pelvis with the apex lying over the left flank and under the left hemidiaphragm. Treatment is by insertion of a rectal tube under direct vision. Decompression is accompanied by the release of flatus and (thankfully) is invariably carried out by the surgical registrar!

QUESTION 150

This is a T1-weighted coronal MR scan of the brain following i.v. gadolinium DTPA in a 56-year-old lady with a progressive spastic paraparesis.

a What is the diagnosis?
b What might you expect to see on CT?
c List three other causes of spastic paraparesis.

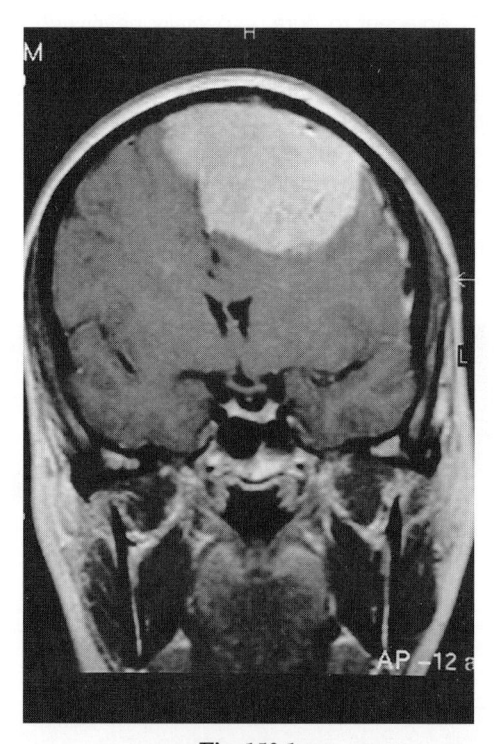

Fig. 150.1

ANSWER 150

a Large parafalcine (parasagittal) meningioma.
b Calcification within the tumour.
 Hyperostosis of the skull vault.
c Multiple sclerosis.
 Cord compression.
 Trauma.
 Cerebral palsy.

Motor neurone disease.
Subacute combined degeneration of the cord.
Tabes dorsalis.
Syringomyelia.
Anterior spinal artery thrombosis.
Friedreich's ataxia.
Hereditary spastic paraplegia.

Discussion

Meningiomas account for 15% of all primary intracranial tumours. They arise from arachnoidal cells and occur adjacent to dura, especially near venous sinuses. Other sites commonly involved are the base of the skull, cerebral convexities, greater and lesser wings of sphenoid, parasellar and parasagittal regions and posterior fossa. Rarely, meningiomas may arise from the lateral ventricles, usually the left.

A parasagittal meningioma will produce a spastic paraparesis with hypertonia, weakness, clonus and extensor plantars. Occasionally the physician may be misled into considering a cord lesion. Meningiomas are relatively slow growing, and may demonstrate internal calcification (20%) and hyperostosis of adjacent bone (18%) on CT. Meningiomas readily take up contrast medium on both CT and MRI. Calcification cannot be appreciated on MRI.

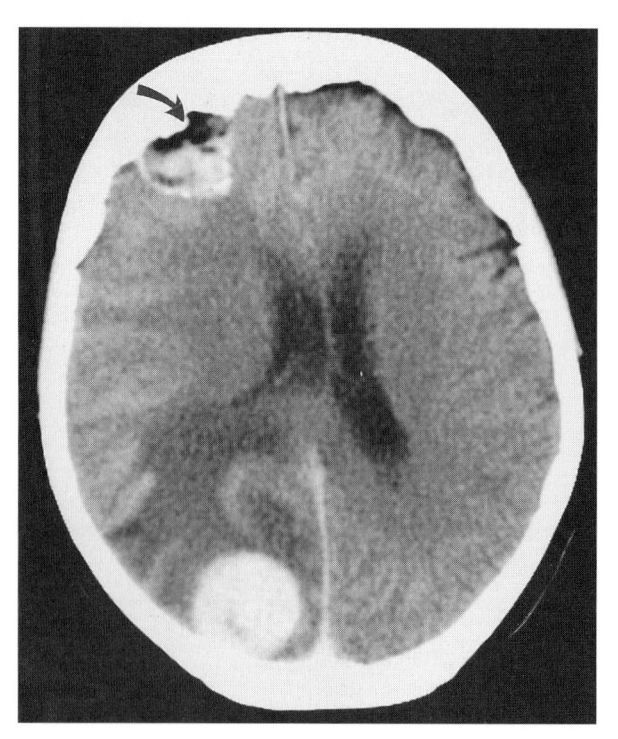

Fig. 150.2
CT brain with i.v. contrast medium. Meningioma of right occipital lobe demonstrating contrast enhancement and surrounding oedema. Note a dermoid tumour in the right frontal lobe with a fat–soft tissue interface (arrow).

QUESTION 151

This is the MRI brain scan in a comatose 53-year-old alcoholic woman.

a What abnormality is demonstrated?
b What is the diagnosis?
c What biochemical abnormality is classically associated with this condition?

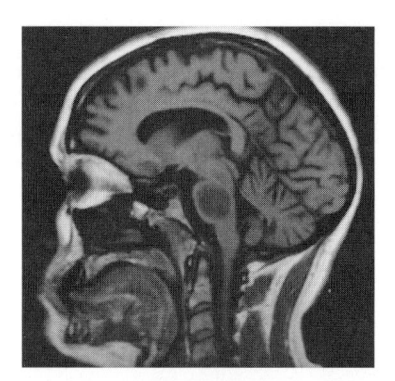

Fig. 151.1a
T1-weighted sagittal image

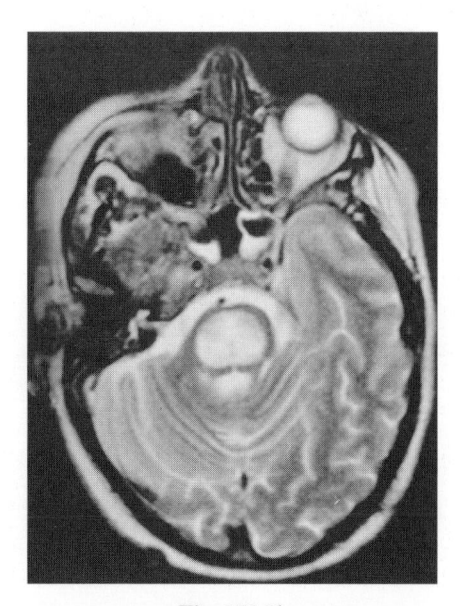

Fig. 151.1b
T1-weighted sagittal image

Answer 151

a Low-signal T1 and high-signal T2 within the pons.
b Central pontine myelinolysis.
c Rapidly corrected hyponatraemia.

Discussion

Central pontine myelinolysis (CPM) is caused by rapid correction of hyponatraemia with hypertonic saline. Myelinotoxins are released in grey matter, causing symmetrical demyelination in the pons. The patient is usually alcoholic. The initial signs of CPM are dysarthria (pseudobulbar palsy), spastic quadriparesis and eventually coma. CPM may be prevented by slow correction of hyponatraemia with isotonic saline. The prognosis is poor, but some patients have made remarkable recoveries with supportive treatment.

QUESTION 152

This is an unenhanced CT scan of the brain in a 75-year-old man with impaired visual fields.

a What abnormality is shown?
   What is the diagnosis?
b What visual field defect does he have?

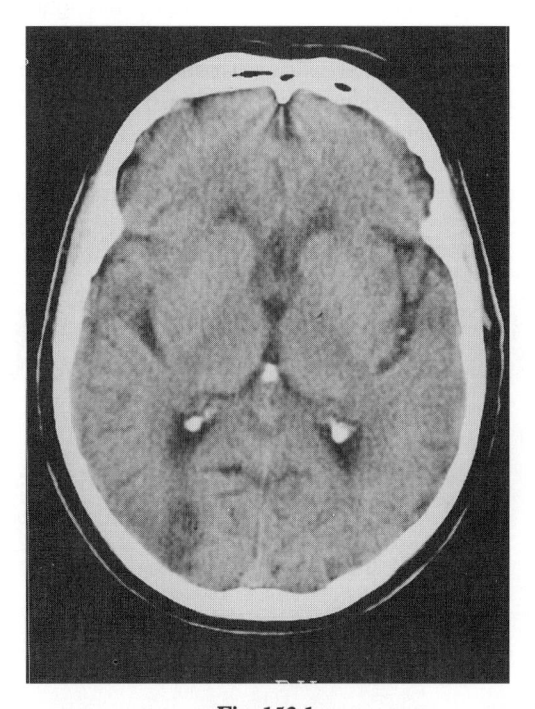

Fig. 152.1

Answer 152

a Peripheral area of low attenuation in the right occipital cortex.
   Infarct.
b Left upper quadrantanopia, or left homonymous hemianopia.

Discussion

The infarct in this case is located in the lateral portion of the right occipital cortex. This area receives fibres from the lower fibres of the optic radiation from the temporal lobe.

A defect of the entire right occipital cortex will result in a left homonymous hemianopia with macular sparing. Bilateral occipital infarcts (Fig. 152.2) characteristically result in bilateral cortical blindness with macular sparing.

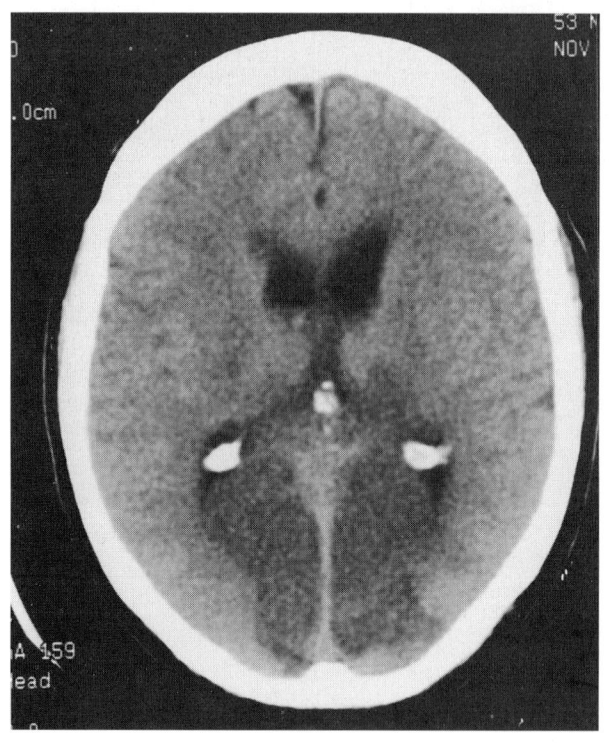

Fig. 152.2
CT brain scan without i.v. contrast. Bilateral occipital infarcts.

QUESTION 153

These two patients suffer from the same disorder.

a What abnormality is shown on the small bowel meal (Fig. 153.1a)?
b What two abnormalities are shown on the CT scan of the chest (Fig. 153.1b)?
c What is the underlying diagnosis?

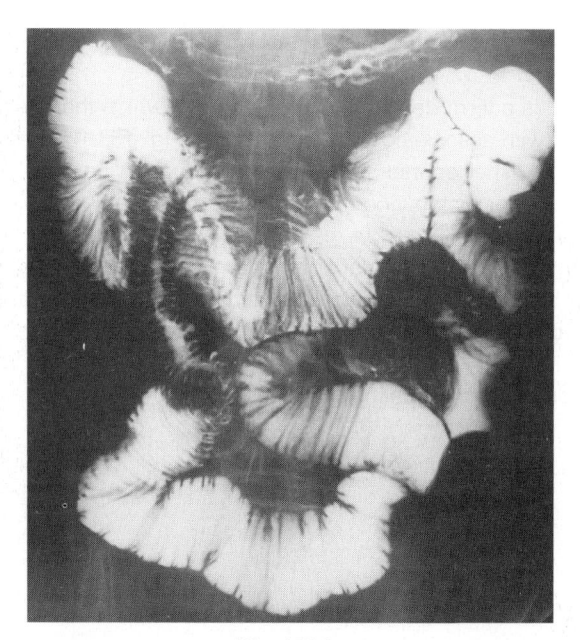

Fig. 153.1a

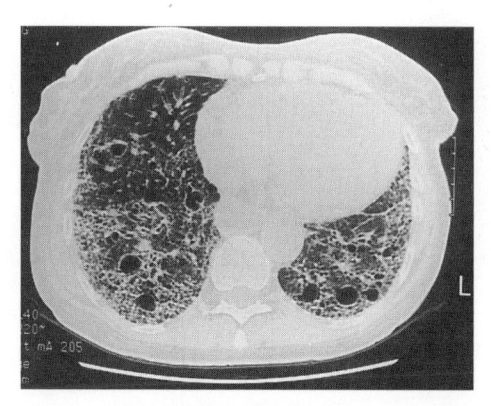

Fig. 153.1b

Answer 153

a 'Coiled-spring' appearance of dilated small bowel.
b Honeycomb lung.
   Oesophageal dilatation.
   Cardiomegaly.
c Scleroderma (systemic sclerosis).

Discussion

'Honeycomb lung' is a term describing fibrotic lung in which there is coarse reticulonodular shadowing with associated cyst formation. In Fig. 153.1b, there is honeycombing in both lungs. The coarse reticulonodular shadowing has a predominantly peripheral and posterior distribution. Furthermore, the oesophagus is dilated, in keeping with scleroderma.

Other causes of honeycomb lung are dermatomyositis, rheumatoid arthritis, histiocytosis X, tuberous sclerosis, lymphangioleiomyomatosis, asbestosis, cryptogenic fibrosing alveolitis, drug-related interstitial fibrosis and sarcoidosis.

See Answer 46 for further information on scleroderma.

QUESTION 154

This 50-year-old man has hypertension.

a What abnormality is shown?
b How can this be treated?

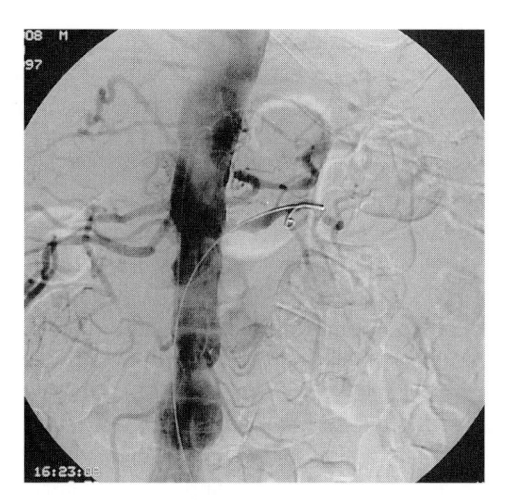

Fig. 154.1

ANSWER 154

a Stenosis of the left renal artery.
b Angioplasty or arterial stent procedure.

Discussion

Renal artery stenosis (RAS) accounts for up to 2% of cases of systemic hypertension. The commonest cause is atherosclerosis. Other causes include fibromuscular dysplasia, neurofibromatosis (mesodermal dysplasia of arterial wall) or congenital causes. Fibromuscular dysplasia gives a beaded appearance to the renal artery, and is the commonest cause of renovascular hypertension in children and young adults, with a female preponderance. Renal artery stenosis (RAS)·may give a delayed nephrogram which becomes increasingly dense over time (due to water reabsorption).

Occasionally ureteric notching is seen, due to collateral vessels. An isotope renogram may show reduced or absent renal perfusion with delayed images. A renal vein renin ratio between the affected and normal kidney equal to or greater than 1.5:1 is a good indicator that the stenotic lesion will improve with surgery or angioplasty. Renal artery balloon angioplasty is highly successful in treating RAS due to fibromuscular dysplasia. Arterial stent procedures have shown considerable promise in the management of renal artery stenosis by enabling the arterial lumen to remain patent. Atheromatous strictures do not respond well to angioplasty, and stenting is particularly useful in these cases (Fig. 154.2).

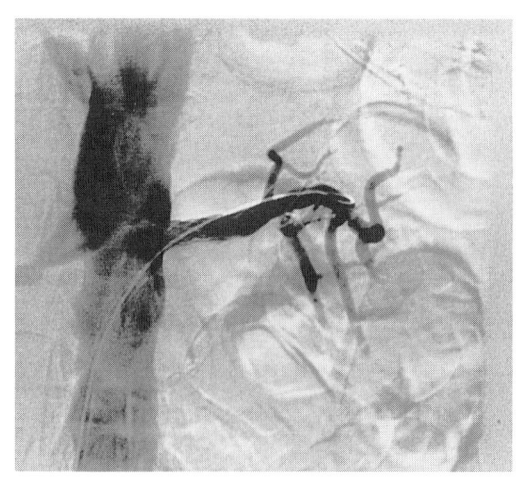

Fig. 154.2
Flush aortogram following left renal artery angioplasty and stent placement.

QUESTION 155

a What two abnormalities are shown in this abdominal radiograph?
b What diagnosis explains these findings?

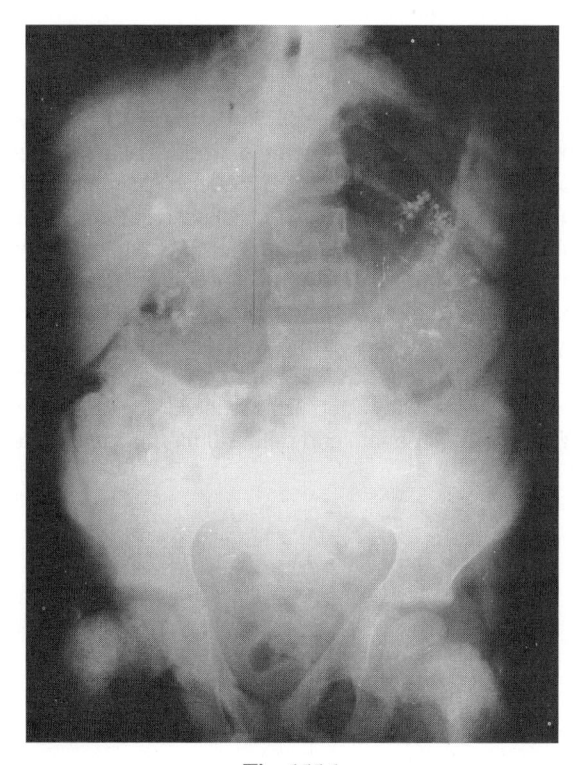

Fig. 155.1

Answer 155

a Nephrocalcinosis.
   Rickets.
b Renal tubular acidosis (distal or type 1).

Discussion

Distal (or type 1) renal tubular acidosis (RTA) is the impairment of hydrogen ion secretion from the renal tubules. An alkaline urine is produced, associated with acidaemia. Presentation occurs in childhood with failure to thrive, polyuria and bone pain. Older children and adults present with weakness due to associated hypokalaemia, renal calculi, bone pain or renal failure. The diagnosis should be suspected when the urine pH exceeds 6 in the absence of urinary tract infection. Severe cases will cause rickets in children or osteomalacia in adults due to impaired phosphate metabolism.

Proximal (or type 2) RTA is due to impaired absorption of bicarbonate from the tubules. It is associated with cystinosis, Fanconi's syndrome and Wilson's disease. The prognosis is good. It *never* results in nephrocalcinosis.

Treatment of RTA is by bicarbonate and potassium replacement therapy.

QUESTION 156

This 70-year-old lady has a painful right foot. She has a leucoerythroblastic picture in the peripheral blood.

a What single abnormality is shown?
b Name two possible causes of her painful foot.
c What is the diagnosis?

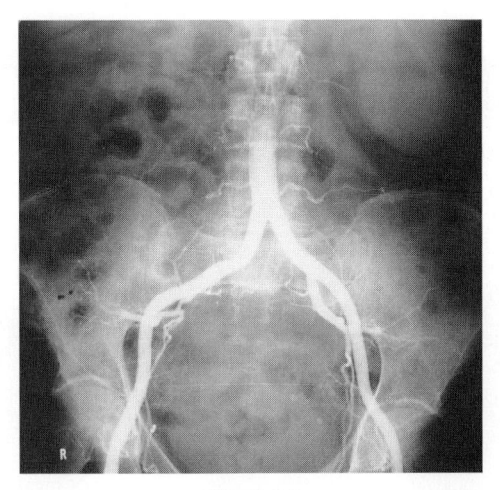

Fig. 156.1

ANSWER 156

a Splenomegaly.
b Gout.
  Arterial ischaemia.
c Myelofibrosis.

Discussion

Myelofibrosis is often preceded by polycythaemia rubra vera. There is an increased predisposition for both arterial and venous thrombosis *in situ*. Another explanation for pain in the foot is gout secondary to hyperuricaemia from increased cell turnover.

QUESTION 157

This is a small bowel meal in a female infant with failure to thrive and iron deficiency anaemia.

a What abnormality is shown?
b What is the diagnosis?
c Name two other symptoms/signs in this condition.

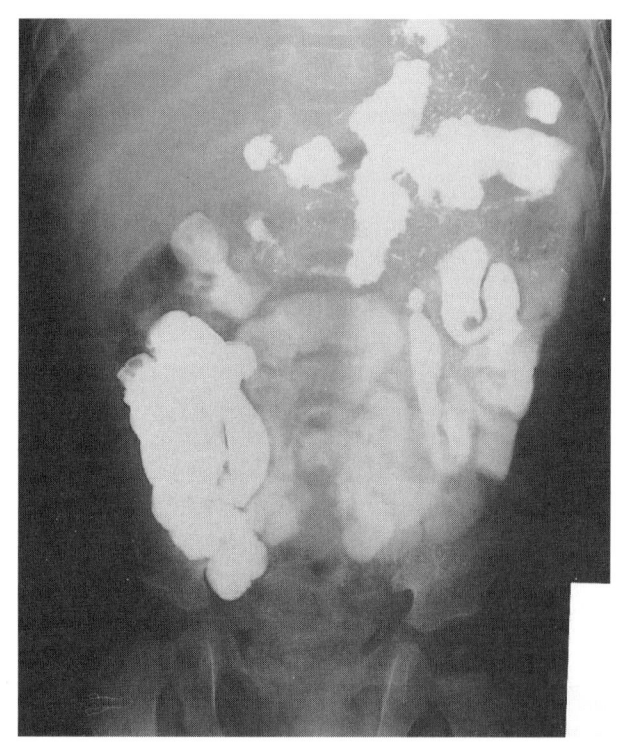

Fig. 157.1

Answer 157

a Small bowel dilatation.
   Featureless tubular bowel (moulage sign).
   Flocculation and segmentation of barium column.
b Coeliac disease.
c Steatorrhoea.
   Abdominal bloating.
   Weight loss.
   Oedema (hypoproteinaemia).

Discussion

Coeliac disease is a chronic intestinal disorder characterized by subtotal villous atrophy caused by intolerance of gluten, a protein found in wheat and rye. Coeliac disease may present at any age and can be totally asymptomatic. Early symptoms include diarrhoea and steatorrhoea, which occur only when the individual is exposed to gluten. Coeliac disease should be suspected in an unwell child with abdominal bloating and wasting who has an adequate diet. A megacolon may occur in children.

In adults a variety of symptoms may disclose the disorder, including weight loss, anaemia, bone pain, oedema and dermatitis herpetiformis. Women tend to present earlier than men due to amenorrhoea or anaemia in pregnancy.

Coeliac disease may cause folate deficiency, hypocalcaemia, hyponatraemia and hypokalaemia. The diagnosis is suggested on barium studies by a dilated featureless bowel. Flocculation and segmentation of the barium column occur because of dilution by small bowel fluid. In adults the ileum takes on the appearance of normal jejunum – 'jejunization.'

QUESTION 158

This is a 62-year-old man with papilloedema and headache for 2 months.
a What abnormality is shown on this contrast-enhanced CT brain scan?
b What important clinical information is needed?
c What is the most likely diagnosis?

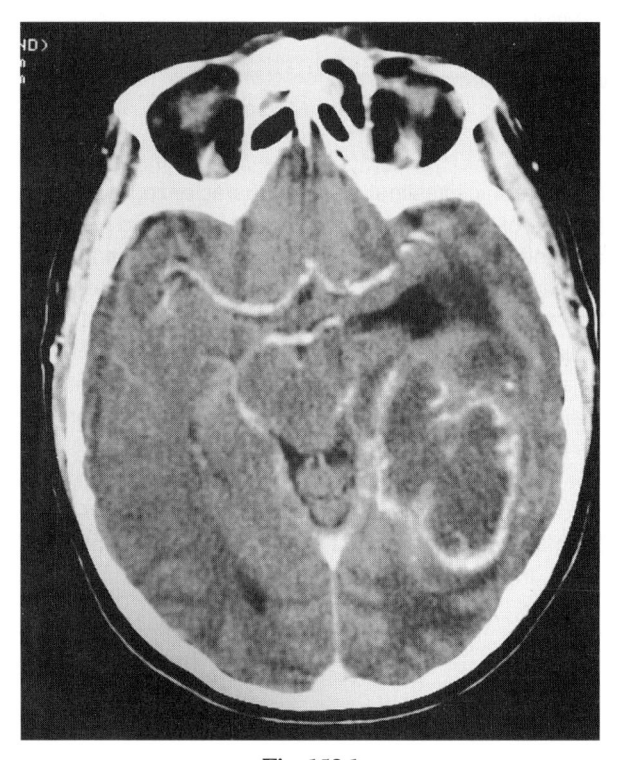

Fig. 158.1

ANSWER 158

a Large low-attenuation cystic mass lesion with peripheral enhancement and deep white matter oedema in the left temporal lobe.
b Presence or absence of fever.
c Glioblastoma multiforme.

Discussion

Malignant gliomas are the commonest primary brain tumours. Glioblastoma multiforme is the most malignant of these and, as its name implies, may have a variety of appearances on CT and MRI. Characteristically there is marked tumour necrosis and surrounding vasogenic oedema. Tumours arise in white matter of the frontal and temporal lobes. The wall of the tumour is irregular and characteristically shows contrast enhancement. These tumours have a dismal prognosis despite radiotherapy. The most important differential diagnosis is cerebral abscess, which is readily treatable. It is essential to elicit a fever in these patients. Cerebral abscesses tend to have a regular, smooth enhancing wall with peripheral oedema (see Fig. 118.1b). Occasionally the diagnosis is not clear and a biopsy may be required.

QUESTION 159

This 47-year-old lady has a chronic medical condition.

a What three abnormalities are shown on this unenhanced abdominal CT (Figs. 159.1a and 159.1b)?
b What specific treatment is she receiving?
c What additional treatment is she receiving?

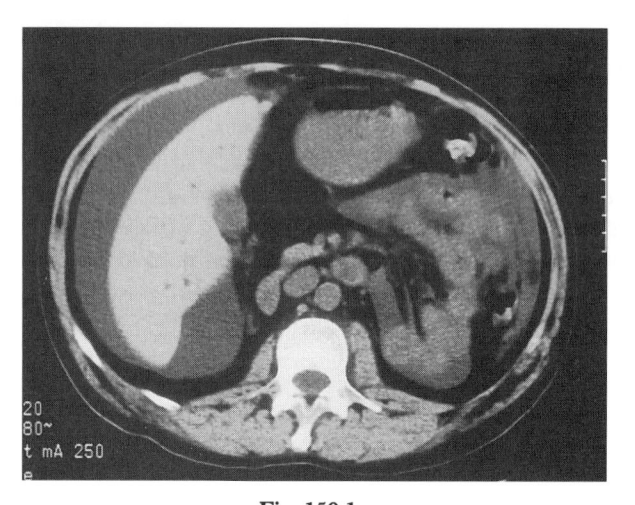

Fig. 159.1a

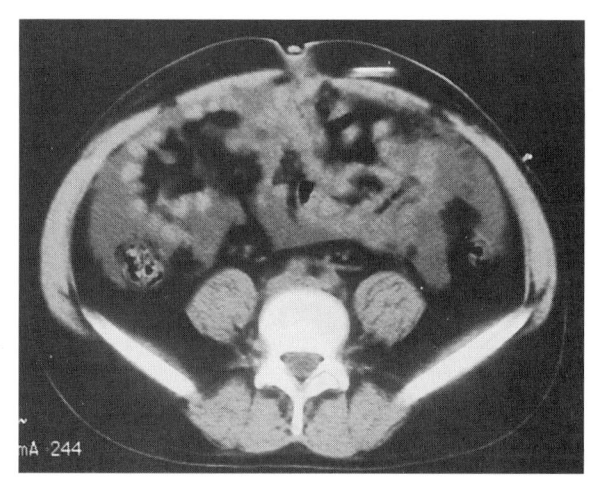

Fig. 159.1b

Answer 159

a Ascites.
Bilateral nephrectomy.
Hyperdense liver.
b Peritoneal dialysis.
c Repeated blood transfusions.

Discussion

There is a high-attenuation linear peritoneal dialysis tube in the subcutaneous tissue of the left anterior abdominal wall (Fig. 159.1b). The ascites is due to dialysis fluid and the hyperdense liver is due to repeated blood transfusions.

Other causes of a dense liver on unenhanced CT are haemochromatosis, haemosiderosis, glycogen storage diseases (may be increased or decreased) and amiodarone treatment.

QUESTION 160

A 40-year-old man has a low-grade fever, abdominal pain and wrist drop.

a What investigation is shown?
b What is the diagnosis?
c List four associated features of this condition.

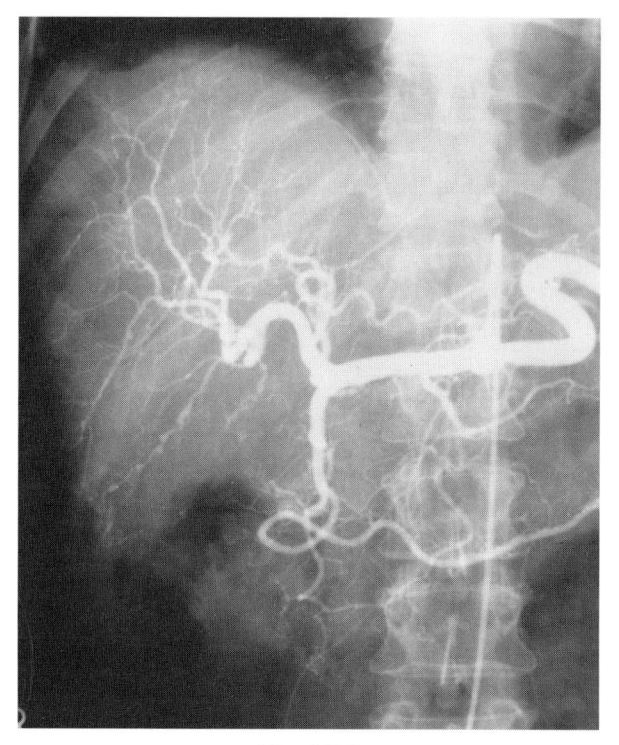

Fig. 160.1

ANSWER 160

a Coeliac axis arteriogram.
b Polyarteritis nodosa (PAN).
c *General*: malaise, weight loss, fever, myositis and arthralgia.
   Renal (80%): hypertension, proteinuria, haematuria and impaired renal function.
   Gastrointestinal: abdominal pain (mesenteric ischaemia), blood loss from gut.
   Cardiovascular (65%): myocardial infarction.

Skin (25%): subcutaneous nodules, urticaria, erythema multiforme, purpura, livedo reticularis
Nervous system: mononeuritis multiplex (motor signs predominating), stroke.

Discussion

Polyarteritis nodosa (PAN) is a multisystem disorder characterized by arteritis of small and medium-sized arteries. Unlike most other collagen vascular diseases, PAN is more common in males (4:1) and may affect one or a combination of all systems. Up to 30% of cases are associated with hepatitis B antigen which, in conjunction with C3 complement, is thought to induce an inflammatory reaction when deposited on the arterial wall. Polymorphs are the predominant inflammatory cell in the arteritis. Repeated inflammation leads to arterial narrowing, thrombosis, infarction and aneurysms, especially at bifurcations.

Patients often present with general malaise, fever and weight loss. Other symptoms are usually present depending on the extent of involvement. The presence of a polymorphonuclear leucocytosis helps to distinguish PAN from SLE, the latter being associated with leucopenia. Biopsies from skin, muscle, liver and kidney are often diagnostic. Electromyography assists in determining a suitable site for muscle biopsy.

PAN has characteristic appearances on hepatic and renal arteriography which may avoid the more invasive renal or liver biopsy. Multiple aneurysms involve the medium-sized hepatic arteries (Fig. 160.2), arcuate and interlobular renal arteries. The nephrographic

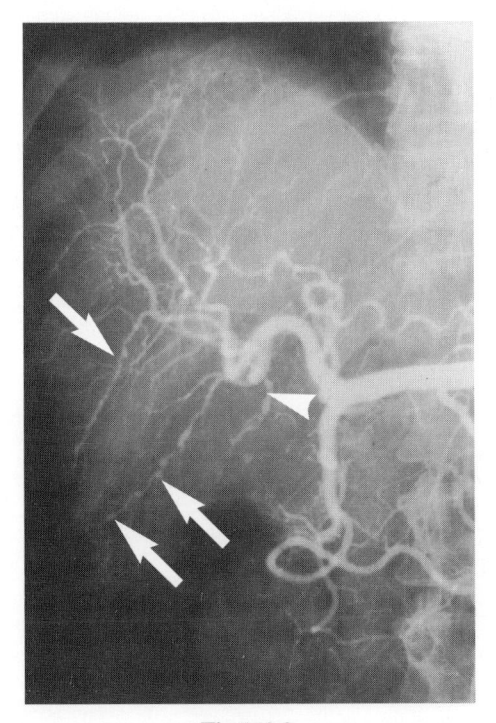

Fig 160.2
Coeliac axis arteriogram in polyarteritis nodosa. Note multiple aneurysms (arrows) in the hepatic arteries.

phase of the renal arteriogram has a 'moth-eaten' appearance due to associated infarction. However, a normal arteriogram does not exclude the diagnosis.

Churg–Strauss syndrome, a variant of PAN, is characterized by asthma, eosinophilia and fleeting pulmonary infiltrates which precede the associated vasculitis. Serum IgE is often elevated.

Treatment with high doses of prednisolone during the early phase of PAN has improved the outlook in these patients. Many patients have no further relapse after initial treatment, especially if PAN is diagnosed early. Immunosuppressives are sometimes required. A poor outcome is more likely in patients with hypertension, aneurysms and renal failure.

QUESTION 161

A 30-year-old woman has a painless neck mass which moves upwards on protruding the tongue.

a What is the diagnosis?

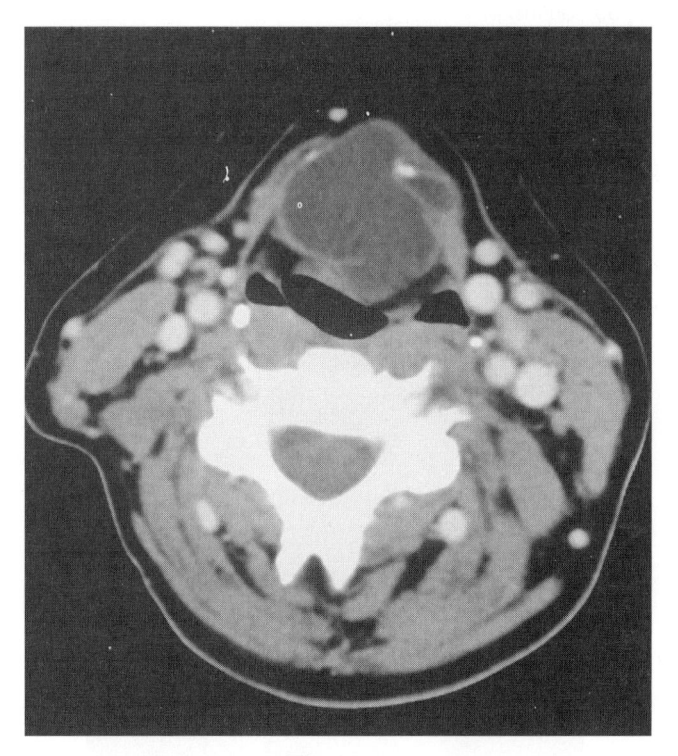

Fig. 161.1

ANSWER 161

a Thyroglossal (duct) cyst.

Discussion

Thyroglossal cysts arise from the remnant of the thyroglossal duct and may occur anywhere along a line between the back of the tongue and the thyroid isthmus. They are frequently found in an infrahyoid or thyroid isthmus location, and tend to be midline structures. The hyoid and thyroglossal cyst move upwards when the tongue is protruded.

QUESTION 162

This young man is HIV-positive. His right wrist has been swollen for 2 months.

a What two major abnormalities are shown?
b What is the most likely diagnosis?
c How would you confirm it?

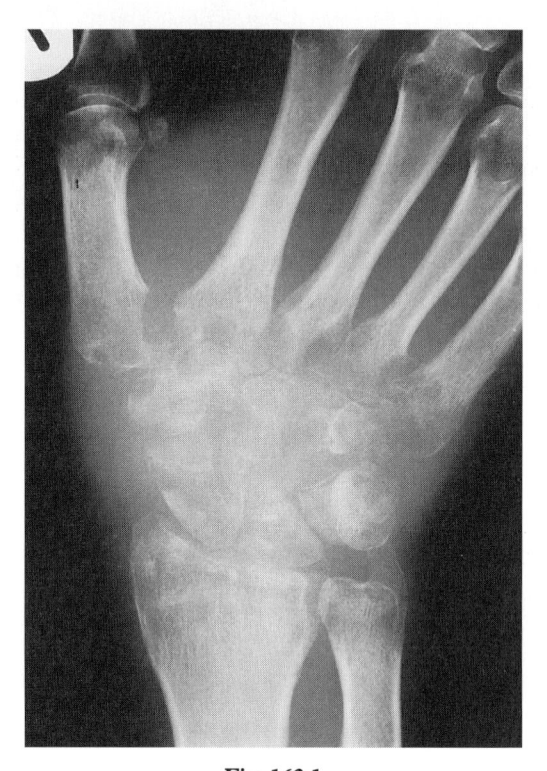

Fig. 162.1

ANSWER 162

a Erosive destruction of the carpal bones and metacarpal bases.
Osteopenia.
Soft tissue swelling.
b Tuberculous arthritis.
c Joint aspiration and culture.

Discussion

Tuberculous arthritis usually has a slow onset and is frequently overlooked as a non-specific synovitis. The swelling is 'spongy', unlike the tense hot joint of pyogenic arthritis. The joint becomes hyperaemic because of this slow process, leading to periarticular osteoporosis. Tuberculous granulomata cover the articular cartilage, finally leading to joint destruction. Unlike pyogenic arthritis, joint spaces are preserved until late in the disease. Infection of the carpus or tarsus can resemble rheumatoid disease, as infection easily spreads in the interosseous spaces. The clue to the diagnosis is the monoarthropathy and HIV positivity, which both raise the index of suspicion that infection is present.

QUESTION 163

This is a coronal T1-weighted scan of the brain in a 12-year-old boy with early-morning headaches and truncal ataxia.

a What is the most likely diagnosis?
b What complication has occurred?
c What urgent treatment is necessary?

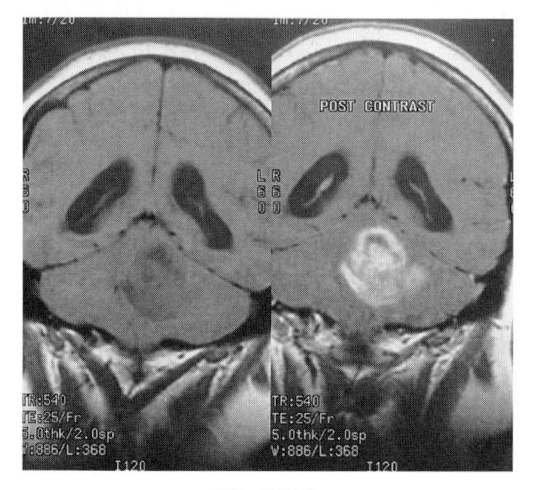

Fig. 163.1

ANSWER 163

a Medulloblastoma.
b Obstructive hydrocephalus.
c Ventricular shunt.

Discussion

Medulloblastomas are malignant posterior fossa tumours arising from the roof of the fourth ventricle; 50% occur in the first decade, when they are predominantly midline in position. There is a second peak in adults, when they may be more laterally placed.

Other posterior fossa tumours occurring in childhood are cerebellar astrocytoma, ependymoma, brainstem glioma and choroid plexus papilloma.

QUESTION 164

This young man is suffering from diabetic ketoacidosis.

a What two abnormalities are shown?
b What is the diagnosis?
c What is the management?

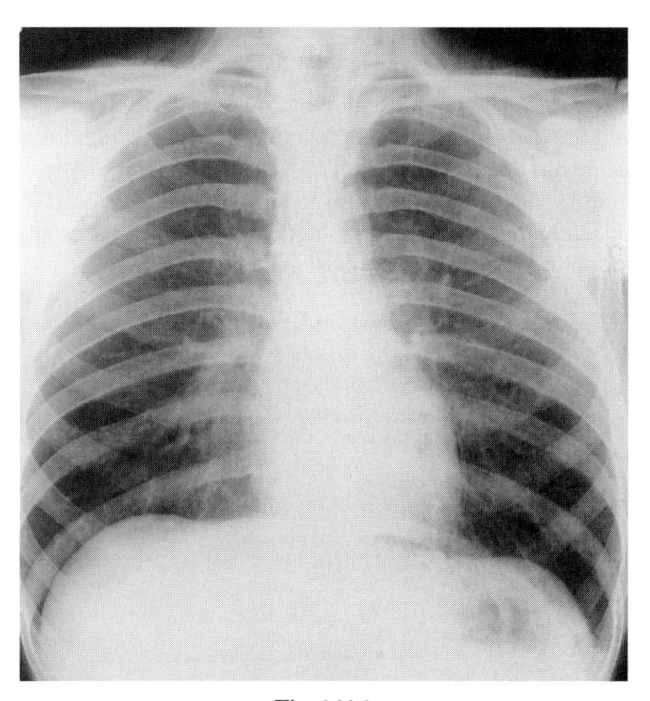

Fig. 164.1

Answer 164

a Subcutaneous emphysema in right supraclavicular fossa.
  Lucent line along left border of mediastinum.
b Pneumomediastinum.
c Nil by mouth.
  Water-soluble contrast swallow.

Discussion

Diabetic ketoacidosis may be complicated by pneumomediastinum. Prolonged vomiting raises intrathoracic pressure, causing either oesophageal rupture or alveolar barotrauma. Air tracks into the mediastinum and fascial planes of the neck. Air may even track into the retroperitoneum or peritoneal cavity and be associated with pneumothorax. The immediate management is to restrict oral fluids until oesophageal perforation has been excluded or confirmed by contrast studies.

QUESTION 165

A 46-year-old man presents with ataxia and dysarthria.

a What is the radiological diagnosis?
b What is the most likely diagnosis?
c Which two investigations would prove most useful?

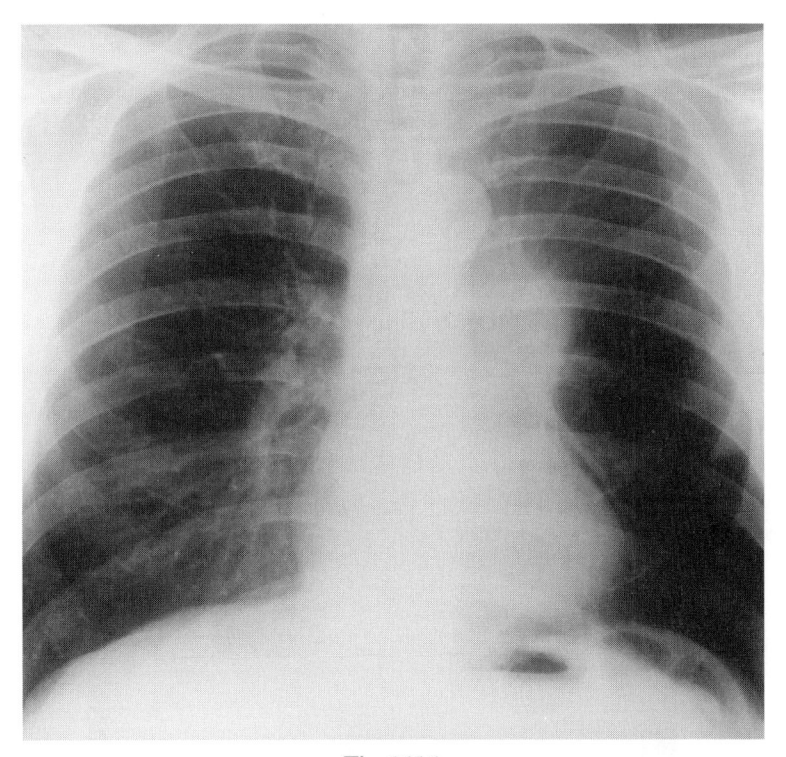

Fig. 165.1

ANSWER 165

a Left upper lobe collapse.
b Cerebellar syndrome associated with carcinoma of the bronchus (left upper lobe bronchus).
c Bronchoscopy.
   CT brain.

Discussion

Cerebellar syndrome of malignancy presents with subacute dysarthria, progressive limb ataxia, diplopia and sometimes vertigo. These symptoms represent non-metastatic manifestations of lung cancer. Cerebellar signs may, of course, be caused by posterior fossa metastases, and it is important to exclude the latter with brain CT.

Other neurological effects of lung cancer without metastases are Eaton–Lambert syndrome, polymyositis, peripheral neuropathy and spinocerebellar degeneration.

Figure 165.1 shows classical left upper lobe collapse. There is a 'veil' of ground glass shadowing in the left upper zone. Note the paucity of vessels in the mid and lower left lung field as the lower lobe hyperexpands to take up the volume vacated by the collapsed left upper lobe.

In a collapse of the left upper lobe, which in adults is invariably caused by bronchial carcinoma, the oblique fissure moves antero-medially (Fig. 165.2).

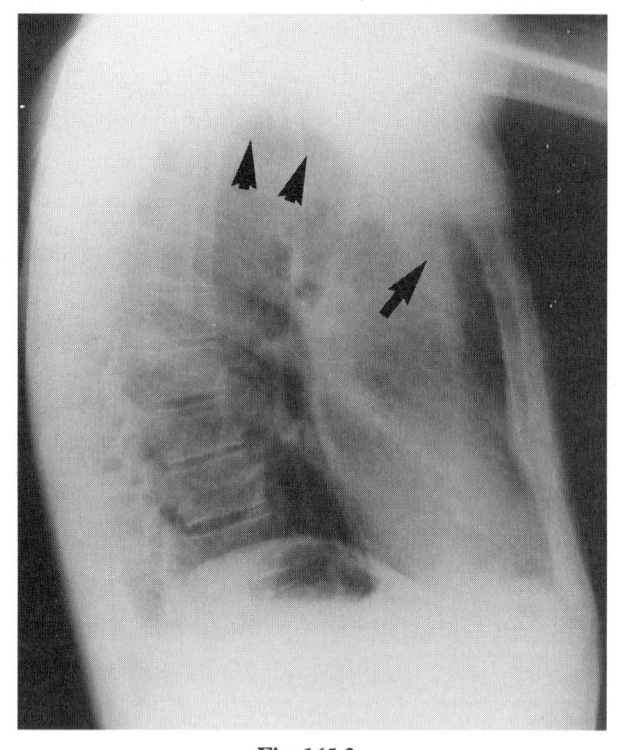

Fig. 165.2
Lateral view. Left upper lobe collapse. Note the tongue of collapsed upper lobe in a retrosternal position (arrow). Note also the hyperexpansion of the left lower lobe (arrowheads).

QUESTION 166

A 53-year-old Asian man has severe backache.

a What abnormality is shown on this MR scan of his lumbar spine?
b What signal change would you expect to see in the L2/3 disc on a T2-weighted image?
c What two investigations are required?
d What is the most likely diagnosis?

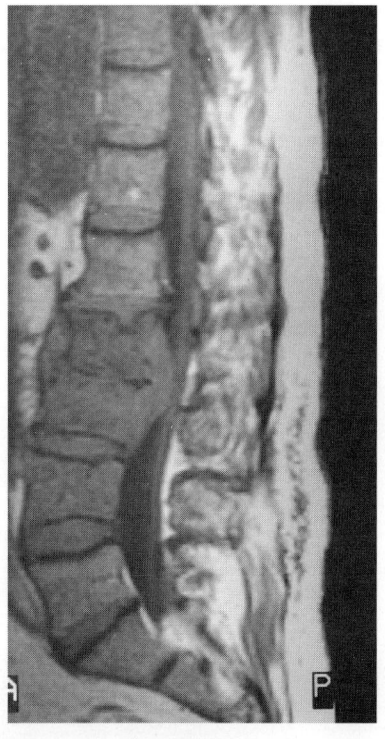

Fig. 166.1a
T1 pre-gadolinium

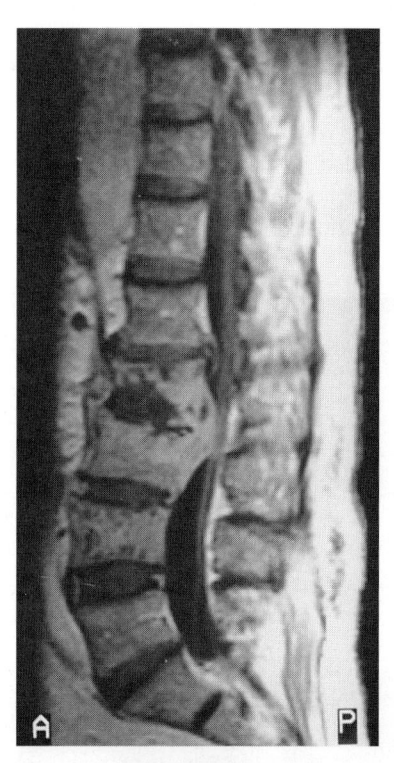

Fig. 166.1b
T1 post-gadolinium

ANSWER 166

a Enhancing extradural mass impinging on the cauda equina.
Destroyed L2/3 disc space.

b High signal due to discitis.
c Chest radiograph.
  Disc aspiration and culture.
d Tuberculous spondylitis (Pott's disease).

Discussion

Tuberculous spondylitis affects less than l% of patients with tuberculosis, but represents up to 60% of all skeletal tuberculosis. It presents with a gradual onset of back pain. Only 50% of patients will have an abnormality on the chest radiograph. Characteristically destruction is insidious, unlike pyogenic infection, where rapid destruction is usual. TB involves the vertebral body and may extend to the posterior elements. Spread is haematogenous via the vertebral venous plexus into the disc, destroying the subchondral end plate. Further spread occurs beneath the longitudinal ligaments to involve contiguous vertebrae.

A T2-weighted image will demonstrate fluid (high signal) in the disc (see Fig. 166.2a) and also in the extradural abscess. Plain radiographs of the spine show end-plate destruction (Fig. 166.2b). Complications of tuberculous spondylitis include acute angular kyphosis or gibbus), psoas cold abscesses (see Fig. 30.2) and cord compression.

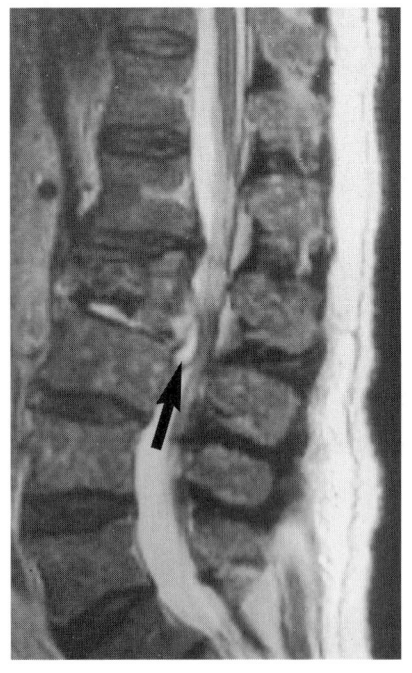

Fig. 166.2a
TB spondylitis. T2-weighted sagittal image. Note fluid (high signal) in L2/3 disc and epidural abscess (arrow).

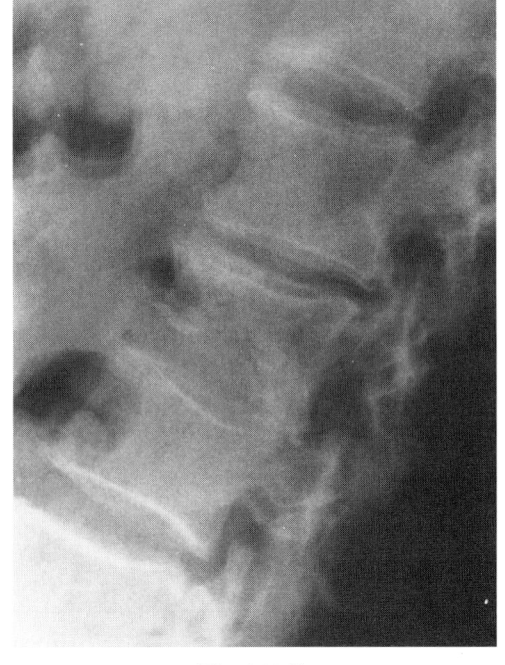

Fig. 166.2b
TB spondylitis. Lumbar spine. There is destruction of the inferior end plate of L2 with wedge collapse of the anterior aspect of L2.

Question 167

This is a barium enema examination in a patient with intermittent left iliac fossa pain. He has a previous history of pulmonary embolus.

a What bowel pathology is shown?
b List three complications.
c What additional feature is present?
d What is the indication for its use?

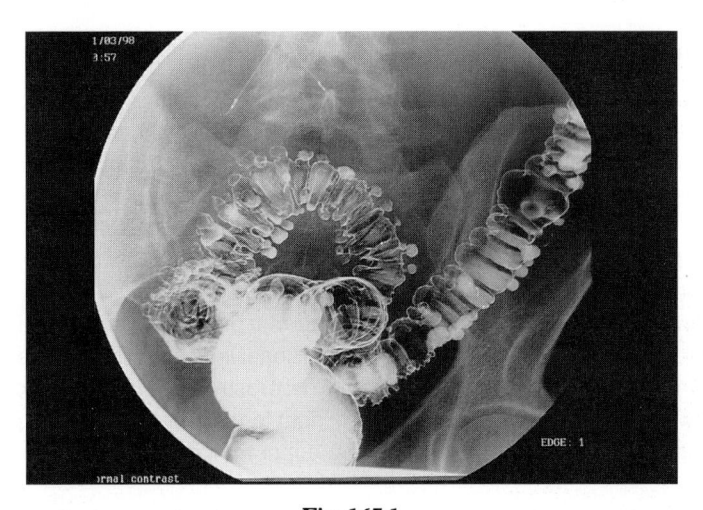

Fig. 167.1

Answer 167

a Diverticulosis of the sigmoid colon.
b Stricture.
  Diverticulitis.
  Pericolic abscess.
  Hepatic abscess.
c An IVC filter is present.
d Iliac or caval thrombus. The IVC filter is placed below the renal veins.

Discussion

Diverticulosis of the colon is very common in Western countries, and is closely associated with a low-fibre diet. Diverticula are outpouchings of mucosa and muscularis mucosa which herniate through the muscularis propria layer. Eighty per cent of patients have disease in the sigmoid colon, in 17% it is global, and in up to 12% it is in the right colon only. Diverticulitis occurs following diverticular perforation with localized pericolic abscess formation. Liver abscesses (Fig. 167.2) may result following entry of infection into the portal vein via the mesenteric circulation.

Vena cava filters are used in patients with recurrent pulmonary emboli or in patients in whom there is a significant risk. There is an additional indication for their use in patients who are unable to receive anticoagulation. The prosthesis is placed below the renal veins following inferior vena cavography. The right femoral or right internal jugular veins may be punctured, and filters may be permanent or temporary.

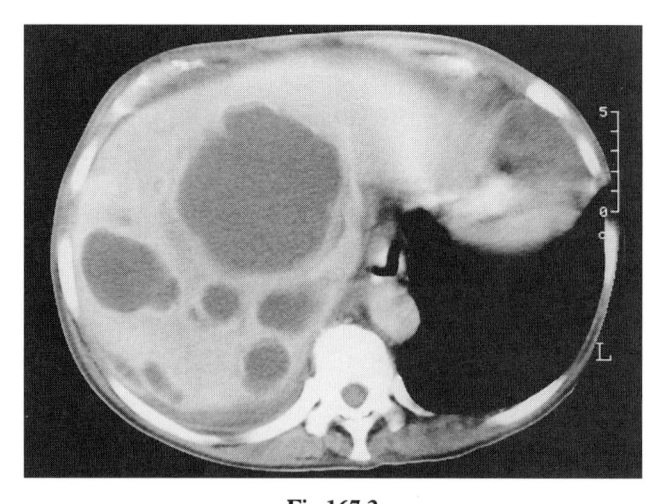

Fig 167.2
CT liver following i.v. contrast medium. Multiple liver abscesses. Note rim enhancement of the abscess walls.

QUESTION 168

This is a contrast-enhanced CT scan of the mediastinum in a 45-year-old woman with unilateral ptosis.

a   What abnormality is shown?
b   What is the most likely diagnosis?
c   List two associated conditions.

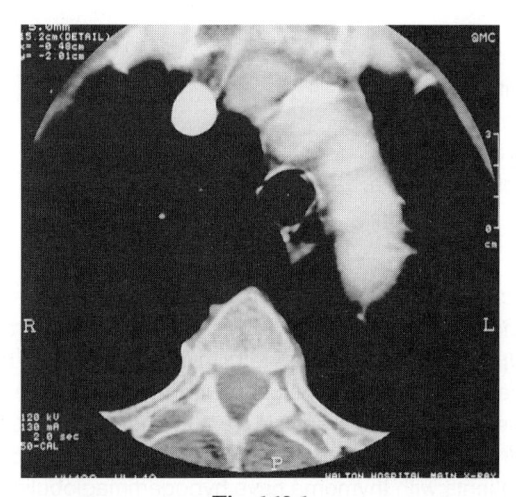

Fig. 168.1

ANSWER 168

a Anterior mediastinal mass located between the left brachiocephalic vein and superior vena cava.
b Myasthenia gravis associated with thymoma.
c Myasthenia gravis associated with:
- autoimmune thyroid disease;
- rheumatoid arthritis;
- SLE;
- Sjögren's syndrome;
- diabetes mellitus;

Thymoma associated with:
- red cell aplasia;
- hypogammaglobulinaemia.

Discussion

Thymomas are the commonest neoplasms in the anterior superior mediastinum, occurring in middle age and having an equal sex incidence. Myasthenia gravis is twice as common in females. Up to 20% of patients with myasthenia gravis have an underlying thymoma. Conversely, up to 50% of patients with thymoma have myasthenia gravis. Fifty per cent of patients with red cell aplasia have thymoma and 5% of patients with thymoma have red cell aplasia; 10% of patients with hypogammaglobulinaemia have thymoma and 6% of patients with thymoma have hypogammaglobulinaemia.

Myasthenia gravis is characterized by weakness and fatigue after limited exercise due to acetylcholine-receptor antibodies. Clinical features include increased muscle weakness following repetitive movements. Ptosis may be unilateral or bilateral, and is accompanied by facial and proximal muscle weakness.

A myasthenic syndrome may be associated with small-cell lung cancer (Eaton–Lambert syndrome). Unlike myasthenia gravis, there is an initial increase in muscle power on repeated contractions. Small-cell lung cancer is often associated with massive mediastinal lymphadenopathy.

QUESTION 169

This 75-year-old man is deaf.

a What is the diagnosis?
b Name two possible mechanisms for deafness.
c Name one intracranial complication of this disorder.

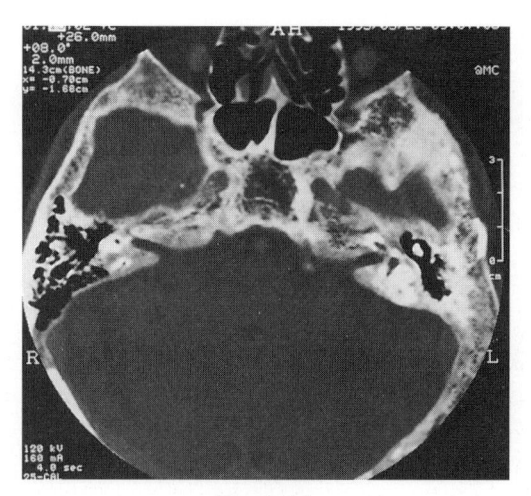

Fig. 169.1

ANSWER 169

a Paget's disease of the skull base.
b Paget's disease of the ossicles.
   Narrowing of the internal auditory canals.
c Obstructive hydrocephalus secondary to platybasia.

Discussion

Paget's disease may cause a mixed hearing loss. The sensorineural component is caused by compression of the auditory nerve in the internal auditory canal. Paget's disease involves the middle ear ossicles, causing fixation of the stapes to the oval window, which results in conductive deafness. Paget's disease involving the skull base may cause narrowing of the optic canals, leading to optic atrophy.

Paget's disease softens bone, leading to basilar invagination and platybasia. This can cause functional obstruction of the aqueduct of Sylvius and obstructive hydrocephalus.

QUESTION 170

This is a CT scan of the chest in a 43-year-old woman.

a What abnormality is shown?
b What is the diagnosis?
c What treatment is necessary?

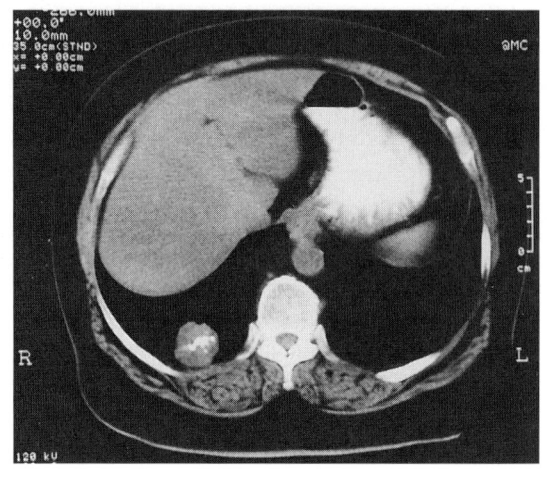

Fig. 170.1

Answer 170

a Lobulated pulmonary mass with internal 'popcorn' calcification in the right lower lobe.
b Pulmonary hamartoma.
c None.

Discussion

Hamartomas are conglomerate masses in which the tissues of a particular part of the body are arranged in a random manner. They are not neoplasms, but tend to contain an excess of one tissue element. A pulmonary hamartoma is a typical example, containing mature hyaline cartilage, connective tissue and smooth muscle. It grows at a rate compatible with the surrounding tissues, unlike neoplasms, which are characterized by excessive growth.

Pulmonary hamartomas may contain fat and fluid, but the main constituent is cartilage, which undergoes 'popcorn' calcification in 15% of cases. Almost all hamartomas are peripherally located and asymptomatic. They are probably present at birth, but will only be diagnosed when seen on routine chest radiographs. Symptoms such as haemoptysis or pneumonia may occur in the rare situations when hamartomas are central and obstruct central airways. No treatment is necessary once a confident diagnosis has been established, but they are removed if the diagnosis is in doubt.

Question 171

This is a contrast-enhanced abdominal CT in a patient with haematuria.

a What is the diagnosis?
b With which syndrome is it associated?
c List three additional features in this syndrome.

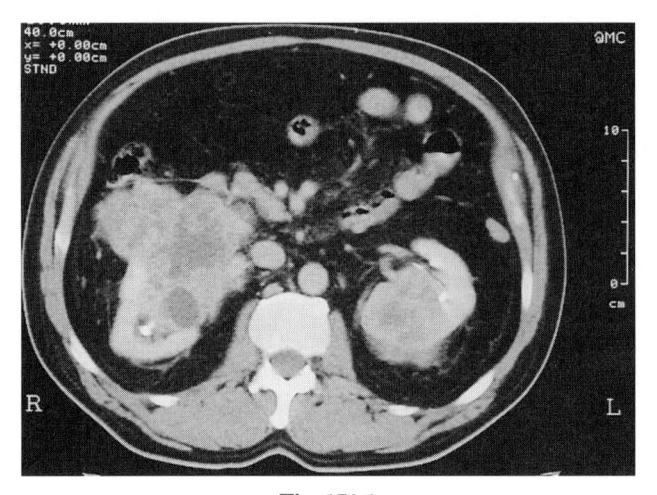

Fig. 171.1

Answer 171

a Bilateral hypernephromas (renal cell carcinoma).
b von Hippel-Lindau syndrome.
c Retinal angiomas.
Haemangioblastoma of cerebellum, brainstem and cord.
Renal cysts and carcinoma.
Cystadenoma of epididymis.
Phaeochromocytomas.
Pancreatic cysts, cystadenoma and cystadenocarcinoma.
Pancreatic islet cell tumour and haemangioblastoma.
Cysts in any organ, especially liver and spleen.

Discussion

von Hippel-Lindau syndrome is an autosomal dominant condition with abnormalities in almost every organ. Pathology of the central nervous system dominates this condition. Classically, patients have haemangioblastomas in the cerebellum (65%), brainstem (10%) and cord (15%); 75% of cases are associated with multiple renal cysts which may be confused with polycystic kidney disease. Hypernephromas occur in up to 45% of cases and are frequently bilateral. Hypernephromas may arise from the cyst wall itself. Renal cell carcinoma without von Hippel-Lindau syndrome is bilateral in 5% of cases.

Other manifestations include retinal angiomas, phaeochromocytoma in up to 17% of cases, cystadenomas of the epididymis, pancreatic cysts and neoplasms, and liver and splenic cysts. Cysts may occur in virtually any organ.

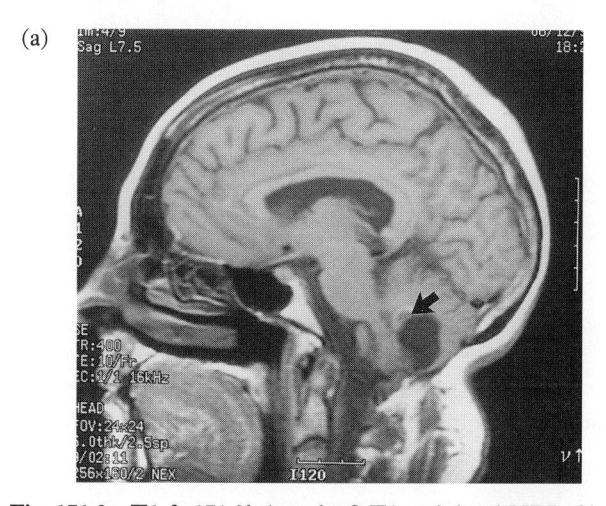

Fig. 171.2a, T1 & 171.2b (overleaf) T2-weighted MRI of brain.
von Hippel-Lindau syndrome. Large cystic haemangioblastoma of the cerebellum. Note the mural nodule (arrow).

(b)

(c)

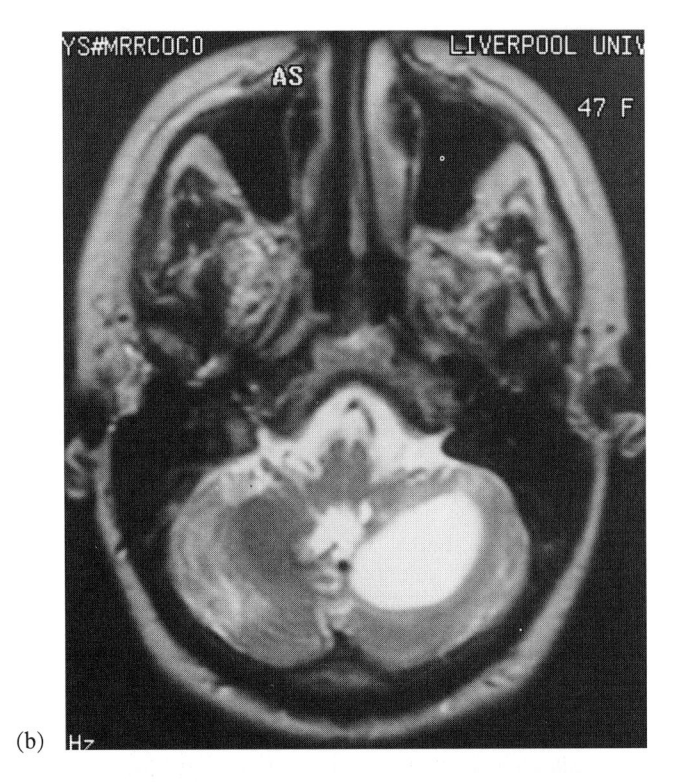

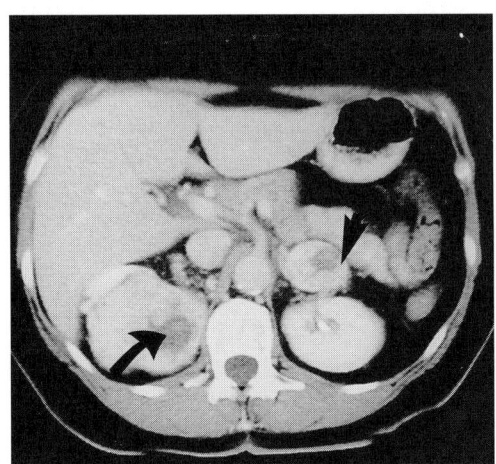

Fig. 171.2c. CT abdomen with i.v. contrast.
von Hippel-Lindau syndrome. Phaeochromocytoma (straight arrow). Renal cell carcinoma (curved arrow).

QUESTION 172

a What is the cause of the appearances on this chest radiograph?
b With which disease is it associated?

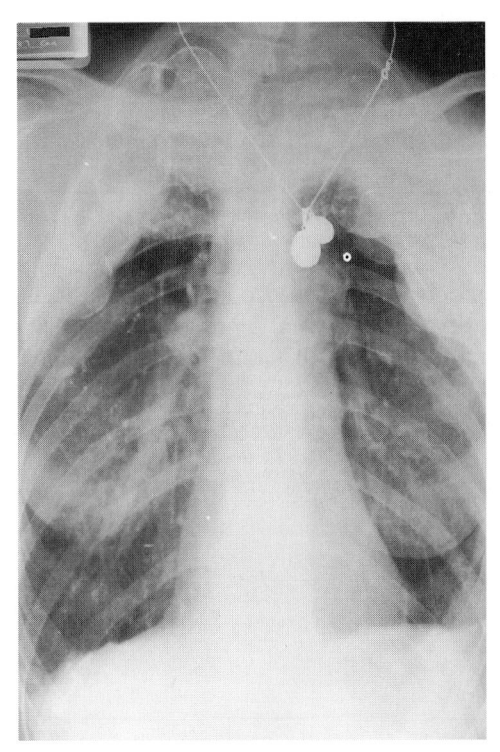

Fig. 172.1

Answer 172

a Plombage.
b Pulmonary tuberculosis.

Discussion

Plombage is a term used to describe filling of the extrapleural space with lucite balls or solid inert material. This was a common surgical treatment for tuberculosis (TB) before antituberculous antibiotics became available. Other surgical treatments for TB included:

- phrenic nerve crush (causing elevation of a hemidiaphragm);
- artificial pneumothorax and pneumoperitoneum;
- thoracoplasty (see Fig. 18.1).

The result of such surgery was to collapse the affected lobe and shorten the disease duration. Evidence of previous surgery is now diminishing. Effective antituberculous chemotherapy was introduced in 1944.

QUESTION 173

This is a T2-weighted MRI brain scan in a 67-year-old febrile woman with recent personality changes and seizures.

a What abnormality is shown?
b What investigations may be helpful?
c What is the diagnosis?

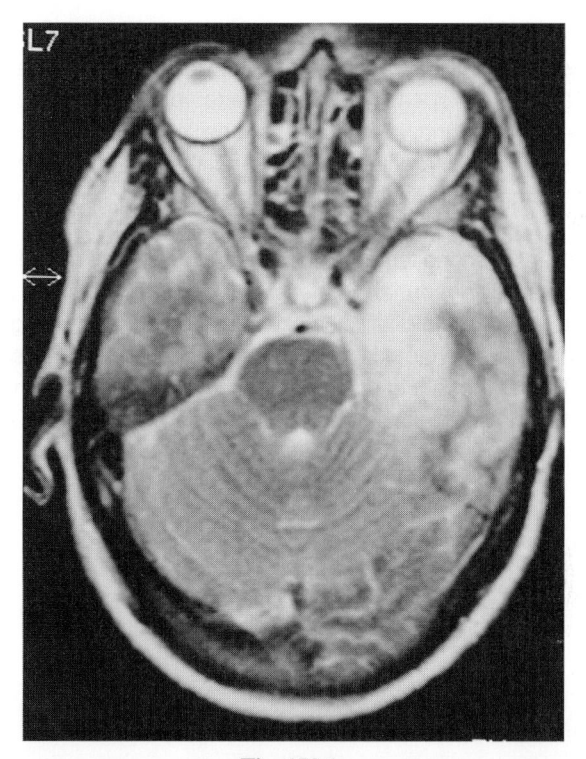

Fig. 173.1

Answer 173

a High signal in the left temporal lobe.
b Lumbar puncture for CSF serology.
 Electroencephalogram (EEG).
c Herpes simplex encephalitis.

Discussion

Herpes simplex encephalitis (HSE) is the commonest infectious encephalitis in the UK. Onset of symptoms is acute, with fever, impaired consciousness, personality changes and seizures. There is a propensity towards the temporal, frontal and parietal lobes in decreasing order of frequency and there may be localizing neurological signs. HSE tends to be unilateral, and characteristically spares the putamen. Pathologically, there is necrosis and oedema which cause a high-signal change on T2-weighted MRI brain scans.

HSE is suggested when the temporal lobes are affected or if red cells are found in the CSF. The EEG is usually abnormal. Sometimes CT demonstrates no abnormality in the face of a positive MRI scan. MRI will also exclude alternative pathology.

Most patients will have serological evidence to suggest previous herpes simplex type 1 infection, and HSE is thought to result from reactivation of dormant virus in the trigeminal ganglion. It has no seasonal pattern and may affect either sex at any age.

QUESTION 174

a What is the most likely explanation for the appearances on this chest radiograph in an asymptomatic 34-year-old woman?

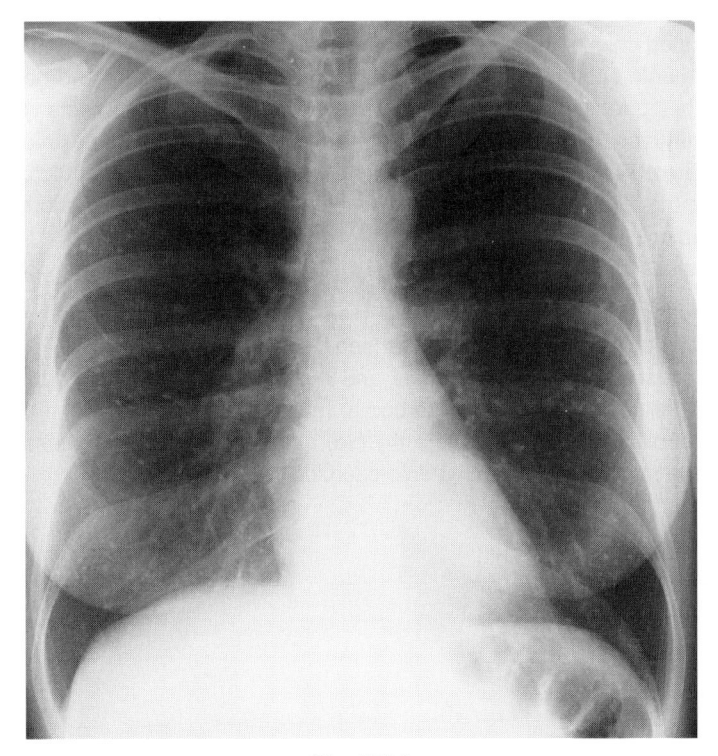

Fig. 174.1

ANSWER 174

a Healed chickenpox pneumonia (varicella pneumonia).

Discussion

Uncomplicated chickenpox mainly affects children. Unlike other viral pneumonias, varicella pneumonia occurs more frequently in adults than in children and has significant morbidity, being fatal in up to 11% of cases. Varicella pneumonia affects young adults, typically immunosuppressed women. Pneumonia is associated with skin and mucosal vesicles. Chest radiography reveals multiple 2–3 mm pulmonary nodules, which coalesce near the hila and lung bases. They disappear in the vast majority of cases. Widespread calcified nodules occur in 2% of cases.

Other causes of pulmonary calcification are:

- *focal causes*: tuberculous granuloma, histoplasmosis, rarely carcinoma (scar carcinoma) and solitary metastatic cancer (see below);
- *diffuse causes*: healed tuberculosis and histoplasmosis, ossific nodules of mitral stenosis, silicosis, metastases (sarcoma, mucinous adenocarcinoma of colon and breast, papillary carcinoma of the thyroid, ovarian cystadenocarcinoma and carcinoid), alveolar microlithiasis, hypercalcaemic state.

QUESTION 175

a What investigation is this?
b What is the diagnosis?
c What is the associated condition?

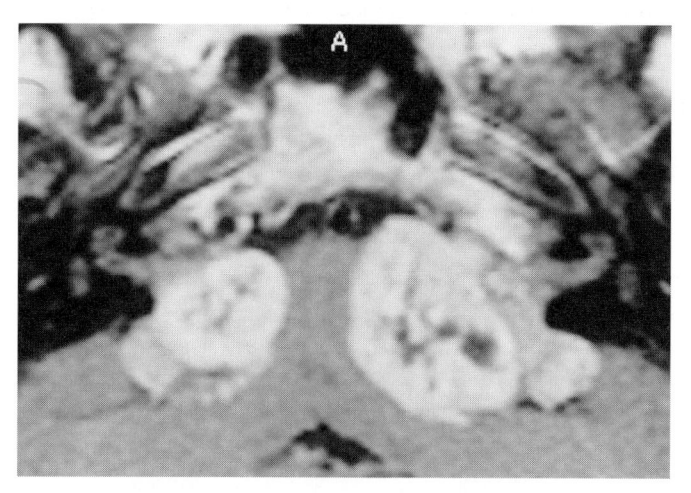

Fig. 175.1

ANSWER 175

a Gadolinium-enhanced T1-weighted MR images through both internal acoustic meati.
b Bilateral acoustic neuromas.
c Neurofibromatosis (central or type 2).

Discussion

Bilateral acoustic neuromas are virtually pathognomonic of central neurofibromatosis. For further discussion see Answer 135.

QUESTION 176

This is a lateral lumbar spine film in a 40-year-old man.

a What term is used for this appearance?
b What other abnormality is shown?
c What is the most likely underlying cause?

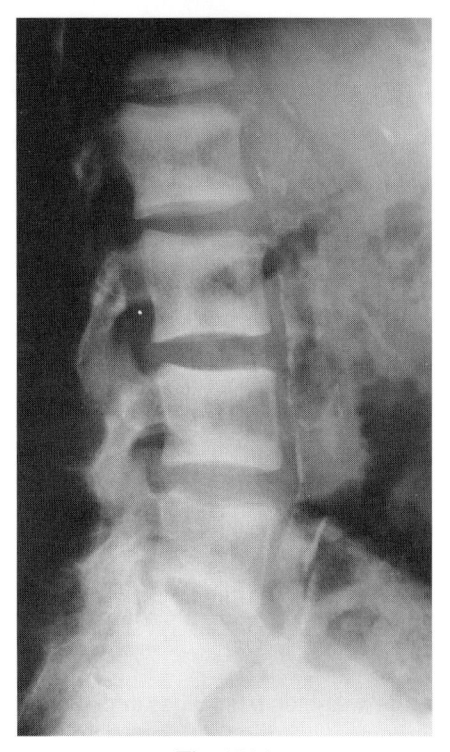

Fig. 176.1

ANSWER 176

a 'Rugger-jersey' spine.
b Heavily calcified aorta.
c Renal osteodystrophy.

Discussion

The term 'rugger-jersey' spine is a term describing sclerosis of the vertebral end plates with intervening bone of normal or reduced density. It is associated with secondary hyperparathyroidism in chronic renal failure.

Renal osteodystrophy is discussed in detail elsewhere (see Answers 25 and 107).

QUESTION 177

A 40-year-old woman who has had recurrent bouts of right upper quadrant pain now presents with generalized abdominal pain and vomiting.

a What is the diagnosis?
b What treatment is indicated?

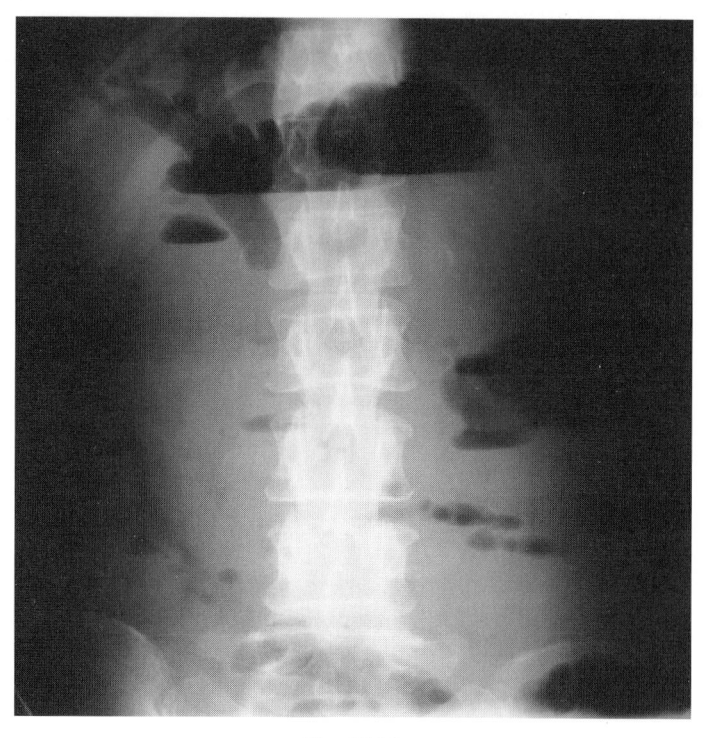

Fig. 177.1

Answer 177

a Gallstone ileus.
b Surgical treatment.

Discussion

Gallstone ileus typically affects middle-aged women, and is a mechanical small-bowel obstruction due to perforation of an inflamed gallbladder by a large gallstone which enters the duodenum via a cholecystoduodenal fistula. It lodges in the ileocaecal valve or in the sigmoid colon – both sites of calibre change within the gut.

Radiologically, gallstone ileus can be confirmed by the presence of small-bowel obstruction and air in the biliary tree. This is shown as air within a tubular branching structure in the right upper quadrant. A calcified gallstone is only visible in 25% of cases. Gallstone ileus requires surgery and carries a high mortality.

Other causes of gas in the biliary tree (pneumobilia) are associated with the following:

- after ERCP or bile duct surgery;
- the elderly (physiological cause due to relaxation of sphincter of Oddi);
- emphysematous cholecystitis;
- perforated duodenal ulcer.

QUESTION 178

This 45-year-old dialysis patient complains of headache.

a What abnormality is shown on this CT scan of the brain?
b What is the diagnosis?
c What is the most likely cause of his renal failure?

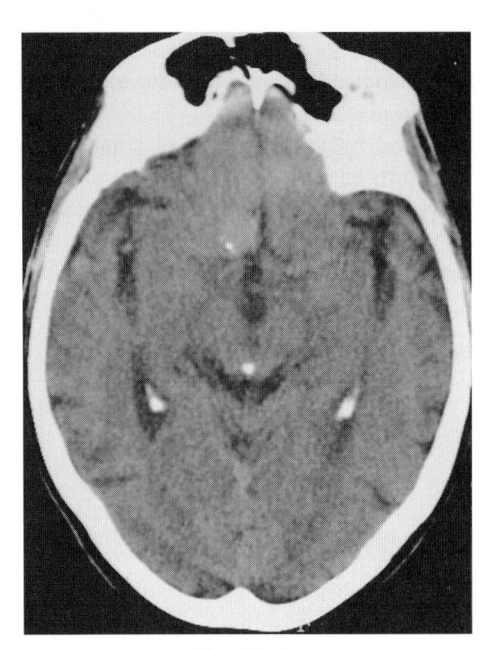

Fig. 178.1a
Pre-contrast

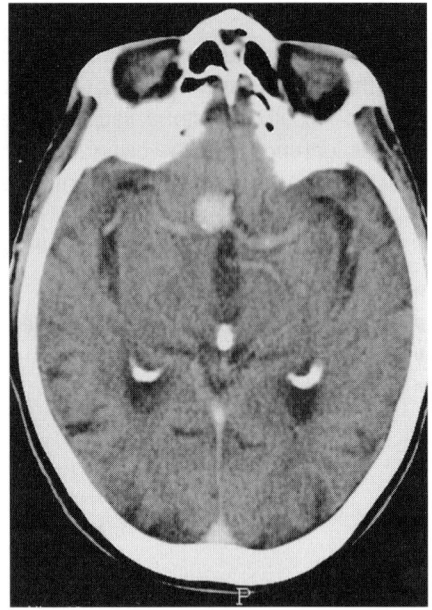

Fig. 178.1b
Post-contrast

Answer 178

a Enhancing calcified lesion at junction of right anterior cerebral and anterior communicating arteries.
b Berry aneurysm of the right anterior cerebral artery.
c Polycystic kidney disease.

Discussion

Ninety-seven per cent of intracranial aneurysms are congenital or berry aneurysms, of which 20% are multiple. They are associated with coarctation of the aorta and polycystic kidneys. Other types of intracranial aneurysms include mycotic aneurysms secondary to infection, arteriosclerotic aneurysms and collagen vascular disease (e.g. Ehlers-Danlos syndrome).

Important sites of subarachnoid haemorrhage from intracranial aneurysms are anterior cerebral (30%), middle cerebral (25%) and posterior cerebral arteries (25%).

Giant aneurysms (larger than 2.5 cm) present with mass effect and affect the internal carotid artery in the middle cranial fossa and basilar, anterior inferior cerebellar and vertebral arteries in the posterior fossa.

Question 179

A 40-year-old Caucasian man developed pneumococcal pneumonia requiring ventilation. Following extubation he remained unwell with failure to improve.

a What three abnormalities are present on thoracic CT?
b What event was elicited in his past history to explain one (and possibly two) of these findings?
c What is the immediate management?

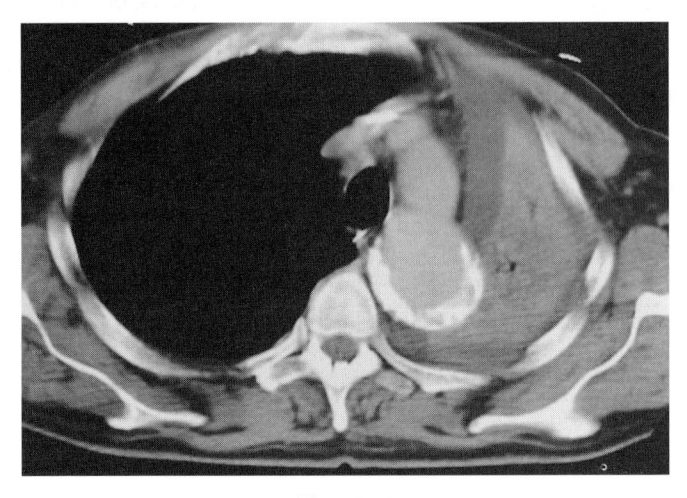

Fig. 179.1

Answer 179

a Calcified saccular aneurysm of the aortic arch.
   Consolidation and collapse of the left upper lobe.
   Pleural effusion.
b Road traffic accident.
c Bronchoscopy and lavage.

Discussion

Deceleration during road accidents causes shearing injuries to the aortic isthmus near the ligamentum arteriosum in the posterior aortic arch. It is at this point that the aorta is relatively unsupported. In patients who do not receive surgery after the trauma, a false aneurysm will develop at this site and become calcified. In this case it is worth considering the possibility of splenic injury or splenectomy at the time of injury – asplenic or hyposplenic states predispose to infection from encapsulated organisms such as pneumococcus.

On CT, there is collapse and consolidation of the left upper lobe. As he has recently been intubated, it is mandatory to bronchoscope him to exclude aspiration of teeth or a component of the endotracheal tube.

QUESTION 180

A 42-year-old man has recurrent nasal stuffiness and arthralgia.

a What abnormality is shown in Fig. 180.1a?
b What abnormalities are shown in Fig. 180.1b?
c What is the diagnosis?
d What other organ may be affected?

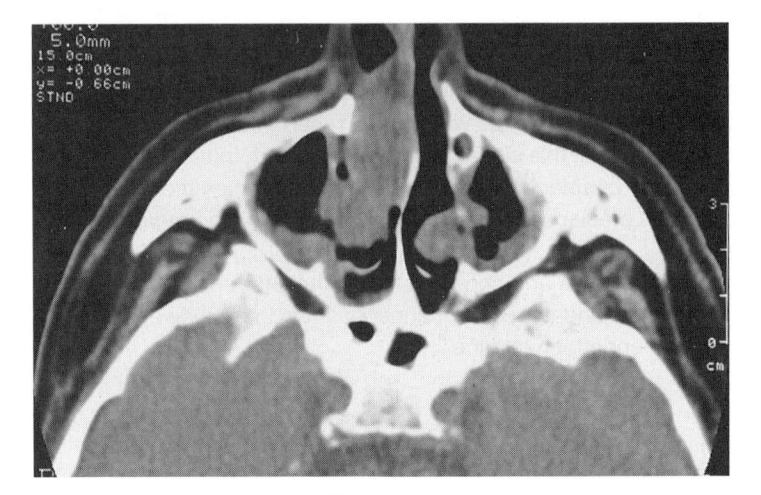

Fig. 180.1a

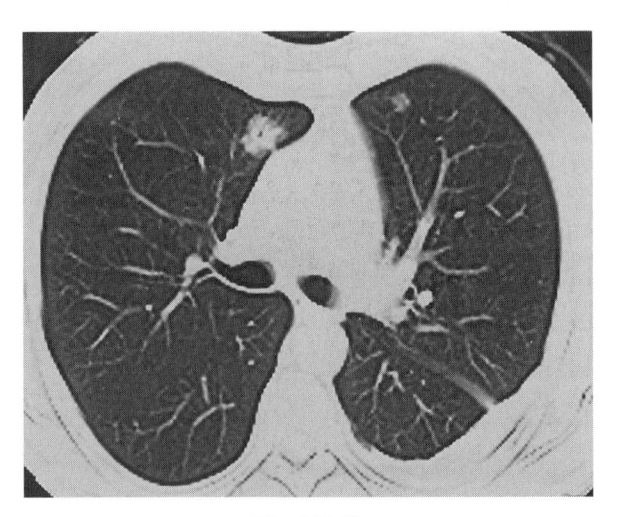

Fig. 180.1b

Answer 180

a Marked mucosal thickening in nasal passages and both maxillary antra with destruction of the medial wall of the right maxillary antrum.
b Bilateral pulmonary nodules. The right pulmonary nodule is cavitating. There is a left pleural effusion.
c Wegener's granulomatosis.
d Renal involvement.

Discussion

Wegener's granulomatosis (WG) is a systemic vasculitis characterized by pulmonary disease, upper respiratory disease and glomerulonephritis. Men are affected more frequently than women, and it may occur at any age. Affected individuals typically present with malaise, fever, arthralgia, sinusitis and a purpuric vasculitic rash. They may have otitis media, causing deafness. Routine urine testing reveals haematuria and proteinuria.

Pulmonary nodules may appear on the chest radiograph (cavitating in up to 50% of cases), and pulmonary haemorrhage occurs secondary to vasculitis which manifests as consolidation. *Pneumocystis carinii* pneumonia may occur as a complication of treatment with cyclophosphamide and steroids (see Fig. 68.1). Antineutrophil cystoplasmic antibody (ANCA) is associated with WG. ANCA has a 95% sensitivity and 80% specificity for WG but can be detected in inflammatory bowel disease. The diagnosis can be made by biopsy of the affected organs.

WG is fatal if untreated. Oral cyclophosphamide and prednisolone is the treatment of choice. Intravenous prednisolone and plasma exchange are reserved for severe disease.

APPENDIX

Computed tomography (CT)

CT uses X-rays to produce axial images which have a much higher contrast between different tissues of the body than occurs in conventional radiography. The basis for CT lies in the ability of different tissues to attenuate (absorb) transmitted X-ray photons, and the construction of images from these different attenuations by means of highly sophisticated computation.

The Hounsfield scale of attenuation ranges from air (–1000 HU) through water (0 HU) to bone (+1000 HU). Soft tissues, such as muscle and kidney, have attenuation values between +30 to +70 HU. Values for fat range from –60 to –100 HU. When images are displayed on 'soft tissue settings', tissues with a *positive* Hounsfield value appear *white*, and those with a *negative* value appear *black*. Soft tissues which have Hounsfield values between +20 and +60 HU appear as varying shades of grey. For example, on conventional soft tissue settings in abdominal CT, the liver will appear grey, abdominal fat and colonic gas will appear black, and bone will appear white. Special 'lung settings' are employed when inspecting lung parenchyma (Fig. A1) and 'soft tissue settings' for the mediastinum (Fig. A2). High-resolution CT (HRCT) is a technique of lung scanning which employs 1-mm sections to improve resolution. It is a particularly useful technique for bronchiectasis and interstitial lung disease.

High-attenuation areas on unenhanced scans are due to either calcification or acute haemorrhage. Cerebral haemorrhage becomes isodense with brain after a period of 2 weeks and hypodense after a further 2 weeks. Iodinated intravenous contrast medium enters blood vessels and soft tissue, thereby increasing their attenuation values and

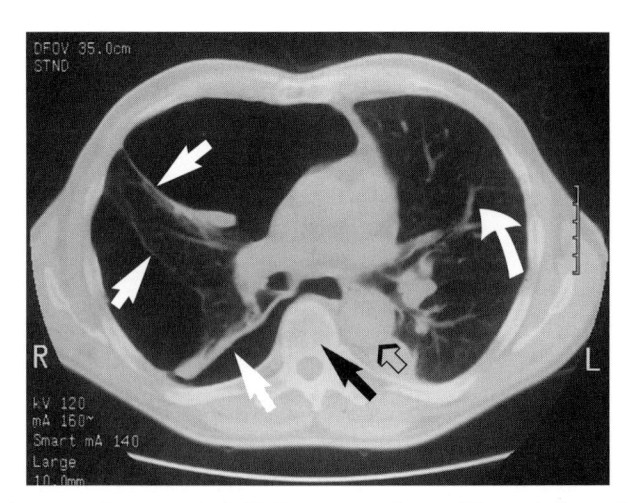

Fig. A1. CT thorax on 'lung setting'. Right pneumothorax. Visceral pleura (white arrows) has separated from the parietal pleura. Bone appears white (black arrow), and the aorta (open black arrow) and branch pulmonary artery (curved white arrow) appear grey.

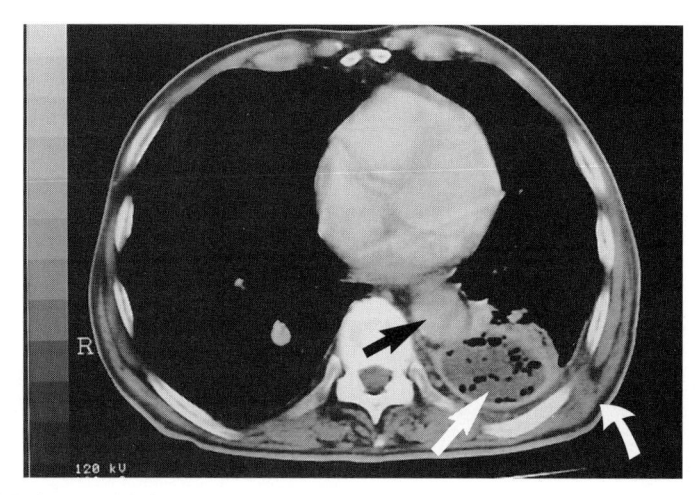

Fig. A2. CT thorax with intravenous contrast medium on 'soft tissue setting'. Left pleural empyema with loculated gas pockets (white arrow). Note that subcutaneous fat (curved arrow) and air within lung appear black on these settings. Note contrast enhancement in the aorta (black arrow).

making structures appear 'whiter'. The uptake of intravenous contrast medium by tissues accentuates differences in attenuation between normal and abnormal tissue. On abdominal and thoracic CT, intravenous contrast medium results in the aorta, IVC/SVC and their main branches becoming 'whiter'.

Magnetic resonance imaging (MRI)

The detailed physics of MRI is complex and beyond the scope of this book. In simple terms, spinning protons in biological tissues have unique physical properties when they are placed in a strong magnetic field and subjected to radiofrequency pulses. These physical properties result in the acquisition of images which have a high degree of tissue contrast.

The advantages of MRI include:

- non-ionizing radiation;
- excellent soft tissue contrast;
- multiplanar images (axial, sagittal and coronal);
- no artefact from bone, making MRI superior to CT in posterior fossa imaging.

The two most important types of image in MRI are obtained with T1- and T2-weighted sequences. T1 images produce excellent anatomical detail. T2 images are sensitive for the detection of pathology (Figs A3 and A4). Fat suppression or 'STIR' sequences are useful for defining pathology in tissues with a high fat content, such as the orbits, bone marrow and subcutaneous fat. This sequence gives fat a low signal, thereby improving the conspicuity of pathology. Intravenous gadolinium DTPA is used to improve the detection of pathology on T1-weighted images. Tissues of *high-signal* intensity appear *white*, *low-signal* intensity appear *black* and *intermediate-signal* intensity appear *grey* (Table A1).

366   Appendix

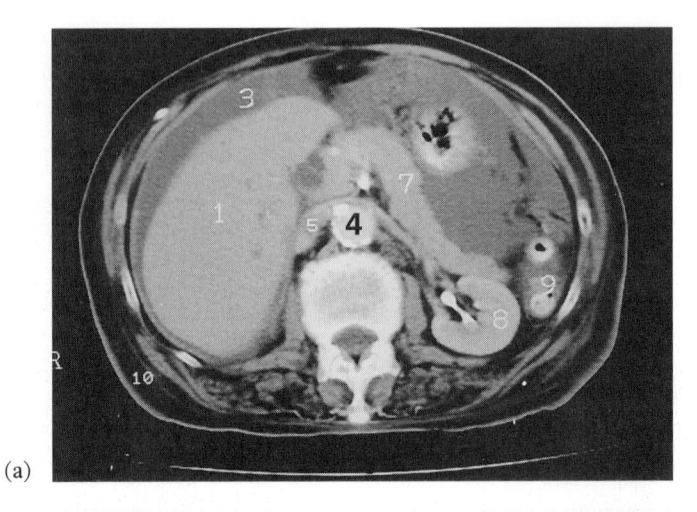

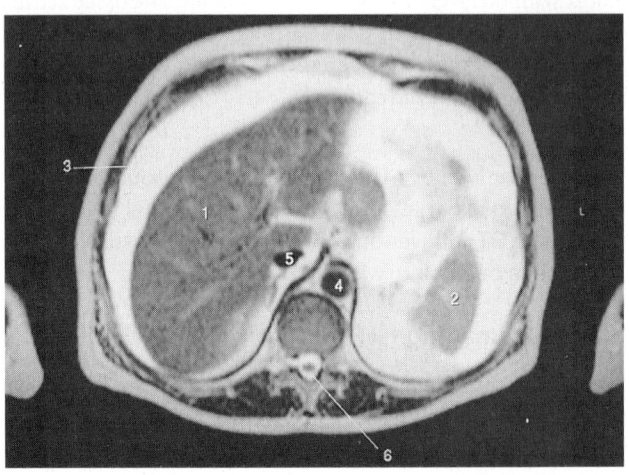

(a)

(b)

Fig. A3. Ascites. (a) CT abdomen. Ascitic fluid has a low attenuation (3). (b) T2-weighted axial MRI abdomen. Ascitic fluid has a high signal intensity (3). 1 = liver, 2 = spleen, 3 = ascites, 4 = aorta, 5 = IVC, 6 = CSF, 7 = pancreas, 8 = left kidney, 9 = descending colon, 10 = subcutaneous fat.

Table A1. Signal differences between T1- and T2-weighted images

	T1	T2
Soft tissue	Intermediate	Intermediate
Fluid	Low	High
Fat	Very high	High
Pathology	Low	High
Pathology after i.v. gadolinium	High	—

Acute haemorrhage may cause a high signal on both T1- and T2-weighted images. After the acute phase, haemoglobin breakdown products cause complex signal changes, making interpretation difficult. For this reason, CT is superior to MRI in the investigation of cerebral haemorrhage.

Figures A4 and A5 demonstrate signal changes in normal and abnormal tissues.

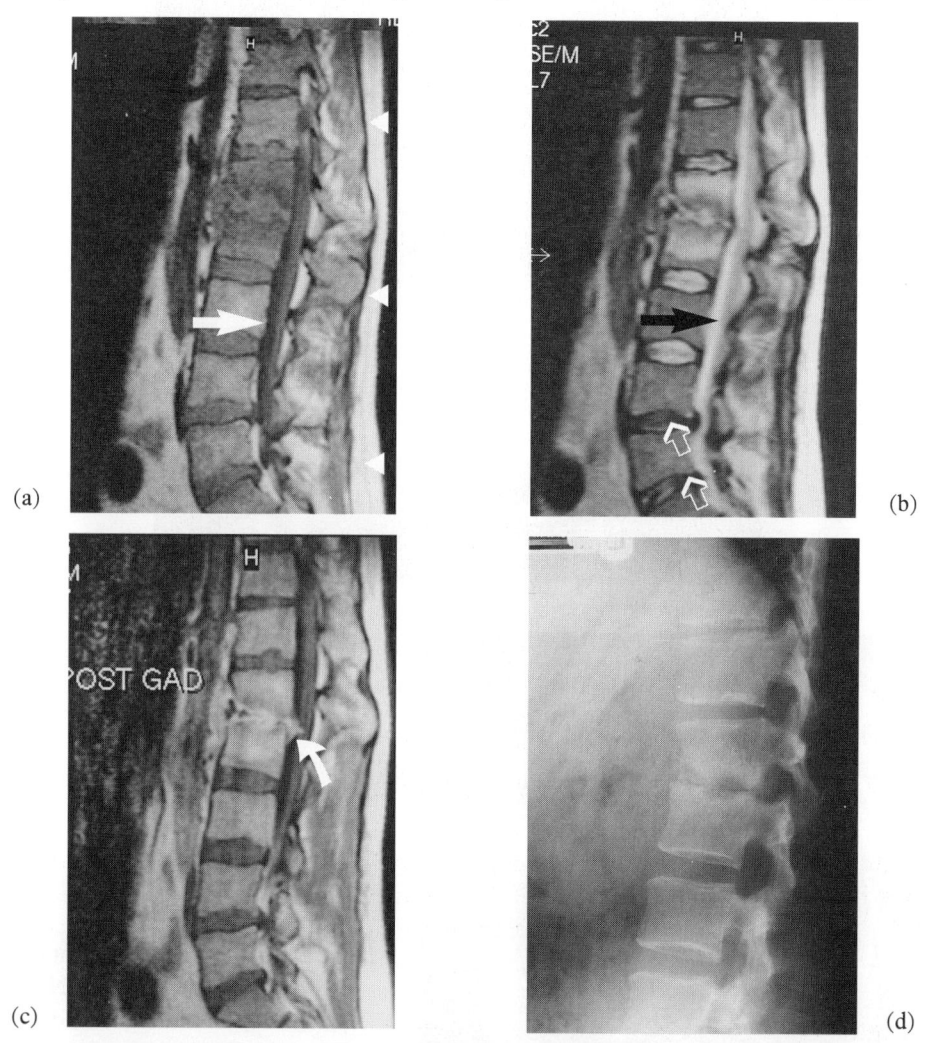

Fig. A4. Pyogenic discitis with epidural abscess L1/2 level. (a) Sagittal T1-weighted unenhanced MRI lumbar spine. Low-signal CSF (arrow) appears black. Note high-signal subcutaneous fat (arrowheads) appearing white. (b) Sagittal T2-weighted MRI lumbar spine. High-signal CSF (arrow) appears white. Note loss of signal signifying dehydration in herniated L4/5 and L5/S1 discs (open arrows). (c) Sagittal T1-weighted MRI lumbar spine following i.v. gadolinium DTPA. There is marked contrast enhancement of the narrowed L1/2 disc and associated epidural abscess (arrow). (d) Lateral lumbar spine. There is end-plate destruction and disc space narrowing at the L1/2 level.

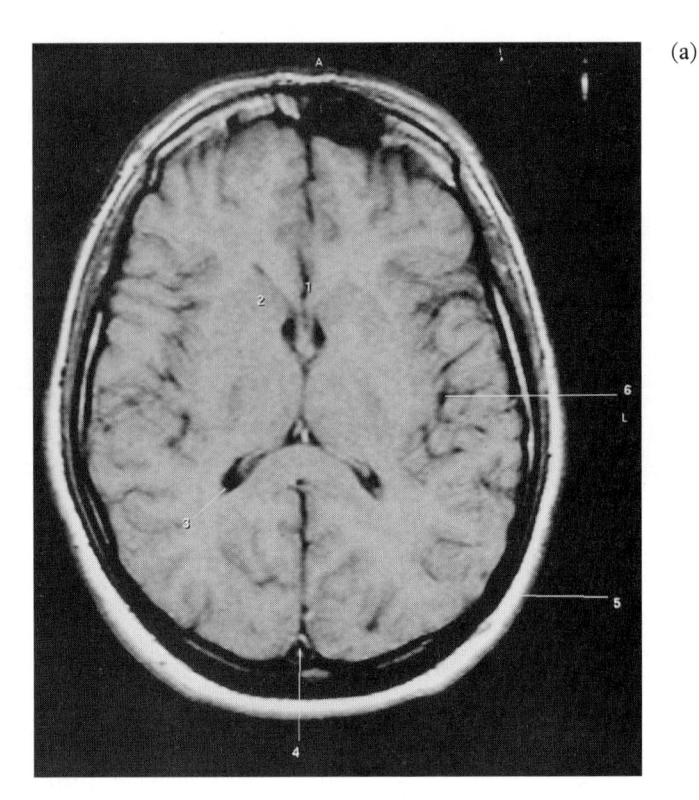

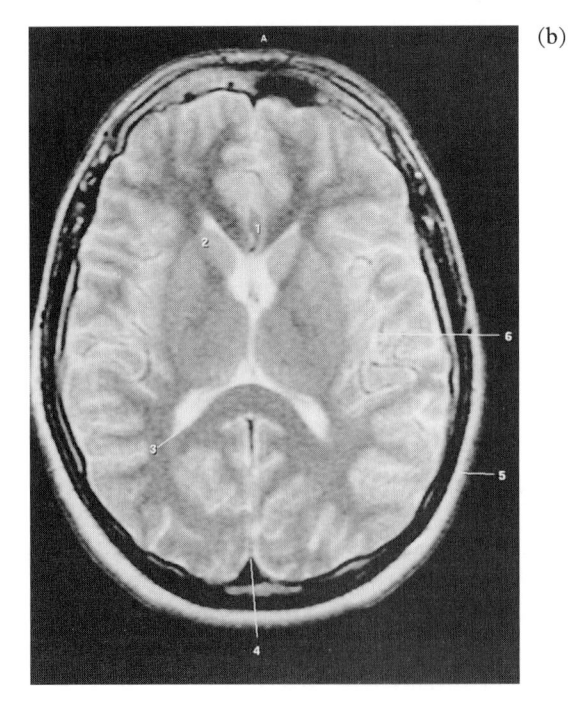

Fig. A5. Normal brain. (a) T1- and (b) T2-weighted axial images at the level of the lateral ventricles. Note the high-signal intensity of CSF on T2. A signal void due to flowing blood (black) is shown within the superior sagittal sinus (4). 1 = corpus callosum, 2 = internal capsule, 3 = posterior horn right lateral ventricle, 4 = superior sagittal sinus, 5 = subcutaneous fat of scalp, 6 = Sylvian fissure.

Nuclear medicine

Technetium (Tc99m), the commonest radionuclide in clinical use, can be used to label a variety of pharmaceuticals which are taken up by metabolically active tissue. Technetium decays with the emission of gamma rays which can be detected with a gamma camera. Isotope studies primarily assess function rather than structure, and have a relatively high sensitivity but a low specificity.

The bone scan is one of the most frequently performed investigations in nuclear medicine. Technetium is labelled to methylene diphosphonate (MDP), which is taken up by osteoblasts in metabolically active bone. Many bone diseases will demonstrate increased osteoblastic activity, making the specificity of the test low. However, given knowledge of the clinical history and pattern of distribution, a diagnosis can be reached in the majority of cases. Bony metastases will give multiple areas of increased tracer activity ('hot spots') throughout the axial skeleton, skull and ribs. A solitary 'hot spot' may be seen with osteomyelitis or primary bone neoplasm. Paget's disease gives a characteristic appearance on bone scanning (Fig. A6). Active arthritic conditions result in increased uptake around joints.

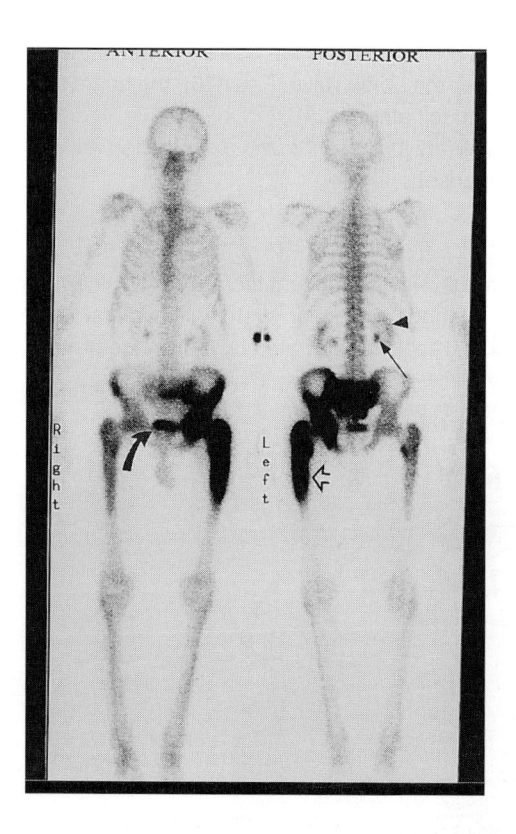

Fig. A6. Paget's disease. Isotope bone scan. There is intense increased tracer activity in expanded bones – left femur (open arrow), left acetabulum, hemipelvis and sacrum. Note tracer activity in the kidney (arrowhead), renal pelvis (arrow) and bladder (curved arrow).

Tracer is eliminated from the body by physical decay of technetium and by excretion of the pharmaceutical. Excretion of MDP occurs via the urinary tract, which is shown on a bone scan by the presence of tracer in the kidneys and bladder.

Technetium may be labelled to other compounds with different pharmacological properties. For example, Tc99m-HIDA is used for bile duct function and Tc99m-DTPA for dynamic renal imaging. Red cells can be labelled with Tc99m and reinjected into the patient in order to investigate the source of gastrointestinal bleeding.

Other radionuclides are used in different applications. For example, gallium (Ga67) is used for inflammation imaging, thallium (Tl201) for myocardial imaging and iodine (I123) for thyroid imaging.

Echocardiography

M-mode echocardiography is a one-dimensional display of the motion of cardiac structures which lie in the path of a rapidly pulsating ultrasound beam. They are readily reproducible and provide ideal examination material.

The image that is produced depends on the position of the probe. If the probe is placed over the mitral valve (Fig. A7), the beam traverses the right ventricle (RV), ventricular septum (VS) and left ventricle (LV), and impinges on the anterior (AMVL) and posterior (PMVL) mitral valve leaflets before finally reaching the posterior wall of the left ventricle (PW). When the probe is placed over the aortic valve (Fig. A10), the beam traverses the right ventricle (RV), aortic valve and left atrium (LA).

Characteristic M-mode echocardiograms likely to present in the examination are presented below with a normal study for comparison.

Normal mitral valve

During ventricular diastole (Fig. A7), the mitral valve opens and the AMVL (black arrow) separates from the PMVL (white arrow). During ventricular systole, the mitral valve closes (curved arrow). Each dot on the vertical scale is separated by a distance of 1 cm.

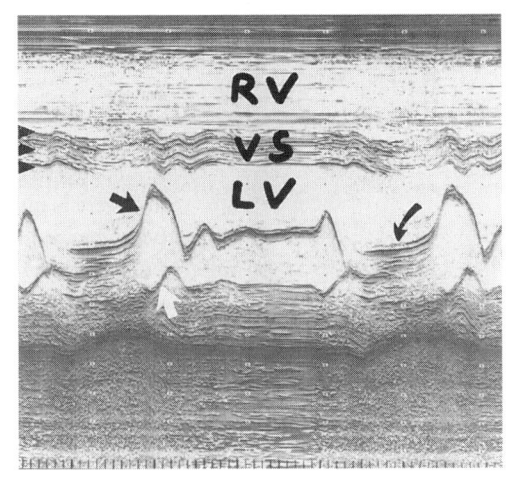

Fig. A7. Bradycardia. M-mode echocardiogram at the level of the normal mitral valve.

Aortic regurgitation

During ventricular diastole, the AMVL and PMVL separate. In aortic regurgitation, the regurgitant jet strikes the AMVL, causing a high-frequency flutter (Fig. A8; curved arrow). Note the dilated LV cavity.

Causes of aortic regurgitation include rheumatic fever, congenital bicuspid valve, infective endocarditis, syphilis, ankylosing spondylitis and other seronegative arthropathies, Marfan's syndrome, rheumatoid arthritis, trauma and hypertension.

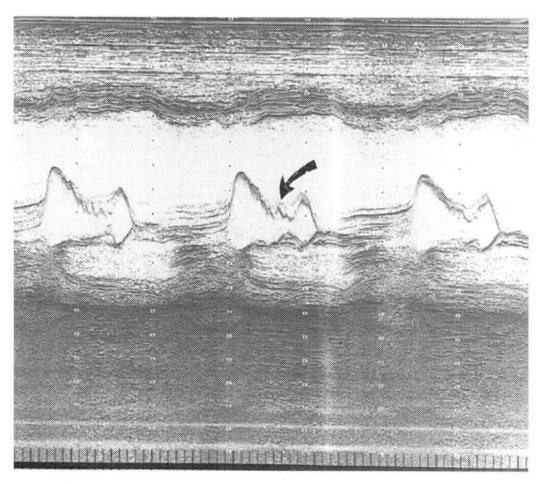

Fig. A8. Aortic regurgitation. M-mode echocardiogram at the level of the mitral valve.

Mitral stenosis

During ventricular systole, the thickened mitral valve closes (Fig. A.9; thick arrow). There

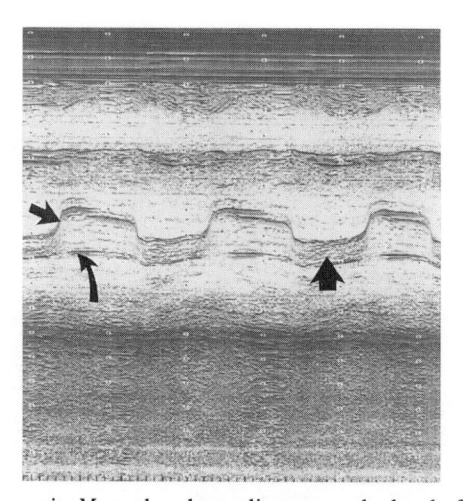

Fig. A9. Mitral stenosis. M-mode echocardiogram at the level of the mitral valve.

is restricted movement of the mitral valve. The AMVL loses its characteristic notch due to a slow closure rate during diastole (thin arrow). The PMVL moves anteriorly during diastole (curved arrow), as it is fused with the AMVL at the commissures. Also note an irregular heart rythym. The third diastolic event has a shorter duration than those preceding it (atrial fibrillation).

M-mode echocardiography is unreliable for assessing the severity of mitral stenosis which is determined by:

- length of mid-diastolic murmur;
- the closeness of the opening snap to the second heart sound;
- the degree of dyspnoea;
- the degree of left atrial dilatation.

Aortic stenosis

The aortic valve is grossly thickened and there is reduced excursion during ventricular systole (Fig. A10). The ventricular septum (VS) is thickened (normal up to 1.2 cm). Note dilatation of the left ventricle (LV) and thickening of the posterior wall (PW) (Fig. A11).

Other conditions likely to be shown in the examination in the form of M-mode echocardiograms are:

- mitral valve prolapse – valve leaflets may be thickened; during ventricular systole, the closed mitral valve bows posteriorly towards the LA;
- hypertrophic obstructive cardiomyopathy (HOCM) – thickened ventricular septum and posterior wall; during ventricular systole there is anterior bowing of the closed mitral valve – this results in narrowing and obstruction of the left ventricular outflow tract;
- pericardial effusion – an echo-free region occurs between the chest wall and the right ventricle (in normal individuals the right ventricular wall merges with the chest wall);
- Valvular vegetations – there are dense echoes on valve leaflets (see Fig. 141.2).

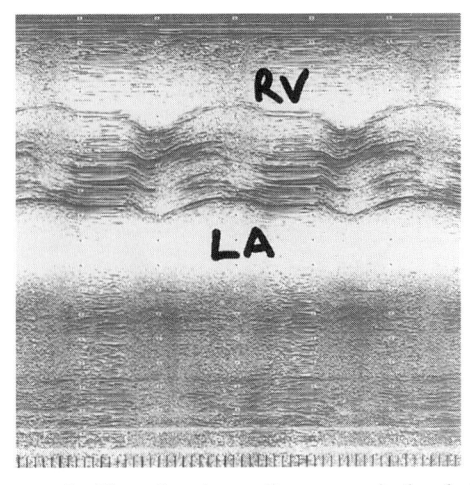

Fig. A10. Aortic stenosis. M-mode echocardiogram at the level of the aortic valve.

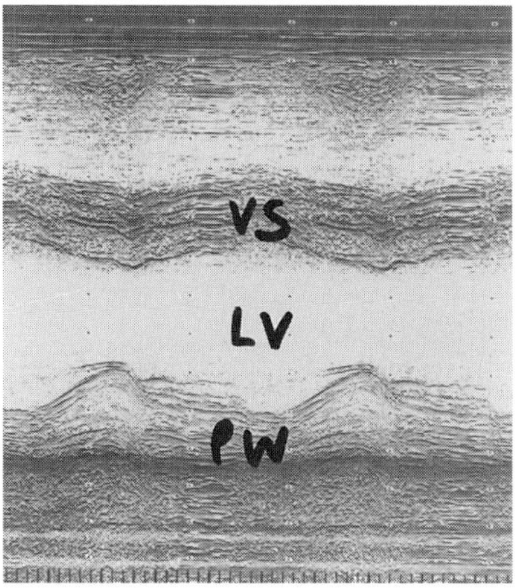

Fig. A11. Aortic stenosis. M-mode echocardiogram at the level of the ventricular chambers.

INDEX

Page numbers in bold indicate that the entry is located in the appendices.

achalasia 225, 245
acoustic neuroma 67, 353
acromegaly 120–1
  chondrocalcinosis 86
adenoma sebaceum 277
ADIPOSE (RPN) 296
adult polycystic kidney disease 57
  berry aneurysm 57, 359
adult respiratory distress syndrome see
    pulmonary oedema
AIDS
  cerebral toxoplasmosis 249
  infections and malignancies 178–9
airway obstruction, causes 78–9
alcohol excess
  avascular necrosis 14–15
  central pontine myelinolysis 307–8
  erosive gastritis 41
  Hodgkin's disease 180–1
  pancreatic pseudocyst 299–300
  renal papillary necrosis 295–6
  subdural haematoma 190–1
alkaptonuria 165–6
allergic bronchopulmonary
    aspergillosis (ABPA) 219
alveolar cell carcinoma 206
alveolitis 49
  miliary shadowing 47
amoebic abscess 193
ampullary carcinoma 14–15
amyloidosis 17
anaemia
  haemolytic 220
  iron deficiency 77, 213, 241
  lead poisoning 139–40
  macrocytic 16–17
analgesic nephropathy 296
aneurysms
  aortic arch 360–1
  berry aneurysm 9, 57, 237–9, 359

  giant 359
  left ventricular 106–7
  multiple, polyarteritis nodosa 324–5
angiodysplasia 281
angiomata, cutaneous 141–2
angiomyolipoma 278
ankylosing spondylitis 105, 161–2
  psoriatic arthropathy 270–1
anticonvulsant rickets 83–4
aorta
  para-aortic soft tissue mass 208
  saddle embolus 221
aortic aneurysm 13
  aortic arch 360–1
  lung collapse 79
  SVCO 156
aortic coarctation 9, 236–7
aortic dissection
  Marfan's syndrome 25
  Stanford A 63
aortic stenosis **372–3**
aortic valve regurgitation **371**
aortography, pulseless disease 53
appendix of modalities 364–73
arachnodactyly 24–5
Arnold–Chiari malformations 109
arterial occlusive disease 53
arteriovenous malformation 9, 117
arthritis
  arthritis mutilans 89–90
  juvenile chronic 75
  pyogenic arthritis 329
  tuberculous arthritis 329
  see also rheumatoid arthritis
arthritis mutilans 270–1
arthropathy, haemophilia 75
asbestos exposure, mesothelioma 39
asbestos-related pleural plaque
    calcification 242
asbestosis 185, 312

ascariasis 204
ascites 322
  in calcific constrictive pericarditis 87–8
  causes 282
  TIPSS 254–5
aspergilloma 37, 118–19
aspergillosis, allergic bronchopulmonary 219
aspiration pneumonitis 33
asthma 218–19
astrocytoma 277, 330
atherosclerosis 314
atrial myxoma 220–1
auditory meatus, acoustic neuroma 67
autonomic neuropathy 17, 225
avascular necrosis
  sickle cell disease 14–15, 69
  XR vs MRI 14, 15

bacterial overgrowth, small bowel 17
Baker's cyst 28–9
bamboo spine 161–2
Behçet's disease, aortography 53
berry aneurysm 9, 237–9
  adult polycystic kidney disease 57, 359
biliary obstruction
  cholangiocarcinoma 284
  and dilatation 115, 174–5
  sclerosing cholangitis 65
bitemporal hemianopia 5
bladder see gallbladder; urinary bladder
Blalock shunt 238
bone metastases 189
  common causes 168–9
  hypernephroma 258–9
  prostate carcinoma 161–2
  super scan effect 289–90
brachial plexus imaging 31
brain see intracranial
brainstem glioma 330

brainstem infarction 230–1
breast carcinoma
  lymph node metastases 26–7, 100, 155–6
  lymphangitis carcinomatosa 159–60
  pulmonary metastases 150
breast prostheses 27
bronchial carcinoma
  airway obstruction 78
  cerebellar syndrome 333–4
  dermatomyositis 33
  lung collapse 78–9, 333–4
  lymphangitis carcinomatosa 159–60
  Pancoast tumour 31
  pericardial effusion 6–7
  SVCO 155–6
bronchial metastases 27
bronchiectasis 157–8
  central 219
bronchogenic carcinoma 185
brown tumour 51
Budd–Chiari syndrome 254–5

caisson disease, avascular necrosis 14
calcific constrictive pericarditis 87–8
calcifications
  asbestos-related pleural 242
  basal cistern 230
  carcinoid 193
  chronic pancreatitis 132
  cysticercosis 21–2
  dermatomyositis 33
  hamartoma 342–3
  holly-leaf 243
  liver 193
  lymph nodes, in silicosis 43
  meningioma 305
  parieto-occipital cortex 141–2
  psoas abscess 60–1
  pulmonary, causes 352
  schistosomiasis 97
  suprasellar 5

Index 377

calcium pyrophosphate dihydrate deposition disease 86
Candida infections
  cystitis 35
  gastritis 41
Caplan's syndrome 43
cardiac enlargement
  chronic renal failure 51
  left ventricular aneurysm 106–7
  pericardial effusion 6
carotid arteriography 9
carpal tunnel syndrome 121
central pontine myelinolysis 307–8
cerebellar astrocytoma 330
cerebellar haemangioblastoma 345
cerebellar syndrome 333–4
cerebral haemorrhage 239
cerebral lesions *see* intracranial
cerebral palsy 305
cerebral toxoplasmosis, AIDS patients 249
Chagas' disease 245
Charcot's neuropathy 108–9, 228
chest wall, mesothelioma 39
chicken-pox-associated pneumonia 351–2
cholangiocarcinoma 65, 284
  extrahepatic 284
cholangiography, percutaneous transhepatic cholangiogram 283–4
cholangitis 208
  primary sclerosing (PSC) 65, 208
cholecystitis, emphysematous 357
cholecystoduodenal fistula 357
cholesterol cyst 5
chondrocalcinosis 86, 121
choroid plexus papilloma 330
choroidal melanoma 235
chronic obstructive pulmonary disease (COPD) 233
Churg–Strauss syndrome 326
Clonorchis sinensis infection 284
cobblestone intestinal patterning 11

coeliac disease 318–19
colloid cyst 59
colon
  familial polyposis coli 183
  sigmoid volvulus 3-3-4
  see also diverticulitis
colon carcinoma 183, 206, 208
  colo-vesical fistula 256–7
  lymphangitis carcinomatosa 159–60
  psoas abscess 61
colo–vesical fistula 256–7
common bile duct *see* biliary obstruction
computed tomography **364–5**
connective tissue disorders 185
  pericardial effusion 6–7
Cooley's anaemia 199
coronary arteries, angina 250–1
cranial nerve palsies 230
craniopharyngioma (cystic) 5
CREST syndrome 95
Crohn's disease 11, 247
  colo-vesical fistula 256–7
  psoas abscess 60
cryptogenic fibrosing alveolitis 185
cutaneous angioma 141–2
cystic bronchiectasis 185
cystic craniopharyngioma 5
cystic dermoid teratoma 13
cystic fibrosis, lymphadenopathy 49
cystic kidney disease, APCKD 57
cysticercosis 20–1
cystinosis 316
cystitis, emphysematous 35
cysts
  Baker's cyst 28–9
  calcified parasitic 21–2
  cholesterol cyst 5
  colloid cyst 59
  enterogenous 269
  liver cyst 193
  pancreatic pseudocyst 299–300
  popliteal cyst 28–9

378 Index

cysts *contd*
  renal cyst 345
  sebaceous cysts 183
  thyroglossal cyst 327
cytomegalovirus infections, gastritis 41

deep vein thrombosis, vs (ruptured) popliteal cyst 29
degenerative joint disease 86
dermatomyositis 33, 312
desmoid tumours 183
diabetes insipidus 5, 170–1
diabetes mellitus 14
  and acromegaly 120–1
  autonomic neuropathy 17, 225
  emphysematous cystitis 35
  fatty infiltration of liver 172–3
diabetic foot 194–5
diabetic ketoacidosis
  ARDS 253
  pneumomediastinum 332
diarrhoea 232, 246
diverticulitis, abscesses 337–8
diverticulosis
  colonic 338
  colo-vesical fistula 256–7
  fistula 35
  jejunal 17
diving, caisson disease 14
Dressler's syndrome, pericardial effusion 6–7
duodenal diverticulosis 17
dystrophia myotonica 164

Eaton–Lambert syndrome 334, 340
Echinococus granulosus, hydatid disease 21, 133–4
echocardiography **370**
  aortic regurgitation **371**
  aortic stenosis **372–3**
  mitral stenosis **371–2**
  mitral valve **370**
Ehlers–Danlos syndrome, berry aneurysms 9

elbow, Charcot's neuropathy 108–9
emboli, systemic 220–1
emphysematous cystitis 35
empyema 143–4, **363**
encephalitis
  AIDS patients 249
  herpes simplex 349–50
endarteritis 231
endoscopic retrograde cholangiopancreatography (ERCP) 65, 115, 131–2, 175
enterogenous cyst 269
eosinophilia, peripheral blood 218–19
eosinophilic granuloma, lungs 171
ependymoma 330
epidural abscess 223
exophthalmos 19, 170–1
extradural haematoma 101–3
extrinsic allergic alveolitis 49
  miliary shadowing 47

familial polyposis coli 183
Fanconi's syndrome 316
fat embolism, trauma 14, 45
fatty infiltration of liver 123–4, 172–3
fibrosing alveolitis 47, 185, 312
fibrosing mediastinitis 208
fibrosis
  bone marrow 210
  interstitial 185, 312
  progressive massive 43
finger clubbing
  myxoma 220–1
  pulmonary osteoarthropathy 129–30
fluorosis 210
Friedreich's ataxia 306
Friedreich's sign, calcific constrictive pericarditis 87–8
fungal mass lesion 37, 118–19, 127–8, 249

gallbladder disease 11, 175
gallstone ileus 356–7

gallstones 175
Gardner's syndrome 183
gastric carcinoma 125–6
   pulmonary metastases 150
gastric resection
   hypochlorhydria 17
   vitamin D deficiency 177
gastric varices 254–5
gastritis
   chronic atrophic 17
   chronic myeloid leukaemia 41
   with splenomegaly 41
gastrointestinal bleeding 279–81
gastro-oesophageal reflux 225
Gaucher's disease 14–15
   splenic enlargement 92
giant cell astrocytoma 277, 330
glandular fever
   miliary shadowing 47
   splenomegaly 92
glioblastoma multiforme 320–1
glioma, brainstem 330
goitre
   intrathoracic 81–2
   SVCO 156
gout 86, 210
Graves' ophthalmopathy 19
gum hypertrophy 83–4
gynaecomastia 27

haematoma
   extradural/subdural 101–3, 167, 190–1
   hepatic 193
   pulmonary 206
haemochromatosis 55, 322–3
   chondrocalcinosis 86
haemolytic anaemia, splenic enlargement 92
haemopericardium 87–8
haemophiliac arthropathy 75
   avascular necrosis 14–15
haemosiderosis 322–3

haemothorax 242
hamartoma
   pulmonary 206, 342–3
   retinal 278
   subependymal 277
hands
   anticonvulsant rickets 83–4
   dermatomyositis 33
   finger clubbing 129–30, 220–1
   Marfan's syndrome 24–5
   pseudohypoparathyroidism 71
   psoriatic arthropathy 270–1
   renal osteodystrophy 215–17
   rheumatoid arthritis 89–90
   scleroderma 94
   thalassaemia major 200
   tuberculous arthritis 329
Hand–Schuller–Christian disease 171
headache
   hydrocephalus 5, 59
   superior sagittal sinus thrombosis 23
heart, septal rupture 264–5
heart block, granulomatous involvement of myocardium 49
heart pacemaker 50
heart sounds, third 87–8
hemianopia 5, 310
hemidiaphragm, tenting 37
Henoch–Schönlein purpura 269
hepatic artery aneurysm 193
hepatic haematoma 193
hepatic varices 254–5
hepatocellular carcinoma 145–6
hepatomegaly, calcific constrictive pericarditis 87–8
hepatosplenomegaly 198–9
hereditary haemorrhagic telangiectasia 241
heroin addiction 222
herpes simplex infections
   encephalitis 349–50
   gastritis 41

hilar lymphadenopathy
  bilateral 49
  in sarcoidosis 49
hilar mass, with lung collapse 78–9
hip, avascular necrosis 14–15, 69
histiocytosis, Langerhans' 171, 185
Hodgkin's disease 180–1, 301–2
homocystinuria, marfanoid features 24–5
Horner's syndrome 31, 109
horseshoe kidney 116
humerus
  avascular necrosis 69
  brown tumour 51
hydatid disease 21, 133–4, 193
hydrocephalus, obstructive 5, 9, 117, 230, 330
  colloid cyst 59
  Paget's disease 112–13, 341
  tuberous sclerosis 277, 312
hydronephrosis 208
  causes 272–3
hydropneumothorax 285–6
25-hydroxycholecalciferol, defective production 84
hypernephroma
  bone metastases 258–9
  renal cell carcinoma 153–4, 344–5
hyperparathyroidism
  chondrocalcinosis 86
  chronic calcific pancreatitis 132
  primary 210
  renal osteodystrophy 51, 355
  super scan 290
hypertrophic pulmonary osteoarthropathy (HPOA) 129–30
hypochlorhydria, gastric resection 17
hypoparathyroidism 71

ileo-colic intussusception 268–9
immunocompromised hosts, infections 41

infantile shock, renal papillary necrosis 295–6
infective endocarditis 92, 237–9, 287–8
inferior vena cava filter, pulmonary embolism 337–8
interstitial fibrosis 185, 312
intimal flap, aortic dissection 63
intracranial lesions
  abscess 127–8, 321
  acoustic neuroma 67, 353
  AIDS-associated 249
  brainstem glioma 330
  choroidal melanoma 235
  cyst 5, 22, 59
  glioblastoma 320–1
  haematoma 101–3, 167, 190–1
  infarction 106–7, 230–1, 309–10
  medulloblastoma 330
  metastases 127–8
intrathoracic goitre 81–2
intussusception 268–9
iris, hamartoma, neurofibromatosis 275
iron deficiency anaemia 241, 77, 213
  child 213
  gastric carcinoma 125–6
  post-cricoid pharyngeal web 77
iron deposition
  CT appearances 55, 322
  MRI appearances 55
ivory vertebrae 293, 301
jejunal diverticulosis 17
joint hypermobility 25
jugular venous pressure, calcific constrictive pericarditis 87–8
juvenile chronic arthritis 75
juxta-articular erosions, fingers 209–10

Kaposi's sarcoma (KS) 206, 249
Katayama fever 97
kidney
  medullary sponge kidney 297–8
  see also renal

knee
  arthrography 28–9
  radiography 74, 85
  tabes dorsalis 228–9
Kussmaul's sign, calcific constrictive pericarditis 87–8

Langerhans' cell histiocytosis 171, 185
lead poisoning 139–40
left atrial hypertension 221
left ventricular aneurysm 106–7
left ventricular failure, pulmonary oedema 260–1
leiomyoma, oesophagus 211–12
leprosy
  lepromatous 202
  tuberculoid 202
Letterer–Siwe disease 171
leukaemia
  chronic lymphatic, lymphadenopathy 49
  chronic myeloid 41
  splenic enlargement 41, 92
leukoerythroblastic anaemia 210
Lisch nodules 275
Lisfranc deformity 195
liver
  calcification 193
  fatty infiltration 123–4, 172–3
  iron deposition, CT and MRI appearances 55, 322
liver cyst 193
liver metastases 235
  ocular melanoma 235
Looser's zones 51, 177
lung, see also pulmonary
lung cavities
  new mass lesion 37, 206
  tubercular 110
lung collapse
  bronchial carcinoma 78–9, 333–4
  secondary to metastatic lymph nodes 26–7

lung honeycombing 184–5
  eosinophilic granuloma 171
  scleroderma 311–12
  tuberous sclerosis 278
lung perfusion defects 2
lung tumours see bronchial carcinoma; pulmonary metastases; small cell carcinoma
lymphadenopathy
  bilateral hilar 49
  calcification in silicosis 43
  lung collapse 79
  metastatic to, breast carcinoma 26–7
lymphangioleiomyomatosis 311–12
  see also lung honeycombing
lymphangitis carcinomatosa 159–60
lymphoma 206, 249
  bilateral hilar lymphadenopathy 49
  ivory vertebrae 293, 302
  retroperitoneal fibrosis (RPF) 208
  splenic enlargement 92
lymphomatoid granulomatosis 206

magnetic resonance imaging **365–7**, **368**
  'flow voids' 23
malabsorption syndrome 16–17
Marfan's syndrome 238–9
  arachnodactyly 24–5
  berry aneurysms 9
mastectomy 26, 99–100
Meckel's diverticulum 214
  intussusception 268–9
mediastinal air, pneumomediastinum 331–2
mediastinal mass 181
  Hodgkin's disease 301–2
  lung collapse 79
  SVCO 156
  teratoma 12–13
  thymoma 13, 339–40
  tracheal deviation 81–2
Mediterranean anaemia 199
medullary sponge kidney 297–8

medulloblastoma 330
melanoma 193
    choroidal 235
    pulmonary metastases 150
meningioma 275, 305–6
    spinal 266–7
meningitis
    AIDS-associated 249
    tuberculous 230–1
mesenteric vessels
    bleeding 279–81
    thrombosis 69
mesothelioma, asbestos-related 39, 243
metabolic alkalosis 197
metacarpal index 24–5
metacarpal shortening 71
metaphyseal bands 139–40
middle ear infections 23
miliary metastases 150
miliary shadowing, causes 47
milk alkali syndrome 298
mitral valve
    normal echocardiogram **370**
    stenosis **371–2**
mosaic oligaemia 1, 2
mucinous carcinoma 193
multiple myeloma 189
multiple sclerosis 147–8, 223, 305
myasthenia gravis, and thymoma 339–40
mycetoma 37, 118–19
Mycoplasma infection 223
myelitis, transverse 222
myelofibrosis 209–10, 293–4, 302, 317
myeloproliferative disorders, super scan 290
myocardial infarction
    pericardial effusion 6–7
    septal rupture 264–5
myotonic dystrophy 164
myxoma 220–1

needle biopsy, hazards 39
nephrocalcinosis 297–8, 315–16

neurofibromatosis 67, 239, 353
    acoustic neuroma 67
    cord compression 274–5
neuropathic spine and hip 228
non-Hodgkin's lymphoma 181
    SVCO 156
NSAIDs
    avascular necrosis 14
    erosive gastritis 41
nuclear medicine **369**
nystagmus, acoustic neuroma 67

ocular melanoma, with liver metastases 235
oesophagus
    carcinoma 212, 225, 245
    corkscrew 225
    dysmotility 95
    dysphagia 77, 211–12, 224
    leiomyoma 211–12
    perforation 331–2
    rupture 262–3
    varices 226–7
ophthalmopathy, Graves' disease 19
optic atrophy 4
optic glioma 275
optic nerve compression 19
optic neuritis, in MS 147–8
oral contraceptives, sagittal sinus thrombosis 23
orbital prosthesis 235
Osler–Weber–Rendu syndrome
    berry aneurysms 9
    hereditary haemorrhagic telangiectasia 241
osteitis fibrosa cystica (brown tumour) 51
osteoarthritis, erosive 270–1
osteodystrophy *see* renal osteodystrophy
osteoma of mandible and skull 183
osteomalacia

osteomalacia *contd*
　rickets 83–4
　super scan 290
　vitamin D deficiency 177
osteopetrosis 210
osteosarcoma 193
　hydropneumothorax 285–6
osteosclerosis 69, 209–10
　sickle-cell disease 69
　and splenomegaly 292
ovarian carcinoma
　lymphangitis carcinomatosa 159–60
　pulmonary metastases 150

pacemaker 50
Paget's disease 112–13, 210, 290, **369**
　hydrocephalus, obstructive 112–13, 341
　ivory vertebrae 293, 301
Pancoast tumour 31
pancreas
　calcification 15
　iron deposition 55
pancreatic carcinoma
　lymphangitis carcinomatosa 159–60
　portal vein 227
pancreatic pseudocyst 299–300
pancreatitis
　ARDS 253
　chronic 132, 296
parathyroid adenoma, neurofibromatosis 275
parathyroid hormone
　hyperparathyroidism 51
　in pseudohypoparathyroidism 71
parieto-occipital cortex, tramline calcifications 141–2
paroxysmal nocturnal dyspnoea 220
pelvis, Paget's disease 112–13
Pemberton's sign, stridor 81
peptic ulceration 233
percutaneous transhepatic cholangiogram 283–4

pericardial effusion
　cardiac enlargement 6–7
　CT vs US 72–3
pericarditis
　calcific constrictive 87–8
　infective causes 87–8
　tuberculous 87–8
　viral 7
peripheral blood eosinophilia 218–19
Perthe's disease, avascular necrosis 15
phaeochromocytoma 345–6
　neurofibromatosis 275
pharyngeal web 77
pituitary fossa enlargement 5
pleural effusion 2
　breast carcinoma metastases 100
　empyema 143–4
　mesothelioma 39, 243
　with pericardial effusion 73
pleural metastases 39
pleural plaque calcification, asbestos-related 242
plombage 347–8
pneumatosis cystoides intestinalis 95, 232–3
pneumobilia, causes 357
pneumomediastinum 252, 331–2
　causes 263
　oesophageal rupture 262–3
pneumonia
　chicken-pox-associated 351–2
　pneumococcal infections 69, 360–1
　Pneumocystis carinii-associated 138, 178–9
　Wegener's granulomatosis 362–3
pneumonitis
　aspiration 33
　overspill 245
pneumothorax 24–5, 138, 185, 252
　hydropneumothorax 285–6
　spontaneous 150, 332
　tension 187
polyarteritis nodosa 324–5

polycystic kidney disease, berry
    aneurysms 9, 57, 359
polycythaemia 220
polycythaemia rubra vera 14, 210, 227, 317
popliteal cyst 28–9
portal hypertension 227
    avascular necrosis 14–15
    splenic enlargement 92, 300
portal vein
    pancreatic cancer 227
    thrombosis 227
post-cricoid pharyngeal web 77
posterior fossa tumours 330
Potts' disease 336
pregnancy
    fatty infiltration of liver 172–3
    headache 23
    sagittal sinus thrombosis 23
prostate carcinoma
    bone metastases 27, 161–2
    ivory vertebrae 293, 301
    lymphangitis carcinomatosa 159–60
prostate-specific antigen (PSA) 161
pseudogout 86
pseudoobstruction 17
pseudo(pseudo)hypoparathyroidism 71
pseudotumour, haemophiliac 75
pseudoxanthoma elasticum, berry
    aneurysms 9
psoas abscess
    calcification 60–1
    Crohn's disease 60
psoriatic arthritis 89–90, 270–1
pulmonary arteriovenous malformation (AVM) 241
pulmonary artery enlargement 2
pulmonary calcifications, causes 352
pulmonary metastases 206
pulmonary fibrosis 185
    asbestos-related 243
    neurofibromatosis 275

scleroderma 95
pulmonary infarction 206
sickle lung 69
pulmonary infiltrates, dermatomyositis 33
pulmonary mass
    causes 206
    hamartoma 206, 342–3
    multiple abscesses 206
    thyroid metastases 150
pulmonary oedema 220–1, 252–3
    bat's wing 260–1
    fat embolism 45
    left ventricular failure 260–1
pulmonary osteoarthropathy (HPOA) 129–30
pulmonary thromboembolism 1, 122
    inferior vena cava filter 337–8
    with/without infarction 2
pulmonary tuberculosis 47, 110, 347–8
pulseless disease, aortography 53
pyelonephritis 296
pyloric stenosis 197
pyogenic abscess 249

radiotherapy, avascular necrosis 14
Rathke's pouch, craniopharyngioma (cystic) 5
Raynaud's phenomenon 95
rectal adenoma 151–2
renal, see also hypernephroma
renal angiomyolipoma 278
renal artery balloon angioplasty 313–14
renal artery stenosis 313–14
renal cell carcinoma 153–4, 258–9, 344–6
renal cyst 278, 345
renal failure
    chronic 51, 215
    ineffective 1-hydroxylation 84
renal obstruction, horseshoe kidney 116

renal osteodystrophy 210, 215–17
  in chronic renal failure 51
  hyperparathyroidism 51, 355
  rugger-jersey spine 354–5
  super scan 290
renal papillary necrosis 295–6, 298
renal polycystic disease, APCKD 57, 359
renal scar, ^{99m}Tc-DMSA scan 135–6
renal transplantation, avascular necrosis 14
renal tubular acidosis 298, 316
retinal angioma 345
retinal hamartoma 278
retroperitoneal fibrosis (RPF) 208
retroperitoneal mass 208
rheumatoid arthritis 89–90, 185, 206, 217, 239
  avascular necrosis 14
  knee appearances 75
  ruptured popliteal cyst 28–9
rib notching, causes 238–9
rickets
  anticonvulsant-associated 83–4
  renal tubular acidosis 316
  see also renal osteodystrophy
rugger-jersey spine 354–5
sacroiliitis 11, 105, 161–2
  psoriatic arthropathy 270–1
sagittal sinus thrombosis 23
Salmonella infections 69
sarcoidosis
  granulomatous involvement of myocardium 49
  miliary shadowing 47
  splenic enlargement 92
  staging 49
sarcoma 206, 286
  Paget's disease 112–13
schistosomiasis 97–8
schwannoma 275
  acoustic 67
scleroderma 217, 233

small bowel 17, 94, 311–12
sclerosing cholangitis 208
  ERCP 65
sclerosis
  lumbar vertebrae 228
  metastatic prostate cancer 27
  osteosclerosis 69, 209–10
  systemic 17, 94, 311–12
sclerotic change 14–15
sebaceous cysts 183
sella turcica enlargement 121
shoulder, Charcot's neuropathy 108–9
sickle cell disease 199, 210
  avascular necrosis 14–15
  renal papillary necrosis 295–6
sigmoid volvulus 33–4
silicosis 185
  lymph node calcification 43
  lymphadenopathy 49
  miliary shadowing 47
  progressive massive fibrosis 43
small bowel
  atony, dermatomyositis 33
  bacterial overgrowth 17
  cobblestone patterning 11
  coeliac disease 318–19
  fistula formation to psoas muscle 60
  Meckel's diverticulum 214
  pneumatosis cystoides intestinalis 95, 232–3
  pseudoobstruction 17
  scleroderma 17, 94, 311–12
  strictures 11, 17
small cell carcinoma
  Eaton–Lambert syndrome 334, 340
  lymph node metastases 155–6
  lymphadenopathy 49
  Pancoast tumour 31
spastic paraparesis 305
spinal artery thrombosis 306

spinal cord
  compression 305-6
  haemangioblastoma 345
  neurofibromatosis 274-5
  syringomyelia 108-9
  transverse myelitis 222
spinal meningioma 266-7
spine
  bamboo 161-2
  Charcot's neuropathy 228
  endplate destruction 336
  ivory vertebrae 293, 301
  rotting-fence 215-16
  rugger-jersey 354-5
  wedge compression collapse 302
spleen
  infarction 69
  varices 226-7
splenomegaly 91-2, 209-10, 227, 300
  erosive gastritis 41
  Gaucher's disease 92
  glandular fever 92
  haemolytic anaemia 92
  infective endocarditis 92
  osteosclerosis 292
spondylosis 165-6
squamous cell carcinoma 205-6
  bladder 97
  lymph node metastases 155-6
  oesophagus 212
Stanford classification, aortic dissection 63
steroid-associated arthropathy, avascular necrosis 14-15
stomach *see* gastric
stridor, dyspnoea 81-2
stroke 237-8
Sturge-Weber syndrome 142
subarachnoid haemorrhage 9, 117
  berry aneurysm 57, 359
subclavian 'steal' syndrome 53
subdural haematoma 101-3, 167
  alcohol excess 190-1

superior sagittal sinus thrombosis 23
superior vena cava obstruction 239
  sagittal sinus thrombosis 23
  tumour 155-6
superior vena cava syndrome 81-2
syphilis (tabes dorsalis) 228-9
syringomyelia 108-9
  neuropathic shoulder 229
systemic lupus erythematosus 14
  splenic enlargement 92
systemic sclerosis 17, 94, 311-12

Taenia solium, cysticercosis 20-2
Takayasu's arteritis, aortography 53
^{99m}Tc scan, mesenteric bleeding 279-80
^{99m}Tc-DMSA scan, kidney 135-6
^{99m}Tc-HMPAO scan 247
^{99m}Tc-MDP, super scan 289-90
^{99m}Tc-pertechnetate scan 214
  thyroid disorders 292
teratoma 13
testicular cancer
  lymph node metastases 155-6
  pulmonary metastases 150
thalassaemia major 199-200
thrombosis
  DVT 29
  mesenteric, sickling crisis 69
  superior sagittal sinus 23
thymoma 13
  and myasthenia gravis 339-40
thyroglossal cyst 327
thyroid disorders
  adenoma 292
  Graves' ophthalmopathy 19
  intrathoracic goitre 81-2, 149-50
  ophthalmopathy 19
  pericardial effusion 6-7
  ^{99m}Tc scan 82, 291, 292
thyroid mass 81, 149-50
toxic megacolon 246
toxoplasma abscess 249

toxoplasmosis 20–2
tracheal deviation, mediastinal mass 81–2
transjugular intrahepatic portosystemic stent shunt (TIPSS) 254–5
transverse myelitis 223
trauma, fat embolism 14, 45
tuberculoid leprosy 202
tuberculomata 21
tuberculosis 193
   complication of silicosis 43
   miliary 47, 230
   plombage 347–8
   primary pulmonary 230
   reactivation 110, 230
tuberculous abscess 206, 249
   calcified psoas muscle 60–1
tuberculous arthritis 329
tuberculous cavities, new mass lesion 37
tuberculous empyema 143–4, 242
tuberculous meningitis 230–1
tuberculous pericarditis 87–8
tuberculous sacroiliitis 105
tuberculous spondylitis 335–6
tuberous sclerosis 277, 312
Turner's syndrome 238–9

ulcer
   aphthous 11
   'rose-thorn' 11
ulcerative colitis 246–7
   ERCP for biliary obstruction 65
urinary bladder
   cancer, hydronephrosis 272–3
   carcinoma 208
   colo-vesical fistula 256–7
   gas, lumen/wall 34–5
   squamous cell tumours 97
uterine carcinoma, lymphangitis carcinomatosa 159–60

varicella pneumonia 351–2
varices 300
   gastric 254–5
   hepatic 254–5
   oesophagus 226–7
   spleen 226–7
vasculitis, systemic 363
venography, deep vein thrombosis 29
ventilation–perfusion (V–Q) scans, mismatch 3
ventricular septal defect 237, 239
vertebrae
   ivory 293, 301
   Romanus lesion 162
   see also spine
vertebrobasilar ischaemia 53
villous adenoma of rectum 151–2
vitamin B_{12} deficiency, bacterial overgrowth 17
vitamin D deficiency
   anticonvulsant-associated rickets 83–4
   osteomalacia 177
vitamin D insensitivity, X-linked 83–4
volvulus 33–4
von Hippel–Lindau syndrome 344–5

Wegener's granulomatosis 79, 137, 206, 362–3
white-cell scan 247
Wilson's disease 316
   chondrocalcinosis 86

X-linked vitamin D insensitivity 83–4